MARATHON MEDICINE

Edited by

Dan Tunstall Pedoe

*A book based on a symposium sponsored by the
British Heart Foundation and the Flora London Marathon,
and held at the Royal Society of Medicine, London,
on 13–15 April 2000*

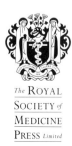

The ROYAL
SOCIETY of
MEDICINE
PRESS Limited

NB - wasn't published until April 2001

1 Wimpole Street, London W1G 0AE, UK
207 E Westminster Road, Lake Forest, IL 60045, USA
http://www.rsm.ac.uk

These proceedings are published by the Royal Society of Medicine Press Ltd with financial support from the sponsor. The contributors are responsible for the scientific content and for the views expressed, which are not necessarily those of the sponsors, of the editor, of the Royal Society of Medicine or of the Royal Society of Medicine Press Ltd.

British Library Cataloguing in Publication Data
A catalogue record for this book is available from the British Library
ISBN 1-85315-460-1

Phototypeset by Toby Matthews, London
Printed in Great Britain by Ebenezer Baylis, The Trinity Press, Worcester

Authors and Chairpersons

Sir Roger Bannister CBE
NEUROLOGIST, FORMER MASTER OF PEMBROKE COLLEGE, OXFORD, UK

Professor Claude Bouchard
EXECUTIVE DIRECTOR, PENNINGTON BIOMEDICAL RESEARCH CENTER,
HUMAN GENOMICS LABORATORY, BATON ROUGE, LOUISIANA, USA

Christopher Brasher CBE
FOUNDER & PRESIDENT, THE LONDON MARATHON

Dr Richard Budgett
DIRECTOR OF MEDICAL SERVICES, BRITISH OLYMPIC MEDICAL CENTRE, LONDON, UK

Dr Alan Donnelly
SENIOR LECTURER, DEPARTMENT OF PHYSICAL EDUCATION AND SPORTS SCIENCE, UNIVERSITY OF LIMERICK,
LIMERICK, IRELAND

Dr Randy Eichner
PROFESSOR OF MEDICINE, HEMATOLOGY-ONCOLOGY SECTION,
UNIVERSITY OF OKLAHOMA HEALTH SCIENCES CENTER, OKLAHOMA, USA

Dr Lawrence Folinsbee
ENVIRONMENTAL MEDIA ASSESSMENT BRANCH, NATIONAL CENTER FOR ENVIRONMENTAL ASSESSMENT, US
ENVIRONMENTAL PROTECTION AGENCY, RESEARCH TRIANGLE PARK, NC, USA

Dr Gerrit Van Hall
THE COPENHAGEN MUSCLE RESEARCH CENTER, RIGSHOSPITALET (UNIVERSITY HOSPITAL), COPENHAGEN,
DENMARK

Professor Adrianne Hardman
DEPARTMENT OF PHYSICAL EDUCATION, SPORTS SCIENCE AND RECREATION MANAGEMENT,
LOUGHBOROUGH UNIVERSITY, LEICESTERSHIRE, UK

Dr Jørn Helge
THE COPENHAGEN MUSCLE RESEARCH CENTER, RIGSHOSPITALET (UNIVERSITY HOSPITAL), COPENHAGEN,
DENMARK

Professor Mike Lambert
DIRECTOR OF HIGH PERFORMANCE CENTRE, MRC/UCT BIOENERGETICS OF EXERCISE RESEARCH UNIT,
FACULTY OF HEALTH SCIENCES, UNIVERSITY OF CAPE TOWN,
SPORT SCIENCE INSTITUTE OF SOUTH AFRICA, NEWLANDS, SOUTH AFRICA

Dr Barry Maron
DIRECTOR, HYPERTROPHIC CARDIOMYOPATHY CENTER,
MINNEAPOLIS HEART INSTITUTE FOUNDATION, MINNEAPOLIS, MINNESOTA, USA

Dr David Martin
EMERITUS PROFESSOR, DEPARTMENT OF CARDIOPULMONARY CARE SCIENCES, GEORGIA STATE UNIVERSITY,
ATLANTA, GEORGIA, USA

Dr Alan Maryon-Davis
SENIOR LECTURER IN PUBLIC HEALTH MEDICINE,
DEPARTMENT OF PUBLIC HEALTH SCIENCES, KING'S COLLEGE LONDON, LONDON, UK

Professor Ron Maughan
PROFESSOR OF HUMAN PHYSIOLOGY, DEPARTMENT OF BIOMEDICAL SCIENCES,
UNIVERSITY MEDICAL SCHOOL, FORESTERHILL, ABERDEEN, UK

Professor William Morgan
DIRECTOR, EXERCISE PSYCHOLOGY LABORATORY, DEPARTMENT OF KINESIOLOGY,
UNIVERSITY OF WISCONSIN-MADISON, MADISON, WISCONSIN, USA

Professor Eric Newsholme
EMERITUS PROFESSOR OF BIOCHEMISTRY, MERTON COLLEGE, OXFORD, UK

Professor Timothy Noakes
MRC/UCT BIOENERGETICS OF EXERCISE RESEARCH UNIT, FACULTY OF HEALTH SCIENCES, UNIVERSITY OF
CAPE TOWN, SPORT SCIENCE INSTITUTE OF SOUTH AFRICA, NEWLANDS, SOUTH AFRICA

Dr Bente K Pedersen
DEPARTMENT OF INFECTIOUS DISEASES, RIGSHOSPITALET (UNIVERSITY HOSPITAL), COPENHAGEN, DENMARK

Mr Trevor Prior
CONSULTANT PODIATRIST, ST LEONARD'S PRIMARY CARE CENTRE, LONDON, UK

Professor Peter Radford
PROFESSOR OF SPORT SCIENCES, DEPARTMENT OF SPORTS SCIENCES, BRUNEL UNIVERSITY,
WEST LONDON, UK

Professor Peter Raven
DEPARTMENT OF INTEGRATIVE PHYSIOLOGY,
UNIVERSITY OF NORTH TEXAS HEALTH SCIENCE CENTER, FORT WORTH, TEXAS, USA

Dr William O Roberts
MINNHEALTH FAMILY PHYSICIANS, WHITE BEAR LAKE, MINNESOTA, USA

Professor Bengt Saltin
THE COPENHAGEN MUSCLE RESEARCH CENTER, RIGSHOSPITALET (UNIVERSITY HOSPITAL), COPENHAGEN,
DENMARK

Professor Craig Sharp
PROFESSOR OF SPORT SCIENCE, DEPARTMENT OF SPORT SCIENCES, BRUNEL UNIVERSITY, WEST LONDON
AND HONORARY RESEARCH FELLOW, UNIVERSITY OF STIRLING, UK

Dr Susan Shirreffs
LECTURER IN PHYSIOLOGY, DEPARTMENT OF BIOMEDICAL SCIENCES, UNIVERSITY MEDICAL SCHOOL,
FORESTERHILL, ABERDEEN, UK

Dr Martyn Shorten
MANAGING PARTNER, BIOMECHANICA, PORTLAND, OREGON, USA

Dr Michael Stroud
SENIOR LECTURER IN MEDICINE & NUTRITION, CONSULTANT GASTROENTEROLOGIST
INSTITUTE OF HUMAN NUTRITION, SOUTHAMPTON UNIVERSITY HOSPITALS TRUST, SOUTHAMPTON, UK

Dr Dan Tunstall Pedoe
MEDICAL DIRECTOR OF THE LONDON MARATHON,
CONSULTANT CARDIOLOGIST, ST BARTHOLOMEW'S & HOMERTON HOSPITALS, LONDON, UK

Professor Clyde Williams
PROFESSOR OF SPORTS SCIENCE, DEPARTMENT OF PHYSICAL EDUCATION,
SPORTS SCIENCE & RECREATION MANAGEMENT, LOUGHBOROUGH UNIVERSITY, LEICESTERSHIRE, UK

Dr Roger Wolman
THE ROYAL NATIONAL ORTHOPAEDIC HOSPITAL, LONDON, UK

Contents

Preface

SIR ROGER BANNISTER CBE

NEUROLOGIST, FORMER MASTER OF PEMBROKE COLLEGE, OXFORD, UK

The marathon has rightly earned its popular appeal in sport. It remains the modern Olympics' historic link with ancient Greece, commemorating Pheidippides' run from Marathon to Athens announcing the Greek victory over the Persians at Marathon. Reputedly after announcing 'Rejoice, we conquer', he dropped dead.

The marathon is indisputably the greatest test of endurance running in the Olympic programme. More deaths and disasters have occurred in the marathon than in any other Olympic event. Glorious failure in the marathon is more often remembered than victory, as in the harrowing photographs of Dorando Pietri at the London Olympics in 1908 and Jim Peters in the Commonwealth games in Vancouver in 1954.

Over the past half century, as public interest in taking part in marathons has burgeoned, aided by the New York marathon and the London marathon developed by Christopher Brasher, serious medical thought has been given to making the marathon safer. This book explores every legitimate assistance that can be given to runners. For example how can sufficient energy be provided, how much fluid and electrolytes are needed, how can body temperature be controlled, which design of shoe is most efficient?

Dan Tunstall Pedoe — cardiologist, Medical Director of the London marathon and an experienced distance runner — has coordinated and edited these proceedings. This book will enlighten, instruct and delight all of us who are enthralled by this extraordinary sporting event.

Introduction

CHRISTOPHER BRASHER CBE

FOUNDER AND PRESIDENT OF THE LONDON MARATHON

I have seen 14 Olympic marathons, an event confined by reputation to elite athletes only. However, in 1979, I took a bus to the start of the New York City marathon which, at the age of 55, was the first marathon in which I participated. I could not believe that some of the men and women, who were of all shapes and sizes, on that bus were about to embark on the toughest event in the Olympic calendar. But they started and they finished many hours later in Central Park.

It was only then that I began to realize the power of the human mind over seemingly weak bodies. It is sometimes a frightening power that drives a person well beyond the bounds of reason. It is important to understand the human body under stress so that, with knowledge, it can match the human spirit. And where better to turn than this volume, distilled from the views of a galaxy of experts assembled in London in the first year of the new millennium by Dan Tunstall Pedoe? Has there ever been a more distinguished band of sports medical experts assembled in one place? That is what makes this book so valuable.

Marathon myths and marathon medicine

DR DAN TUNSTALL PEDOE

MEDICAL DIRECTOR OF THE LONDON MARATHON,
CONSULTANT CARDIOLOGIST, ST BARTHOLOMEW'S & HOMERTON HOSPITALS, LONDON, UK

This book is more than a volume of conference proceedings — it is an update on the sports medicine of marathon running.

The Marathon Medicine meeting was held to celebrate the 20th running of the mass participation modern London marathon and the millennium, and to update the science explored in the seminal New York Academy of Sciences 1977 publication based on the 1976 conference *The marathon: physiological, medical, epidemiological and psychological studies*[1]. It was an excellent opportunity to combine the expertise of the past with scientific developments of the last 25 years and, although not rivalling the New York conference in size, invite an international faculty (some of whom were at the 1976 conference) to share their knowledge with each other and, through this publication, the readers. Each speaker was asked to review progress in his or her field over the past 25 years.

As a runner for 45 years and medical director of the London marathon for 20, it was a self-indulgence to be able to invite so many international experts to talk on subjects that are of such topical interest in 'exercise medicine'. Many of the areas are controversial and have been prone to 'medical myths'. Some of these myths will be discussed in this chapter, and a few topics included in the book will be mentioned here.

Marathon deaths: can marathon runners kill themselves with over-exertion?

As a cardiologist, I am intrigued by the origin of the modern marathon race, as a product of the myth of a professional Greek runner (a hemerodromoi) bringing the news to Athens of the victory over the Persians at the battle of Marathon and dying from a ruptured heart. It was popularized by Robert Browning, a Victorian poet whose poem is said to have gripped the imagination of the Anglophile founder of the modern Olympics, Baron de Coubertin.

> *Till in he broke 'Rejoice we conquer!' Like wine through clay.*
> *Joy in his blood bursting his heart,*
> *He died — the bliss!*

(Robert Browning, 1879)

The death of Pheidippides, also known as Phidippides (discussed in Dr Martin's chapter), although lacking any contemporaneous or even credible historical accounts, is widely quoted as the first reported sudden cardiac death in sport. It appears, along with famous pictures of collapsing marathon runners, to have given rise to an expectation that marathon runners are close to death.

In 1980, when planning the first London marathon as an open-entry people's race without medical screening, there were press reports of sports medicine specialists claiming '*Unfit runners will kill themselves in the London marathon*'. This is a popular misconception, based on a misunderstanding of the term 'fitness' and regarding it as meaning freedom from disease. Fitness means that a person is trained for a specific task and is capable of performing it. A fit, aerobically trained marathon runner may be quite unfit for repeated episodes of intense anaerobic exercise such as in a hard game of squash racquets, and a sprinter would not be fit to run a marathon. However, the term 'fitness' is used rather non-specifically to mean someone who takes regular exercise and is not unwell. A fit person may or may not have heart disease. An 'unfit' person may or may not have heart disease, but is more likely to have coronary artery disease than an aerobically fit person (see Professor Hardman's and Dr Eichner's chapters), and is at greater risk of sudden death on exercise than a fit person if he or she has heart disease. Most deaths of marathon runners are from heart disease or heat problems such as heat stroke or hypothermia, and do not occur simply from exhaustion, which recovers rapidly.

The myth of Pheiddipides was given credibility by the Victorian and early 20th century view (when undiagnosed heart disease was common) that exertion was bad for the heart and might even be fatal (also mentioned in Professor Radford's chapter). The current view is that marathon running does not confer immunity to coronary heart disease as proposed by Bassler in the 1976 New York conference[2], but that aerobic exercise has significant effects in reducing coronary risk (see Professor Hardman's chapter).

The London marathon, with no deaths in the first nine years, has now in its full 20 years had five deaths from severe heart disease in 450,000 runs and one death from subarachnoid haemorrhage. It has also had five successful cardiac resuscitations (see Dr Tunstall Pedoe's chapter on *Morbidity and mortality in the London marathon*)[3].

The mortality risk for running the London marathon on a 'time of exposure basis' after the 19th race has been calculated to be half that of riding a motorcycle for the same length of time, slightly more than twice that for riding a bicycle based on European Transport Union statistics, and one-seventh the risk of travelling in a car[3]. In other words the risk of death was the same for two hours on a motorcycle, four hours of running the London marathon, 14 hours cycling and 28 hours in a car. The death in 2000 from subarachnoid haemorrhage makes these figures about 10% less favourable to marathon running, but still shows a low level of risk, comparable to familiar daily activities. Table 1 shows the amended risks including 2000 data.

Table 1 *London marathon deaths compared with European Transport Union travel risks*
Modified from[3].

Mode of transport	Deaths/ 100 Mkm	Deaths/ 100 Mh	Deaths/ 100 y	Normalized death risk/time exposed
London marathon (1981–2000)	28	280	2.5	7.8
Motorcycle	16	500	4.4	14
Bicycle	6.3	90	0.9	3
Car	0.8	30	0.3	1
Airline	0.06	36.5	0.35	1
Rail	0.04	2	0.02	0.06

Thus, 'unfit' runners have not killed themselves in the London marathon; runners with heart disease, however, have but this was due to the severe heart disease in combination with the exertion of running the marathon, not purely the exertion of running the marathon. Would compulsory cardiac screening of all entrants be sensible? This question is posed repeatedly, especially after a tragedy[3]. Screening to prevent one death in 80,000 runs, with runners coming from all over the world, would be a logistic nightmare. The expensive tests are not very specific nor necessarily sensitive enough to detect all causes of sudden death. In addition, there is no internationally recognized form of certification that would be recognized. The emphasis has to be on runners taking responsibility for their own safety[3].

Exertion-related cardiac deaths with no obvious cardiac pathology, so called idiopathic ventricular fibrillation, do rarely occur. The death of a young woman, Anna Loyley, at the end of the Bath half marathon in 1998 is an example of this rare phenomenon[3]. Idiopathic ventricular fibrillation deaths also occur during normal daily activity including sleep, but there may be an increased risk with exertion. They are thought to have a metabolic basis; to most cardiologists it seems inconceivable that the 'normal heart' can rupture or even fibrillate purely from prolonged exertion, but this remains a semantic argument until the causes of idiopathic ventricular fibrillation are discovered.

Whether or not exertion exhausts the normal heart and causes it to fail also remains controversial. Rare cases of exertional pulmonary oedema in young people and athletes appear to be due to pulmonary capillary damage rather than true heart failure and only seem to occur under exceptional circumstances[4]. A recent study of prolonged severe exertion in half-ironman and ironman triathlons suggests a reversible degree of cardiac 'fatigue', or left ventricular dysfunction which fully recovers within 48 hours[5]. This conclusion was based an echocardiographic findings, with cardiac enzyme values suggesting possible myocardial damage. It is of theoretical but probably not of any great clinical significance.

Unless they had heart disease, unfit runners would have great difficulty killing themselves with exhaustion. They would seize up with cramp. But there is another mechanism. A fit or unfit runner who is unwell with a viral infection and runs a marathon can suffer from myocarditis or develop immune suppression leading to death. This is one of the reasons why every entrant to the London marathon receives written medical advice (see Dr Tunstall Pedoe's chapter on *Morbidity and mortality in the London marathon*). Although we do not wish unwell runners to take part, we have to face increasing risks of this happening because of the modern type of entrant. It is a myth that all runners are fit athletes, or even that they are necessarily free from illness. Many have complex motivation and are running for money.

Reasons for running a marathon

There are many reasons for running a marathon, particularly one with a great deal of media coverage and exposure (Table 2). Most involve the marathon as a way of raising self-esteem. A mass marathon may include the supreme international athletes who 'stretch the envelope' of human performance. It also includes a spectrum of runners, ranging from the fit, young club runner to the relatively unfit, possibly coronary prone middle-aged runner who has taken up marathon running to re-establish his or her virility, reduce (hopefully) chances of coronary disease, or as a reaction to a 'dare' or personal bet from an acquaintance. It is now attracting thousands of charity runners who run for sponsorship and the glory of the amount of money that they raise for the charity, which gave them an entry. In the 2000 London marathon, >70% of participants were running to raise money for charity and many were running with a medical problem or disability. Perhaps following the lead in the London marathon this appears to be a growing phenomenon worldwide.

All entrants to the London marathon are expected to be fit and well on the day of the race and to withdraw if they are not; the medical director must be informed if they have a medical problem that may require attention should they become a casualty. This is discussed in the chapter *Morbidity and mortality in the London marathon*. A few examples of groups of participants running the marathon with a medical condition or disability are briefly outlined in Table 3.

Table 2 *Some reasons for running a marathon*

- To prove you can do it — as a challenge to runners in their 30s and 40s that their physical powers are not declining, and as proof that an illness or disability is not really a handicap
- To prove you can do it better than last time (traditional runners)
- To become 'fitter', improve body image (and reduce coronary risk)
- To raise money for a charity (and possibly get publicity and kudos for doing so)
- As a form of self-promotion or promotion of some disability such as multiple sclerosis or even political promotion (End World Hunger, Save the Rhino etc)
- Exhibitionism (outlandish costumes etc)

Table 3 *Medical conditions in the London marathon*

- Cardiac: post-myocardial infarction, post-coronary artery surgery, heart transplant, hypertension
- Endocrine (treated): thyroid disease, Addison's disease, diabetes mellitus
- Respiratory: asthma
- Gastrointestinal: colectomy
- Neurological: motor neurone disease, epilepsy, paraplegia (wheel chair athletes)
- Pregnancy
- Cancer and leukaemia (in remission)
- Ocular: blind runners
- Musculoskeletal: lower and upper leg amputees with and without crutches

Disabled runners

Increasing numbers of runners and walkers who are either disabled or have medical conditions that are not normally associated with superior fitness are entering these races (Table 3). Some with considerable public relations support are giving their own disability and favoured charity media exposure.

The only separate category in the London marathon is for wheelchair athletes, who do not strictly qualify for a foot race but, after considerable media and political pressure, were given entry to a separate race held with the marathon. The marathon course was originally closed to all vehicles to protect the runners. It was re-opened to racing wheelchairs, which can reach speeds of up to 40 mph on downhill slopes and have covered the marathon distance in 90 minutes. They do not mix easily with large numbers of tired, uncoordinated runners who are expected by the wheelchair competitors to move out of their way. Their involvement needs careful planning.

Illness denial

The wish for sufferers from these conditions to reject the passive 'invalid role' and take part in a challenging activity is in many ways admirable. However, it can sometimes verge on naivety or even foolhardiness. Some feel they have a right to take part whatever the consequences for themselves or for the organizers. Some examples, admirable or foolhardy, depend on your viewpoint.

Heart disease

An engineer in his 60s who regularly runs marathons completed the 20th London in four hours and 15 minutes (aiming at four hours) despite triple vessel coronary disease, previous myocardial infarction, treated hypertension and hyperlipidaemia, episodes of well tolerated ventricular tachycardia and a previous transient ischaemic attack. He had been told that he should not be competitive if he decided to run. He believes his health would be far worse if he did not run regularly, and runs two or more marathons a year.

One runner has claimed that he is an 'ex-heart patient' having had triple coronary bypass grafts >15 years ago (a time at which many grafts become blocked). He raises money for the British Heart Foundation.

Motor neurone disease

One runner with motor neurone disease, who had never run further than five miles, also took part. Despite increasing disability, he completed the marathon distance with his wife and an attendant runner (to help him up if he fell as he was not able to pick himself up), knowing he would be too disabled to try again.

Multiple sclerosis

In 1999, a 50-year-old woman came to London from New York with multiple sclerosis. She had a large support team and completed the course on crutches in 30 hours, averaging <1 mph. Was she really part of the event?

Lung transplant

A sad example from New York in 1999 was of a young man with pulmonary cystic fibrosis who was president of the Norwegian Achilles club (a club for the disabled and survivors of the life-threatening disease), had survived bilateral lung transplantation, and was the first Norwegian success for this operation. He had run the New York marathon in a special category before his transplant and had become a celebrity as a spokesman for the disabled and even had a book written about himself. He felt sufficiently recovered to take part in 1999 and came with a medical support team. After the race he noticed pain and swelling in his left big toe, which later spread to his ankle. On the flight home two days after the marathon, he became breathless and was admitted to hospital in Copenhagen. Despite intensive treatment, he died four days after the marathon with multiple organ failure from a β-haemolytic streptococcus septicaemia. The immune suppressant effects of prolonged exercise (see Dr Pedersen's chapter) added to immune suppression from his lung transplant anti-rejection medication appear to have led to this unfortunate outcome.

Pregnancy

This happier example took place in London. A woman wrote to me saying she would be running at 27 weeks of her pregnancy and had the full support of her obstetrician! She completed the course in three hours and 45 minutes (normally three hours and five minutes) carrying 18 lb (8 kg) extra weight, and luckily it was not a hot day as foetal welfare might have suffered.

Acquired 'illness'

Fractured ribs and pneumothorax

A man in his late 70s had a heavy fall at five miles and, despite severe pain and increasing breathlessness, finished the course and was sent to hospital where he was found to have rib fractures and a major pneumothorax.

Fractured femur

A young man trained for the first London marathon but developed pain in the groin, which became severe and impeded his training to the extent that did virtually none for the last three weeks before the race. He did not wish to miss the inaugural run and managed to cover 18 miles before the pain became too much for him. He was admitted to hospital and X-ray showed an obvious femoral fracture but luckily without significant displacement. He had obviously been training and competing with a fatigue fracture of some weeks' duration, as early fatigue fractures do not show on plain X ray. He spent several weeks in hospital recovering.

Of the London examples only the pregnant woman wrote to me of her condition. Usually out of 30,000 entries I receive about 12 letters informing me of conditions such as diabetes and epilepsy. Obviously other runners did not regard themselves as having a 'problem' and either thought the request for information did not apply to them or else felt their entry would be rejected on medial grounds. We do not do this, but put the responsibility on the runner and his or her own medical advisor.

More worrying is that runners publicizing their illness rejection (eg the 'ex'-heart patient) or publicizing the large sums of money they are raising for charity are unlikely to follow medical advice if they are taken ill in the few days before the marathon and withdraw. Being a wimp when in the full glare of publicity may be sensible but is not easy.

Marathon collapses

Myths surround not only Pheidippides but also other collapses. The two most famous are of Dorando Pietri (see Dr Martin's chapter) in the 1908 London marathon and Jim Peters in Vancouver in 1954. Peters brought the best time for the marathon down from two hours, 26 minutes and seven seconds (2:26:07) to 2:17:39, a reduction of 6% between 1952 and 1954, achieving four of the six best marathon times over that period. In the 1954 Vancouver Commonwealth Games marathon under unfamiliar hot conditions, he was leading by 10 minutes but collapsed several times in the stadium just short of the finish and had to be taken to hospital. It has been reported that the aid stations were abandoned along the route, as the staff was anxious to see the 'mile of the century' (the first of many), in this case the duel between Landy and Bannister, the first two four-minute milers. Subsequent medical rumour was that Peters developed renal failure from his heat stroke and was advised not to run. Sir Roger Bannister has given me copies of Peters' medical admission notes and some correspondence about his collapse and electrocardiograms (ECGs). It is difficult to define heat syndromes (discussed in Dr Roberts' chapter). Sir Adolphe Abrahams, the founder of British sports medicine, at the time wrote that Peters had suffered heat exhaustion not heat stroke, and that some temporary ECG abnormalities (ventricular bigeminy and ST and T wave abnormalities) were of no account and did not indicate a primary cardiac cause for his collapse. Peters wisely decided to retire because future championship races were scheduled for hot environments. This has become a recurring problem for athletes from temperate climes.

The example of Peters not drinking enough water (or not taking it as was a long tradition in running as described by Professor Radford) led to tremendous emphasis on fluid intake immediately before and during endurance events. The pendulum swung to an opposite extreme — encouragement in mass marathons in the early 1980s for runners to supercharge with fluids before the race and the claim that a cup of strong coffee (supplied by a sponsor) just before the race helped prevent the wall (glycogen depletion) were observed to have disastrous effects on some runners. In New York, where runners have to make their way to the start 20–30 minutes before the start, agonized male runners were seen to be urinating over the edge of the bridge into the Bay. In London, there were queues of runners hit by 'runners trots' and bladder distension waiting for toilets as early as three miles into the race. More recently, excess water drinking along the route, particularly by women runners, has led to water intoxication (hyponatraemia) becoming an important cause of collapse in some marathons (see Dr Eichner's and Professor Maughan's chapters).

Another famous collapse that promoted a myth was that of Alberto Salazar, a world record holder at the distance who sweated profusely while running even in mild conditions and who has collapsed after major effort on more than one occasion. He collapsed at the end of the Boston marathon after a very close finish. Although it was not a particularly cold day and he was running at a five-minute mile pace, generating a calculated minimum of a kilowatt of heat, he was said to have collapsed from hypothermia — this was reported in many newspapers worldwide. The myth arose because he had an oral temperature taken after sucking ice in the recovery tent.

The problems of defining the causes of exercise-associated collapse and through which orifice the most meaningful body temperature can be recorded are covered in Dr Roberts' chapter.

Greek myth of Atalanta and the superiority of female runners

Atalanta was the tomboy daughter of a man who wanted a son. She became a runner who beat all comers and was promised in marriage to any man who could outrun her. She was eventually beaten by a male suitor who sprinted ahead of her dropping golden apples (supplied by the Goddess of love), which she stopped to pick up. He won the race and claimed her as a bride.

The 1960s saw the pioneers of women's marathon running scandalizing race officials by entering what had previously been a male preserve. They amazed spectators first by completing the distance and then by often appearing to be in much better shape at the finish than members of the 'weaker sex'. Perhaps inspired by the Greek myth of Atalanta, various medical men pronounced on the phenomenon and predicted that women were probably better suited to endurance exercise than men. Since their bodies were designed for the prolonged hard labour of childbirth, they were metabolically better adapted for endurance running. In 1962, Charlie Robbins pronounced that, since marathon running was not a test of strength but of heart and lungs, women would be better at this than at shorter distances. The 1970s and 1980s saw women's world records improving at a greater rate than men's and provoked a statistical prediction in 1992 that women would be running faster than men over the distance[6]. This was based on assumptions that the rate of improvement, which had apparently remained constant for many decades, would continue, and ignored the physiological superiority in the average male athlete over the average female athlete not only in strength but in body composition, cardiovascular and respiratory indices, haemoglobin and aerobic power.

Obviously outstanding female athletes will be superior to most men — thus, what are the differences in performance of the elite men and women and the average male and female marathon runner? Do they support the concept of women performing proportionately better at marathon distances and longer? Analysis of world record performances from 100 m sprint to the best marathon performances show that the opposite appears to be true. The world 100 m male time is 7.2% faster than that of the female, 200 m male time is 10.6% faster than the female time, 400 m is 10.2% faster, and 800 m, 1,500 m, 10,000 m and marathon are all 11.9–12.0% faster, and the half-marathon 12.4% faster in males. In the US list of age-best marathon times for men and women (discussed in Professor Sharp's chapter) there is a lot of scatter, but the average difference clusters around 15% between the ages of 20 and 50 years and, perhaps because of the paucity of post menopausal female runners or the effect of the menopause itself, the difference increases from 20% at 55–60 years to >30% over 60 years.

How do the elite runners compare with the general run of marathon runners? Experience in the London marathon has been that the modal times for men and women differ by about 30 minutes (12–5%) with women <40 years being equivalent to men >60 years in finishing times (personal data).

Perhaps some of the older women's sprint world records are tainted by the suspicion of being drug enhanced, and 12% is the true unaided difference between elite men's and women's running speed and 15–20% for the average runner. These figures do not provide any evidence of female superiority at marathon running, although there have been exceptional performances by women in ultra distance cycling, swimming and fell running. Possible metabolic differences are discussed in Professor Saltin's chapter on Muscle metabolic factors decisive for marathon running, who indicates that elite women are closer to men in the use of substrate.

It therefore seems inherently unlikely that in the mid-21st century men will have to resort to golden apples to run as fast as women. The statistical prediction of 1992 seems less and less tenable.

Ageing and running

Some physiologists have seen ageing as a form of disuse atrophy. Decline in performance is blamed on lack of training ('If you don't use it, you lose it'). Professor Sharp discusses in his chapter the biological phenomena and the average decrement in performance in the marathon with age.

From personal experience of 45 years' running, vanity at being able to outpace your students and maintain performance for many successive years gives way to sudden plunges in performance, and the realization that returning after injury or illness becomes increasingly difficult. Recovery from minor injury or a lay off takes longer as does recovery from a hard run. The series elastic element and agility as well as strength seem to decline. The biology of ageing is complex and is more like a terraced hillside than a steady slope in the individual. The number of runners who can and still wish to run marathons in their 80s is very small, and many super vets started running late in life. Perhaps there is over-use atrophy as well as disuse atrophy.

Benefits and risks of exercise — are these exercise myths?

Mass marathon running is a late 20th century phenomenon and has provoked extreme and disparate views from those promoting and those incredulous of the benefits of exercise. In the 1970s and 1980s, it rapidly became a paradigm for the health and fitness movement and was promoted as a 'health event'. Participants were expected to banish the risk of coronary artery disease by burning excess calories and setting a lean and hungry, low fat body composition, reduced low density lipoprotein cholesterol, increased high density lipoprotein cholesterol example to the 'loafers'. These products of modern civilization, the obese television spectator 'sportsmen', were products more of inadequate caloric expenditure than excessive caloric intake, and were at high risk from coronary artery disease. Running a marathon was even proposed as the ultimate 'graduation ceremony' for successful cardiac rehabilitation following myocardial infarction and, despite the morbidity of the marathon run itself as opposed to the healthy effects of training, was promoted as a 'health event'. Some hospitals treating large numbers of runners would question this promotional description which obviously is at the mercy of the weather conditions. Extravagant claims were made for running including the famous claim by Bassler that no marathon runner had ever died from coronary disease[2]. Jim Fixx, a writer and journalist, claimed almost complete immunity from coronary disease for those who ran enough, but unfortunately died from coronary disease himself and like Bassler his claims were discredited.

Running became a media-led, trendy activity, which it was claimed improved life expectancy and sexual activity. The 'locker room look' became fashionable even among those who rarely raised a sweat. There were 'born again' exercising journalists promoting running and 'couch potato' journalists denigrating running, both groups sometimes promoting extreme views or indeed myths.

Joggers and particularly marathon runners have been ridiculed by their detractors for performing repetitive, brain-numbing exercise as they '*hammer hammer hammer down the hard high road*' (an Edwardian music hall song about a lame horse) in the perhaps vain hope of prolonging their lives by a small margin but in the actuality of a real risk of developing significant overuse injuries. Many are not anatomically designed for marathon running, whether from leg length discrepancies or foot strike errors. The human foot has evolved to cope with varying terrain not tar macadam and an unvarying camber, and the running shoe has evolved from a sandal or thin moccasin to the plimsoll of the 1950s to, in some cases, an imitation of a 1960s American car — overweight with a heavily damped ride and designed for protection rather than agility. Most are designed for the average jogger rather than the elite runner, but despite fashion dictates there is science behind the design (see Dr Shorten's chapter).

The combination of endurance exercise and primitive low glycaemic diets has been described as a Palaeolithic prescription for longevity. Marathon runners have been described as being exercise addicts hooked on endorphins and, despite the 'as you can tell by their faces', not enjoying what they are doing (discussed in Professor Morgan's chapter). Exercise has been proposed as a cause of infections and even cancer by biochemists researching in free oxygen radicals, and as a ready excuse for promoting dietary supplements such as large doses of vitamins, minerals and herbal concoctions.

The paradigm of marathon running has now been dethroned by health promoters with the perhaps slow realization that it will always be a minority activity, not achievable by many who need to take more exercise to benefit rather than be frightened by the excessive demands of a marathon run. Instead of promoting extensive and intensive exercise, health promotion has moved beneficial exercise down a gear, and endorsed brisk walking and other less intense activities (see Professor Hardman's chapter).

Heat stress and air pollution

Medical charities have not been reticent in involving themselves with advice about running. Whereas the British Heart Foundation endorses regular aerobic exercise for the heart and circulation (most easily achieved by jogging, walking or cycling), spokespersons for the British Lung Foundation and Cancer charities have publicized the problems of runners exposing themselves to air pollution and ultra violet light during summer heat waves, making it sound as though running outside is dangerous.

I will briefly comment on the relevance of laboratory measurements to actual runners' experiences. Although these factors depend on the climate, which can be assessed by meteorological and air pollution observations, each runner has his or her own microenvironment and can control it to some extent, making theoretical measurements difficult to apply. Their clothing and whether or not they run in the sun, in the shade, close to other runners or on their own dictates this. A close pack of sweating runners may increase the local air temperature and humidity significantly and prevent some of the cooling effects of air movement. On a hot day, it may be possible to maintain a noticeably faster pace on the shady side of the street rather than on the sunny side. The cooling effect of heavy rain, especially with coincident wind, is also very local as are the effects of water sprays and water poured over the body.

In addition, there are many unanswered questions about air pollution. Unfortunately, Dr Folinsbee was taken seriously ill shortly before the conference and his contribution was presented by Professor Raven at the Marathon Medicine meeting. I wished to know whether or not there were any data on runners accumulating long-term problems from exposing their airways to large amounts of pollutants, both from the increased air volumes and lack of protection from the nasal filtering mechanism during exercise-induced mouth breathing. No data appear to exist, but judging by the numbers of runners using nasal dilating strips (which must have a negligible effect in preventing mouth breathing while running a marathon) many of them must have the same anxiety. We wish Dr Folinsbee well.

These and many other topics such as whether or not runners are born or made (genetic basis and possible African superiority) are covered by the authors, who generously give us the science rather than the myths of marathon medicine.

Acknowledgements

I would like to thank the Royal Society of Medicine (RSM) for responding so readily to and supporting my proposal for this conference and book, in particular Marty Adair and Jack Tinker. I also thank the other members of the planning committee — Richard Budgett, Ron Maughan, Craig Sharp, Alan Storey, Clyde Williams — and the RSM Press for all their work. Sadaf Hashmi at the RSM Press deserves a special mention. The conference and book would not have been possible without generous financial support from the London marathon and the British Heart Foundation.

References

1 The marathon. *Ann N Y Acad Sci* 1977; **301**.

2 Bassler TJ. Marathon running and immunity to atherosclerosis. *Ann N Y Acad Sci* 1977; **301**: 579–92.

3 Tunstall Pedoe DS. Sudden cardiac death in sport-spectre or preventable risk. *Br J Sports Med* 2000; **34**: 137–140.

4 Tunstall Pedoe DS. Heart or lung failure: what causes exertional, high altitude, and cold immersion pulmonary oedema? *Br J Sports Med* 1995; **29**: 218–20.

5 Whyte GP, George K, Sharma S *et al.* Cardiac fatigue following prolonged endurance exercise of differing distances. *Med Sci Sport Exerc* 2000; **32**: 1067–72.

6 Whipp BJ, Ward SA. Will women soon outrun men? *Nature* 1992; **355**: 25.

Endurance runners in Britain before the 20th century

PROFESSOR PETER RADFORD

PROFESSOR OF SPORT SCIENCES, DEPARTMENT OF SPORTS SCIENCES, BRUNEL UNIVERSITY, WEST LONDON, UK

The 'marathon' appeared on the modern athletics programme for the first time in 1896. However, long-distance races were part of the sporting culture long before then. It is impossible to say with certainty when the common people of Britain began their love affair with running. We know that in Scotland running was sufficiently well established as a sport for an annual race to be organized as early as 1507, which still continues[1]. In the midlands of England, John Dover's annual Cotswold Games may have begun as early as 1605 and continued for nearly 250 years[2]. In Kent, Sir Dudley Digges gave money for annual prizes for men and women runners to race for from 1638[3] — these continued for more than 200 years. This chapter will focus on the long-distance athletics culture that flourished in Britain in the 18th and early 19th century.

In any discussion of long-distance events, care must be taken when describing the competitors as either 'runners' or 'walkers', as many of the races were so long that competitors both ran and walked, and there was often an indistinct line between the two. The term 'pedestrian' was not in common use before the 19th century, so 'foot race' and 'foot racer' will be used throughout the chapter to describe events and the people who competed in them.

Foot races in the 18th century

Two distinct categories of foot races have been identified from contemporary 18th century newspapers, magazines and diaries:

- annual, calendar events, in which the races were part of a local fair. There were prizes and/or money for the winners and sometimes the runners-up; twice as many girls and women took part in comparison to boys and men. These races were usually relatively short, not exceeding half a mile, and will not be discussed further in this chapter
- especially arranged races, usually for wagers or for stake money — 287 of these events have been recorded (Table 1). From these events, 263 different performers (248 men and 15 women) have been identified although not all by name. These data form the basis of this chapter.

Table 1 Reported foot race wagers, and the number of participants, in 18th century Britain

	Females	Males
1700–24	3	9
1725–49	3	17
1750–74	4	42
1775–99	3	206
	Total=13	Total=274

The rise in reported events for males may be explained either by a progressive increase in the number of races during the century or by more races being reported, but more information is needed to resolve this. One inescapable feature of these data is that, unlike in local fairs, racing for wagers was mainly a man's activity.

The distances of 19 (7%) of the men's, and most of the women's, events could not be identified. Of the remaining 255 male events, only 21 (8%) were sprint events up to 440 yards, 146 (57%) were ≥10 miles, 83 (33%) were ≥25 miles, and 60 (24%) were >50 miles (Figure 1). As most events were more than 10 miles long, this was clearly an 'endurance' rather than a 'sprint' culture. Ninety per cent of these events were 'solo', ie the athlete competed against a previously agreed time and not against another competitor. The object was not to beat a fellow athlete but a fellow wagerer. The other 10% were usually 'matches', in which two foot racers competed against each other, but as a general rule, the further the distance, the less likely it was that the event would be arranged as a match.

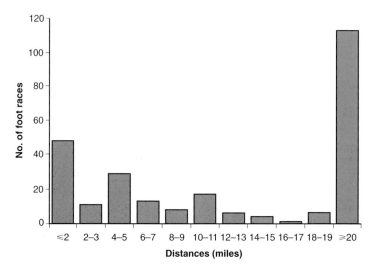

Figure 1

Distances of male foot races (n=255) in 18th century Britain

The competitors

Analysis of the foot racers in events ⩾10 miles long reveals that they came from every part of society and were of all ages. Not surprisingly, there were letter-carriers, porters, running footmen, chairmen, shepherds, farmers, pig-drovers, lamp-lighters, blacksmiths, sawyers and labourers, whose daily activities would have helped prepare them for their competitions. In addition, there were tradesmen, carpenters, shoemakers, cloggers, butchers, millers, barbers, horsehair-weavers, basket-makers and breeches-makers. There were also brewers, innkeepers, pie men, meal men, servants and ostlers, and those involved in finer and more delicate work such as hairdressers, tailors, peruke makers, stay makers and watch-case makers. Among the women, one was a peddler and another was described as a 'broom' girl.

At the upper echelons of the social scale there were many foot racers among the gentlemen, army officers, honourables and lords — a royal prince almost got involved too. The Duke of York — famous for marching his men to the top of the hill and marching them back again — agreed to race six miles for 200 guineas in January 1788, but failed to turn up for the start and lost his stake money. It seems that the whole of British society took part. This was not a sport for the privileged few but genuinely a sport of the people.

Some foot racers were very experienced and had remarkably long careers. Pinwire (or Pinwherie), for example, was said to have competed in 102 races in the five years up to 1733[4]. There are records of 16 of Foster Powell's performances spanning 24 years, 24 of Captain Barclay's spanning 17 years, and 19 of Abraham Wood's spanning 15 years. The careers of the latter two bridged the 18th and 19th centuries.

Nearly 80% of the foot racers, however, appear in the records only once.

Ages of competitors

There are many references to 'old men' and 'young men', and occasionally to 'boys', but there is a lack of detailed information. The ages of 25 males have been identified, revealing that nearly two-thirds were aged 50 years or over (Figure 2).

The youngest boy was 12 years old, who ran three-and-a-half miles in 1792. The oldest was Richard Brown, reported to be 114 when he ran 24 miles in eight hours in 1794. Next in longevity was Donald McLeod, who was variously reported to be 102 and 104 when he ran 10 miles in two hours and 23 minutes in 1790. McLeod incidentally had walked from London to Inverness and back again the previous year, a distance of 1,148 miles, and astonished everyone with his 'hilarity of disposition' and 'healthful appearance' in doing so[5].

It is even more difficult to establish the ages of the women during this period. Mary Wilkinson was reported to be 90 years when she went 259 miles from County Durham to London in five days and three hours in 1764. 'Lady Butterfield' said she was 74 years when she challenged 'any woman in England seven years younger, but not a

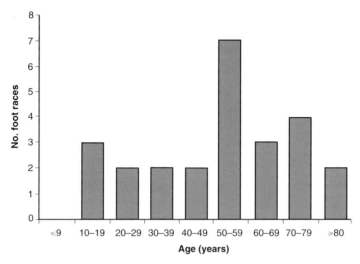

Figure 2

Age of male foot racers (n=25) in 18th century Britain

day older', because she would not 'undervalue' herself[6]. It was a 'young woman', however, who went 72 miles in one day in 1765.

An open and accessible sport

The 'athletic class' had not yet appeared in the 18th century, and foot racing was accessible to all regardless of age, gender, nationality, race, class or physical shape, condition or ability. Anyone could take part in a race, and at any time. As there were no clubs, governing bodies and written rules, people could do as they pleased. To enter into a wager, its terms had to be agreed with another person and a trustworthy third party had to be sought to hold the money. It was wise to put the articles of agreement into writing and appoint one or more race officials to arbitrate in case of disagreement. That done, you could make up any rules you liked.

Events in the 18th century were not only concerned with physical ability but also about people pitting their wits, knowledge and experience against each other. Setting the terms of the wager, its distance, route, terrain, time of day and date for completion was as much a mind-game as it was a test of physical ability.

Body size and shape

In 1788, the crowd was astonished by a young man named Evans because he was so short — he ran 10 miles in 55 minutes and 18 seconds. John Hoole, another 10-miler, drew attention because he was 'very short in stature, and remarkably bandy legged'. There were also big and strong men like Mr Shadbolt, a publican from Ware in Hertfordshire who was known locally as 'Goliath'. He wagered to run and push his cart 24 miles from Ware to Shoreditch Church, which he did in about six hours. Many fat men also took part. Mr Hardwicke, for example, won a wager to run 25 miles from Worcester to Birmingham in 1790 when he completed it in six and three-quarter hours. The papers called this 'remarkable' because of his 'gross habit of body and unwieldy size'[7].

Fat men could also race on equal terms with thin men if they could find a willing partner. In Bedford in 1790, John Thong wore a specially made pad weighing 58 lb in his five-and-a-half mile race against John Jordan, in order to make their two weights equal. In 1796, the same principle was used to adjust for age. Luke Ashmore, aged 25 years, wore a 35 lb weight in his 10-mile race against George Gooding to allow for Gooding's extra 35 years. The 60-year-old man won by three minutes.

Carrying extra weight did not seem to be a barrier to foot racing. In 1760, a porter covered nearly 20 miles in three-and-a-half hours carrying 50 lb of half-pennies. 56 lb (25.3 kg) was a particularly 'popular' weight to run with. In 1763 a man covered seven miles in 45 minutes carrying 56 lb of fish on his head. Another man ran four miles in 59 minutes with a 56 lb weight on his shoulders in 1788. In 1793 a runner named Chambers went from Birmingham to Coventry (18½ miles) in three hours and 57 minutes carrying a 'Scotchman's pack' that weighed 56 lb in Birmingham but, due to the rain, was 60 lb when he arrived in Coventry.

Fun and games

These 18th century long-distance foot races should not all be thought of as gruelling, no-fun events. For example, in 1775, John Green wagered to go seven miles in one hour on the Artillery Grounds in London while eating a cold fowl and drinking a bottle of wine. In 1792, John Barrett took only 53 minutes to run the same distance, eat ½ lb of beef-steak and drink a pint of wine. No wonder the crowds, sometimes in their thousands, were attracted to these events! Lieutenant Colonel Thomas Thornton completed a 50-mile wager in 1787 accompanied by his favourite pointer which, not surprisingly, 'indicated his joy with a prodigious bark' when it was all over[8]. A few years later, in 1791, Cotterel ran 20 miles against a horse. In 1793, a wager was made to go 10 miles from Piccadilly to Hounslow in three hours, going backwards for one stride on every fourth stride. In 1797, William Hearn ran a coach wheel 22 miles in three hours. Everybody could find an event to suit themselves. An elderly man with a wooden leg offered to run any man in the kingdom 'of whatever age, weight and size' provided he could choose the ground[9].

Fitness and training

In an age before the internal combustion engine and electricity, common sense tells us that people, on average, must have had a higher level of daily exercise than those 200–300 years later, and that this lasted most of their lives. When Captain Barclay's father was a member of parliament in the 1790s, he used to walk 510 miles from Stonehaven, Scotland to Westminster, England. There are countless other examples, particularly of poor people, who walked regularly from necessity. For instance, it was calculated that one man in Lincoln had walked at least 45,760 miles over the previous 40 years just to go to the market.

In addition, there were well-known professional trainers who would prepare foot racers for their wagers. They looked after the athletes' diet and the state of their skin, and supervised their sweats and purges. They would also organize their 'breathings', and prescribe the right quantity and quality of exercise. Training would typically last three weeks, but could be three times longer if necessary. Methods of training were shared between the trainers of runners, boxers, racehorses and cock feeders. Some trainers achieved national fame and were in great demand. For example, Jackey Smith in Yorkshire and Old Ben in Lancashire who were both farmers; Ripshaw the gaoler in Ipswich; and Bill Warr, the ex-prize-fighter from Bristol who operated in London. In 1806 their methods moved from the old oral tradition to the printed page when Sir John Sinclair published the findings of his national survey into training methods for sport[10].

Risk

The bravery of those who took on the endurance events, particularly in the first half of the 18th century, should not be underestimated. Plutarch and Lucian's story of how Philippides (also called Pheidippides) ran from Marathon to Athens and then fell down dead was well-known by all educated men and women[11], as was Plutarch's story of Euchidas who ran 125 miles in one day, handed over the sacred torch, and then died[12]. It was so well-known that athletes could outstrip their own strength and die from overexertion, that those who engaged in such activities were thought to be foolhardy. In the 25 years between 1733 and 1758 alone, stories circulated of the imminent or actual deaths of: John Appleby, Pinwire and Woolley Morris after they had run in 10-mile events; Griffith Morgan (often known as Guto Nithbran) after a 12-mile event; and Stephen Morris after he had run 38 miles of a 40-mile event[13]. These reports were consistent with the prevailing medical view expressed by Robert Burton in 1651 who stated, 'Nothing better than exercise (if opportunely used) for the preservation of the body: nothing so bad if it be unseasonable, violent, or overmuch'[14].

By the end of the 18th century, however, more men and women raced long-distance and survived to tell the tale. In the last quarter of the 18th century, newspapers began to write more positively about endurance athletes, repeatedly reporting how little fatigued they were and how they completed their events with 'apparent ease'. However, fear of overexertion had such a grip of the popular imagination that it continued despite the evidence. In 1793 when Foster Powell, the best known endurance athlete of his age, died unexpectedly in his 50s, newspapers reported that his death was due to his exertions in a 394-mile event nine months earlier. In December 1798, *The Sporting Magazine* attempted to discourage a young Scottish man from attempting a 50-mile event by writing: 'we recollect more instances than one of Gentlemen having lost their lives by breaking a blood-vessel, from too great an exertion'[15]. The following month, they reported, with a barely concealed note of 'I told you so', that a young 20-year-old who ran a 50-mile wager in nine hours and 18 minutes had 'dropped down, and was taken home in a chaise as a dying man'[16].

The reality behind the newspaper stories was not always as bad as it seemed. Five years after the papers reported that Pinwire 'cannot live', they reported his performance in a 12-mile race[17]. Further information about Foster Powell also revealed that his cause of death had more to do with a 'swelling in his neck, which had been unskilfully treated' than the long delayed effects of overexertion[18].

Specialization

The 18th century was an age that generally distrusted extremes in anything, even in sport. Those who competed in one sport often competed in another. Even those who were specialist foot racers often 'ran' an extraordinary range of distances. Foster Powell, for example, took part in events from one mile to 400, Abraham Wood from 440 yards to 40 miles, and Captain Barclay from 440 yards to 70 miles. Thus, many athletes were all-rounders in their sport, training and lifestyle. There were, nevertheless, some specialists. Pinwire was a 10-mile specialist as was Joe, the head ostler at Mr Fozzard's in Park Lane, London. Joe was in his 40s when he ran 10½ miles in 57 minutes. Richard West, from Old Windsor, was a specialist at distances from 40 to 60 miles; he was in his 50s when he beat Foster Powell over 60 miles, within six hours. William Aspinal, from Pontefract, who was at his best in his 40s, seldom ran below 100 miles.

How good were the competitors?

The world of 18th century long-distance foot racing was based on different assumptions from our own. There were neither records nor personal bests. The reason for this was that running as fast as possible was not the point of their races. This is a major difference as compared with the late 19th and 20th centuries. There was no need to run faster than the time set for the wager. Indeed there were well-known medical reasons for not doing so. For the few regular racers there was the additional reason of not revealing how fast you could run, as this would affect the next wager you might make. Bets were also laid on the result of races while they were in progress, another reason for not revealing too much too soon.

Nevertheless, evidence from a few established athletes suggests that some were very good indeed. In separate reports, six years apart, Pinwire was reported to have run 10 miles in 52 minutes and 3 seconds in 1733, and 12 miles in 64 minutes and five seconds in 1738–9. Just after the turn of the century, Captain Barclay completed 110 miles in a time-trial in heavy rain and muddy conditions. His time of 19 hours and 27 minutes was reported to be 'the best on record'[19]. Clearly, there were some outstanding and well-trained endurance athletes in the 18th century.

Accuracy of reports

Distances could be measured accurately if it was worth doing, and sometimes there were reports that the courses were measured 'accurately', often with an agricultural chain. In most cases, it did not matter whether or not the course was measured precisely. For example, it was well known that the 'Four Mile' course at Doncaster was 408 yards short. Many events, however, used well-known landmarks such as Mr Mullins's wager in 1765 to go from Shoreditch Church to St George's Church in the Borough, and back (about 13 miles) in 50 minutes. The convention was to touch the church door, so in this case the distance was very precise even if it was not measured.

Time keeping could also be relatively accurate, particularly over longer distances, but the only important time was that set for the wager. It was the wager that was timed and not the athlete. The athlete's time was unimportant and, as it was usually only an approximation, could seldom be relied on. For example, in Mr Mullins' wager, mentioned above, it did not matter what his actual time was so long as both sides agreed which side of 50 minutes it was. In this case he got in about three-and-a-half minutes ahead of his target time, but this was only a rough estimate, not an official time. To avoid disputes, the convention was to set several watches in a sealed box and place it at the finish under the supervision of the stake-holder. Specialist watchmakers such as Mr Bramble from Oxford Street, London, were sometimes used to provide specially selected and regulated watches.

Reporting the wager was often the worst part. Newspapers relied heavily on correspondents from the general public, or another newspaper. There were few specialist correspondents, nor any respect for other people's copy. Errors inevitably crept in and were often copied and repeated, but these were sometimes corrected in later editions. Details are often tantalizingly sparse, but they did improve later in the century, and it is occasionally possible to get some sort of 'triangulation' on a result from different reports that are clearly independent.

'Marathon' times

Those brought up on the 20th century version of foot racing find it difficult to think of races without considering times, personal best performances and records. It is clear that asking about the 'times' of 18th century athletes is something of an anachronism, especially when enquiring about 'marathon times' because the marathon itself did not have a standardized distance until 1924. Nevertheless, there were many performances over distances between 20 and 30 miles. If those involving men who were fat, very old or carrying heavy weights, and those who were obviously walking, are disregarded, four events can be identified from which we can make an estimate of time. These events took place in the London area.

1712 — a 22-mile race[20]. This was between two professional runners, one English and the other Scottish. It was held on a grass course measuring almost four miles, which was 'measured and cut even'. The winning time was 'two-and-a-half' hours, roughly equivalent to a three-hour marathon.

1740 — a 21-mile wager[21]. This wager by Thomas Calile (Carlisle) was for two hours. It was held on a grass course on a popular sports ground and thus was probably measured. It was roughly equivalent to wagering to run a marathon in two hours and 31 minutes. Calile won. Nine years later, he was reported as winning a 10-mile wager in 55 minutes, a roughly equivalent performance. Based on this evidence he was an experienced and consistent runner.

1753 — a 21-mile wager[22]. This wager was for two hours and was undertaken as a solo performance by Matzee (Matzel), probably an Italian. The course was on the road between two known landmarks. Similar to the 1740 wager, this is equivalent to wagering to run a marathon in two hours and 31 minutes. Matzee won easily. If he had won by the quarter of an hour as the reports say, this would be equivalent to a marathon time of about two hours and 11 minutes.

1769 — a 30-mile wager[23]. A solo performance by a Swiss professional runner, this wager was for 3¼ hours. The course was on the road between known landmarks and was roughly equivalent to wagering to run a marathon in two hours and 45 minutes. He won very easily. If he won by the three-quarters of an hour that the reports say, this would be equivalent to a marathon inside two hours and 10 minutes. He was said to be the best runner in Europe, and this performance was reported as 'the most extraordinary performance of its kind that was ever known'. The reporter seems to have known his athletics.

Regardless of the times they actually ran, the latter three runners had sufficient confidence in their ability to believe they could 'run a marathon' in two-and-a-half hours and two-and-three-quarter hours respectively. Such performances — carried out on their own, in an age before running shoes, and on running surfaces that were unlikely to be even — indicate that there were some good marathon runners in the 18th century. Furthermore, the last two runners were reported to have won very easily.

Foot racers in the early 19th century

The types of events, and the types of competitors that took part in them, in the first 15 years of the 19th century were similar to those in the 18th century; but by then the references were more numerous and gave more detail than before. Doctors and surgeons were increasingly called on to attend events and to supervise athletes during them. Long-distance events retained their fascination and attracted even larger crowds. In many ways the first 15 years of the 19th century were a Golden Age of long-distance foot racing, and the leading long-distance athletes achieved a fame that has seldom been touched since.

Captain Barclay

Captain Barclay became the most famous athlete of his age when he completed one mile every hour for 1,000 hours (nine hours short of six weeks)[24]. The event took place in the summer of 1809 on Newmarket Heath, on a one-mile measured course and in front of thousands of people. His winnings were £16,000, which in absolute terms was unbeaten for more than 150 years, and in relative terms has probably never been exceeded. It was worth 320 times the national average income, and may have been worth more than £4 m today.

George Wilson

George Wilson was a 50-year-old, poor, thin man from Newcastle who attempted to run 1,000 miles on Blackheath Common in 20 days in the summer of 1815[25]. Enormous crowds turned out and innumerable booths and tents were erected to provide food and drink, each with its waiters, musicians and seats facing the action. There were Scottish pipers, jugglers, fire-eaters and a famous elephant. 'Nothing could exceed the bustle and confusion which the heath presented'[25]. The crowd got in his way and trod on his feet, and he had to appoint men with whips and staves to keep his path clear. It was all too much for the local Justices of the Peace who ordered his arrest after he had completed 751¼ miles and was on schedule to complete the 1,000 miles on time.

Foot racers after 1811

From 1811, and certainly from 1815, the national economy went into decline and the social structure of the country began to change. The Luddite disturbances, the Peterloo Massacre, the Cato Street conspiracy, the Chartist movement and the reformed Parliament of 1832 were all indications of a country in social and economic turmoil. Poor men and women began performing long-distance events, for money, of course — 'pedestrianism' had arrived.

Although poor men competing for money had been relatively commonplace, the appearance of poor girls and women was a new phenomenon in Britain. Newspapers and magazines commented on the ease and confidence with which they completed their events, and gave no suggestion that the distances were too long for them or that they were in any way distressed. There are many examples. A large crowd came to see a 30-year-old woman run 40 miles in 1811. Mary Frith, a 36-year-old, attempted to run 30 miles a day for 20 days in 1816; the following year Esther Crozier had completed seven days of her task to go 50 miles a day for 20 days (ie 350 miles), when she gave it up over 'some dispute'[26]. In 1820, a 17-year-old woman attempted 40 miles a day for six days. In 1823, a girl of about 11 years managed to run alongside a professional runner in an 11-mile event despite having to run home with her clogs after two miles and being impeded by a crowd of boys, one of whom she had to fight. In 1823, 'a young woman' in the west of Scotland lost a 15-mile race against 'a lad'. A woman won a 50-mile wager in Exeter in 1826 and, in 1833, a 70-year-old woman attempted to run 96 miles in 24 hours at Paisley, Scotland. After 45 miles, when she was five miles ahead of schedule, she was arrested because the large and unruly crowd had threatened public law and order.

Two of the most remarkable females of this period were Mary McMullen and Emma Freeman.

Mary McMullen

Mary McMullen was a poor Irish woman out of Yorkshire, and was the mother of a family of sons who became itinerant pedestrians in the 1820s[27]. None were as successful as she was. She was in her 60s in 1826-7 when she took part in at least seven events in 15 months, the distances ranging from 20 to 92 miles with a mean distance of 63 miles, and she made her money by taking collections during the events. She, too, could attract large crowds, which often impeded her, sometimes deliberately. Six thousand people came to see her at York.

Emma Matilda Freeman

Emma Freeman was eight years old in 1823 when she completed four events in only nine weeks[27]. The first three distances covered were 30 miles, and the fourth was 40 miles. For the 40-mile event she was wagered to do seven hours and 50 minutes, but there was some doubt about the time. She was known as the 'Pedestrian Girl', and came from Suffolk and seemed to be managed by her parents.

The amateur age

The social upheaval in Britain continued. The new economy demanded more people in the great factory towns and the 'working class' and Victorian England slowly emerged. The old sport was replaced by a new concept led by young, middle-class men in universities. Not only did they devise 'amateur athletics' but also the 'championship meeting'. The prime movers were young men who preferred shorter events. Exeter College, Oxford, led the way, but their innovative cross-country event was only two miles long and the longest event in their inaugural sports was only 440 yards. Later, the championship meeting evolved with a three-mile event and a seven-mile walk but it was not the long-distance foot racing of old.

This new 'amateur athletics' was certainly not based on an endurance culture — it does not really seem to have been based on hard work at all! The men from the universities leading this movement were looking for an afternoon's sport, and in this process the old long-distance running culture lost its pre-eminence. An indication of how such attitudes changed can be found in Stonehenge's 1888 definition of long-distance running as anything 'from one mile upwards'[28].

25

The rich diversity and individuality of the old sport disappeared; the new sport worshipped standardization, regulation and control. Professionals and others whose jobs might have given them an edge were excluded from taking part. So were women. Competing for wagers and betting on the result was prohibited, removing the very reason why most of the old foot racers had competed in the first place. As the old endurance running culture declined, so probably did the athletic standards. In 1888, remnants of the old professional sport still survived alongside the new Amateur Athletics (founded in 1880), and lists of both professional and amateur records were complied. For every event from 10 to 100 miles, the amateur records were always inferior. Yet it was the amateurs who prevailed. The old sport died, and with it, its culture, personalities and achievements.

References

1 Clouston E. Red Socks. *The Scotsman Weekend* 1998 Aug 29: 8–11.

2 Vyvyan ER. *Cotswold games — Annalia Dubrensia*. Cheltenham: Williams & Son, 1878.

3 *Annals of Sporting* 1823; **3**: 174.

4 *The Country Journal, or The Craftsman*; 1733 Dec 22.

5 *The Edinburgh Advertiser* 1789 Oct 16–20.

6 Ashton J. *Social life in the age of Queen Anne, taken from original sources*. London: Chatter & Windus, 1882: 243.

7 *Jackson's Oxford Journal* 1790 Apr 15.

8 *The London Chronicle* 1787 Apr 5–7.

9 *The Sporting Magazine* 1799 July: 217.

10 Radford PF. From oral tradition to printed record: British sports sciences in transition, 1805–1807. *Proceedings of The XIIth HISPA Congress 1989*; Sankt Augustin: Academia-Verlag, 1989: 295–304.

11 Lee HM. Modern ultra-long distance running and Philippides' run from Athens to Sparta. *Ancient World* 1984; **9**: 107–13.

12 Sweet WE. *Sport and recreation on Ancient Greece*. Oxford: Oxford University Press, 1987: 34–5.

13 Radford PF. Escaping the Philippedes connection: death, injury and illness in 18th century sport in Britain. In: Terret T, ed. *Sport and health in history*. Sankt Augustin: Academia Verlag, 1999: 87–100.

14 Burton R. *The anatomy of melancholy (1621)*. London: Chatto and Windus, 1927: 158.

15 *The Sporting Magazine* 1798 December: 165–6.

16 *The Sporting Magazine* 1799 January: 235.

17 *The Warwick and Staffordshire Journal* 1738–9 29 March.

18 *The Sporting Magazine* 1793 Apr: 48.

19 Thom W. *Pedestrianism, or an account of the performances of celebrated pedestrians during the last and present century*. Aberdeen: D Chalmers and Company, 1813: 104.

20 Fiennes C; edited by Morris C. *Illustrated journeys of Celia Fiennes*. London: Macdonald & Co Ltd, 1982: 243–4.

21 *The Sporting Magazine* 1792 Oct: 8.

22 *The Sporting Magazine* 1793 Nov: 97–8.

23 *Aris's Birmingham Gazette* 1769 July 24.

24 Radford PF. Captain Barclay. In: Huntington-Whitley J, ed. *The book of British sporting heroes*. London: National Portrait Gallery, 1998.

25 Wilson G. *A sketch of the life of George Wilson, the Blackheath pedestrian*. London: Hay and Turner, 1815.

26 *The Edinburgh Advertiser*, 1817 Oct 29.

27 Radford PF. Women's foot-races in the 18th and 19th centuries; a popular and widespread practice. *Can J His Sport* 1994; **25**: 58–63.

28 Walsh JH. *British rural sports; comprising shooting, hunting, coursing, fishing, hawking, racing, boating and pedestrianism*. London: Frederick Warne & Co, 1888: 616.

DISCUSSION

Attendee: Can you please tell us about the diet of participants, and the use of port and wine and other stimulants that were taken during these races?

Professor Peter Radford: They were very cautious about what they drank. It was thought that drinking too much was unwise, especially water which in many areas may have been unsafe to drink. Beer was safest, even for women, and in those days children also drank beer. Gentlemen were allowed port and a little wine during their training but that was thought too rich for the ordinary digestive systems. Brandy mixed with water was a commonly used drink during long-distance events lasting many hours or days. With regards to food, Sir John Sinclair carried out a survey of training methods in 1806 and this included items on diet. This revealed that participants were not advised to eat vegetables because they were too watery, or cheese and/or even butter as they went rancid in the stomach. They were not really enthusiastic about carbohydrates, but were about large quantities of meat which had to be undercooked. During long-distance events, cold fowl was consumed.

Attendee: Were participants sometimes rubbed vigorously with loofahs and stiff brushes?

Professor Peter Radford: Yes, in the Victorian age in particular athletes were rubbed with camphorated oil. Trainers were taught how to transfer these fluids onto the athlete at the correct temperature — the trainer held the oil in his or her mouth for several minutes so it reached body temperature, spat it over the athlete to ensure it did not cool down, and immediately started rubbing. An art that has been lost over the centuries!

Marathon running as a social and athletic phenomenon: historical and current trends

DR DAVID MARTIN

EMERITUS PROFESSOR, DEPARTMENT OF CARDIOPULMONARY CARE SCIENCES,
GEORGIA STATE UNIVERSITY, ATLANTA, GEORGIA, USA

In 1976, an international conference was devoted for the first time to the medical and scientific aspects of marathon running. It was held in conjunction with the inaugural New York City marathon run through the city's five boroughs; proceedings of the 77 presentations have been published in the *Annals of the New York Academy of Sciences*[1]. The conference was a logical outgrowth of several factors including:

- a developing general participatory interest in endurance sport, especially jogging and running
- an increasing mass of scientific research investigating performance aspects of long-distance running
- a relative absence of forums for debating findings and discrepancies in such research.

This world of endurance sport — ranging from the highest level of competition by professional athletes to participation by everyday fitness enthusiasts — has expanded over the 24 years since the New York conference, with much laboratory study of how this performance is achieved. For example, there was a 20.6-fold increase in the number of participants for the 1999 New York City marathon than in 1976 — proportionately more women participated in 1999 and there was an improvement in winning finish times, especially for women (Table 1). These trends are seen consistently in many other similar marathons contested worldwide.

Table 1 New York City marathon statistics: 1976 and 1996

	1976	1996
Male participants:		
– No finishers	1,504	22,626
– % of finishers	97.5	71.2
– Winning time	2:10:10	2:09:14
Female participants:		
– No finishers	39	9,160
– % of finishers	2.5	28.8
– Winning time	2:39:11	2:25:06

In London, an international all-women's marathon took place on 3 August 1980, two days after the Moscow Olympic men's marathon. It was won by New Zealand's Lorraine Moller in two hours, 35 minutes and 11 seconds (2:35:11), who later became the only woman to have completed the first four women's Olympic marathons. This led, in 1981, to the mixed race extravaganza known as the London marathon, which has since risen in stature until today it equals the New York City event both in total participants and quality of top-level performances.

The marathon is now as much a social phenomenon as a highly competitive event.

This chapter will briefly review how the marathon foot race originated and how it has gradually evolved into its current status as a global participatory event. It will also discuss how the distance for the London marathon was selected.

Legendary basis for the origin of a 'marathon run'

The word 'marathon' refers to a village in Greece about 40 km north-east of Athens where, according to the well-known chronicler of Greek history, Herodotus[2], King Darius of Persia landed a force of 20,000 men onshore in 490 BC. Darius planned to conquer the Greeks and punish them for helping the Ionians (who lived in western Asia Minor) revolt against his rule. Although the Greeks were directed by the competent General Miltiades, they were outnumbered nearly two to one and needed reinforcements. Cornelius Nepos, a first century BC Roman historian and biographer, reported that 'the Athenians, distressed by this war so near and so great in their own land, sought aid nowhere other than from the Lacedaemonians (Spartans) and sent Phidippides, a runner of that class known as hemerodromoi, to report how urgent was the need of aid'[3]. The hemerodromoi were trained distance runners; Phidippides' name has been variously written as Pheidippides and Philippides.

The exact distance covered by the trained soldier/runner in executing his duties remains unclear. If he first journeyed from Marathon to Athens (40 km) to report the need for more troops, then made a round-trip (480 km) between Athens and Sparta to request troop deployment, returned to Marathon (40 km) to inform Miltiades of his efforts to recruit assistance, and finally made the celebrated 40 km return to Athens, this would total 600 km in just a few days. Ironically, the Spartan support forces did not reach Marathon in time to assist General Miltiades in his struggle, due to their preoccupation with a religious festival[4], but fortunately for the Greeks, they were not needed. Miltiades faced the Persians with his troops and soundly defeated them. The Greeks lost only 192 men in the battle, a small fraction of the 6,400 Persians who died. A large mound, allegedly holding the remains of these 192 Greeks, can still be seen at the site of the old battlefield.

Herodotus does not mention the return journey from Marathon to Athens by this trained runner after the battle, who was sent to announce the news of the victory to the king. According to legend, on arrival, Pheidippides gasped the single Greek word 'NENIKHKAMEN' ('we have won!'), then collapsed and died. Robert Browning, in his famous 1879 poem entitled 'Pheidippides', translated this word as the phrase 'Rejoice, we conquer'[5]. Some authors have wondered why such an exciting ending to this chronicle of events was not reported by Herodotus[6] — perhaps it did not happen! However, the legend lives on.

The first Olympic marathon

When the ancient games of Olympia were reborn in Athens during 1896 in the form of a global sports competition, the organizers believed that Greek enthusiasm for hosting these games would be optimized by the inclusion of a unique athletic event relevant to Greek history. Thus, the legendary run from Marathon to Athens assumed a modern reality as part of the competition programme. The plan was to have a competitive, long-distance foot race of approximately 40 km (about 25 miles) called 'the marathon race', starting at the Marathon battlefield and ending in the Panathenaikon stadium that was rebuilt for these games.

In 1896, two unpaved roads connected Athens with Marathon. The legendary run of Pheidippides from Marathon to Athens could, thus, have taken either route[7]. The longer route, about 40 km (25 miles) in length, was initially flat, extended south along the sun-baked seacoast past the villages of Mati and Raphena, turned west, and eventually crossed the mountains surrounding Athens. The highest point was near the village of Stavros, 240 m (788 feet) above sea level, with the final 10 km being a descent into the city. The shorter route, about 34 km (21 miles), began climbing immediately into the mountains just west of Marathon, reaching an elevation of 350 m (1,150 feet) above sea level in the first nine kilometres (5.6 miles). Descending gently toward the south-west through cool, pine-filled forests, eventually into the suburbs of Kifisia and Amaroussion, the route then entered the city of Athens. Thus, although the latter route had greater total ascent, it was 15% shorter in total distance and runners would have encountered the ascent while still fresh.

The longer 40-km seacoast route was selected for the 1896 Olympic games in preference to the shorter mountainous route, for reasons that remain unknown. Perhaps it was because the distance is also familiar to participating nations that are accustomed to the Imperial measurement system. Forty kilometres is just 234 m (256 yards) short of 25 miles. It was, however, also a fair challenge, as the initial level portion allowed athletes to develop a sense of efficient race pace. After negotiating the mid-course ascent, the long sloping downhill finish allowed a pace increase for the very fit, yet eased the discomfort for those having a bad day.

As the Greeks very much wanted to win this first Olympic marathon race, they held two selection races over the actual course to choose their participants. With only a month to the Olympic race, such a short time period for recovery may have been more of a liability than a benefit as very little was known about training for such events in those days. The first Greek selection race was held on 27 February using the local Julian calendar (10 March using the more global Gregorian calendar). Being an event of the Pan-Hellenic Sport Celebration, the 12 entrants were members of Greek sports clubs. Only the times of the top six athletes are known; the winner of this very first marathon foot race was Kharilaos Vasilakos (3:18:00). Another race was held two weeks later, on 12 March Julian (24 March Gregorian), which was called an Olympic trial and in which 38 athletes competed. These athletes had to produce better winning times than those of the Pan-Hellenic games in order to be selected for the Olympic team. The winner was Ioannis Lavrentis (3:11:27). In fifth position was Spiridon Louis (3:18:27); he was placed on the Greek Olympic team despite finishing outside the time limit, as he was very close behind the fourth-placed trial finisher who was inside the time limit.

Details of the first Olympic marathon have been widely publicized[8]. Spiridon Louis won the race in 2:58:50, cheered on by a full stadium of spectators. Seven minutes and 13 seconds later, Kharilaos Vasilakos entered the stadium, finishing in 3:06:03, and it was bedlam all over again. The time difference between the winner and runner-up remains the largest in Olympic marathon history. As one can imagine, 23-year-old Spiridon Louis was a grand hero, instantly famous, and the Olympic marathon was born.

Present Olympic distance

The first six Olympic marathon courses were all different in length: 40,000 m at Athens in 1896, 40,260 m at Paris in 1900, 39,996 m at St Louis in 1904, 42,195 m at London in 1908, 40,200 m at Stockholm in 1912, and 42,750 m at Antwerp in 1920. At the start of the 1924 Paris Olympic games, it was decided that the distance for subsequent games should be standardized. The International Olympic Committee (IOC) delegated considerable authority regarding details of event preparations to various international sport federations that had developed over the preceding years. The International Amateur Athletic Federation (IAAF), which governed the sport of athletics, was formed two days following the Stockholm Olympic games in 1912.

At the Fifth IAAF Congress in Geneva on 27 May 1921, a list of proposed competitive events was presented to the assembled delegates for approval. The list included the marathon and its length was given as 42.195 km (26 miles, 385 yards) — the same as at the 1908 London Olympic games[9]. No explanation was provided as to why that particular distance was selected, and the Congress delegates offered no debate regarding any other distance. Senn suggests that it may simply have been a combination of influential British membership on the IAAF committee that prepared the track and field agenda[10]. Another contributing element may have been the extensive publicity surrounding the 1908 London Olympic marathon race that gave this edition more identity. There, an Italian, Dorando Pietri, entered the stadium first, collapsed at 26 miles, staggered to his feet, continued around the track, fell a few more times, was assisted to his feet in the process, crossed the finish line, and was disqualified for receiving assistance. The gold medal went to John Hayes of the US.

At the Geneva IAAF Congress, no requirements were mandated regarding the shape of the course (eg loop, point-to-point, out-and-back, starting and/or finishing inside the stadium). The final vote taken was to give discretion to local organizers regarding layout, but to require conformity to the 42,195 m distance[9]. A limit of six runners per team was also mandated and, in 1932, this maximum entry quota was reduced to three, remaining so to this day.

Origin of the London marathon distance

How was the unusual distance of 26 miles, 385 yards selected for the 1908 London Olympic games marathon? It resulted unintentionally following the final details for the royal family to participate in the marathon start and finish[11]. The course route was originally planned to extend eastward from Windsor Castle to White City Stadium, an approximate distance of 26 miles. The royal box at the stadium was on the long straightaway across from the marathon entry tunnel, and athletes were to finish in front of Queen Alexandra. This would be a delight for both athletes and spectators, as the grand finale would be a run of more than one-half a lap around the 536 m (one-third mile) track inside the full stadium.

Initially, the Queen was to send a signal by telegraph to the starter of the race, Lord Desborough of the British Olympic Association, when the athletes were assembled on the street alongside Windsor Castle; Lord Desborough would then fire the starter's pistol. This plan was eventually modified to allow the Princess of Wales to receive the signal from the Queen, who in turn would command Lord Desborough to start the race. The Princess wanted her children (Edward VIII and George VI, both of whom later became King in 1936) to view these festivities, so the starting point was shifted to the castle grounds, on the East Terrace under the windows of the nursery.

Final measurement of the course along local roads from the Windsor Castle starting point to the stadium put the 26 miles point just inside the stadium, on the track near the entry tunnel. The additional distance to the Queen's royal box was 385 yards. As a standard marathon distance did not exist, the distance of 26 miles and 385 yards was used — no attempt was made to change the route and shorten it to achieve a 'rounded' distance such as exactly 26 miles.

Marathon boom: from athletic contest to social activity

The marathon is unique among the running events on the Olympic games programme as it is contested on the roads instead of on the track. It is a profound challenge, so demanding that its competitors virtually exhaust their energy reserves in the process. A serious commitment to extended physical training is only part of marathon preparation; much attention should be given both to energy and fluid intake before and during the event. Until the 1970s, the only people who attempted such an arduous race were serious athletes, mainly men interested in top-level competition. National championships were staged annually in those nations who sent teams to the Olympic games.

From Athens in 1896 and continuing through Atlanta in 1996 (including the 1906 Intercalated Games marathon also sanctioned by the IOC), 1,496 different athletes (1,275 men and 221 women) have started Olympic marathons[11]. Some ran more than one Olympic marathon, totalling 1,795 performances (1,541 by men and 254 by women). More often than not, Olympic marathons have been held in warm, humid, summertime conditions, which has made quality competition difficult. In fact, in the 24 Olympic-level men's marathons held between 1896 and 1996, only 73.5% of the starters have completed the race; one of them (Portugal's Francisco Lazaro in 1912) even died attempting to finish it. The women have fared somewhat better, with 84.1% of starters finishing the four Olympic marathons staged since 1984[11].

The 1970s saw the start of a transition into marathon running by amateur fitness enthusiasts who enjoyed 'following in the footsteps of the stars'. As marathon foot races are conducted on city streets, there is much room for mass participation. One event often mentioned as a catalyst for this upsurge of participation is Frank Shorter's gold medal performance at the 1972 Munich Olympic games. It was televised throughout the US — his victory appeared easy and the media coverage was extensive. Participation in general outdoor endurance sport was also increasing in the US during this period. For example, the number of marathons in the US increased from 46 in 1970 to 144 in 1975. A second catalytic event may have been the 1976 Montreal Olympic games marathon, televised live to prime-time US viewing markets. Once again, Shorter won an Olympic medal but was later upstaged by another American, Boston's Bill Rodgers, in the New York City marathon. Unprecedented attention to endurance running as a participatory sport for the masses occurred with television coverage of this event on its new route — moved from its several laps around Central Park onto the large bridges and city streets of this teeming metropolis. The number of people that completed this marathon increased from 339 in 1975 to 1,532 in 1976.

Other cities began to realize the favourable economical impact of such a large influx of 'marathon tourists'. The 'marathon boom' continues to expand worldwide, with more than 2,000 such events held each year. In the US, its athletics federation has a Road Running Information Center (RRIC) that compiles statistics on various aspects of road racing. Its periodic newsletter provides a view of the growth of activity in that country, where such sport participation is the most extensive. In 1990, for example, 26 US marathons had 1,000 or more finishers and, by 1999, this number had grown to 45. In 1999, three marathons had more than 20,000 finishers (New York City with 31,875, Chicago with 24,604, and Honolulu with 21,211). The estimated number of marathon finishers in the US has grown by 67% since 1990 (260,000 in 1990 vs 435,000 in 1999). In addition, the growth rate of female finishers over the past 10 years has increased more rapidly than the men's rate. For instance, in the US, 19% of marathon finishers were female in 1990 while, by 1999, this had increased to 35%. Similar statistical trends exist in the major European countries and in Oceania.

Explanations for the boom

Explanations for this growth are multifaceted. First, there is the feeling of achievement in training for and successfully completing a marathon. Training requires such commitment that the resulting lifestyle change causes a desire to attempt subsequent marathon races, obsession with which can take on a myriad of forms. Three examples come from the December 1999 Huntsville (Alabama, US) marathon. Norm Frank of Rochester, New York, US, was assigned race number 700 to honour his completion of 700 marathons (his time was 5:34:00). Ed Burnham of Kansas City, Missouri, US, finished his 100th marathon in 5:56:24 at the age of 80 years — beginning his 'career' at the age of 70, this means he averaged 10 marathons per year! Richard Worley of Kingwood, Texas, US, was assigned race number 154 to signify the number of consecutive weeks in which he had completed a marathon (4:14:33).

Second, novice runners, who otherwise would not attempt such an athletic feat, are being encouraged to participate in training programmes oriented around the theme of 'running for a cause'. In the US, for example, the Team in Training raises money for the Leukemia and Lymphoma Society, and there is the Arthritis Foundation's Joints in Motion programme; similarly in the UK, charities such as the National Meningitis Trust and the Sargent Cancer Care for Children have been established. Unfortunately, participation by people who have minimal fitness or who are running with disabilities, while laudable in that they enjoy taking part and providing funding for worthy causes, places a substantial burden on race volunteers, municipal employees and city residents to endure ever-lengthening street closure periods. In 1999 at Honolulu, for example, the final finisher required 14:35:05 to complete the event. This pace of 20:44/km (33:26/mile or 1.8 miles/h) — a very slow walk — is far removed from 'marathon running'.

Third, increasingly popular organized travel tours now contribute from hundreds to thousands of runners to a marathon's entry list. Tour participants enjoy the camaraderie of being with others desirous of combining the goals of touring a far-off destination with entry into the local marathon. However, a major city is not always involved, for instance there is the Antarctica marathon, the Mount Everest marathon and many others.

Fourth, the 'power of promotion' is causing people to sign up for the newest twist — 'theme marathons'. A few examples include the San Diego (California, US) Rock 'n' Roll marathon, with live music at each aid station, and the Tromsø (Norway) Midnight Sun marathon, where participants can run in broad daylight in the middle of the night.

Future achievement

While those behind the elite-level front runners are running ever more slowly, the elite group is running ever more quickly although not necessarily in larger numbers. Figure 1 illustrates the increasing quality of marathon running each year by men since 1924 and by women since 1970. The year 1924 was selected as a starting point for the men's compilation as this was when the now standard distance of 42,195 m (26 miles, 385 yards) was approved for the Olympic games by the IAAF and IOC. Since 1968 for men and 1983 for women, the rate of quickening of the annual fastest marathon performance has reduced substantially. However, both men and women continue to improve, confirmed by the current world best times set in 1999 by both men (2:05:42 by Morocco's Khalid Khannouchi) and women (2:20:43 by Kenya's Tegla Loroupe). Khannouchi became a US citizen on 2 May 2000 but did not compete in the Sydney Olympic games. Loroupe placed 13th.

Applying mathematical modelling techniques to the data illustrated in Figure 1 allows such predictive estimates as the best performance in a given future year, or a theoretical

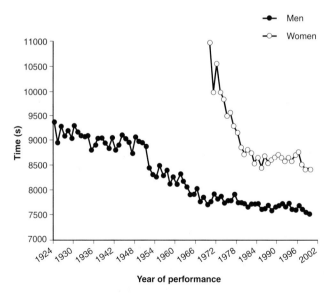

Figure 1

Fastest marathon performance by men and women (1924–99)

Redrawn from[11].

Table 2 *Sub-2:20:00 (men) and sub-2:55:00 (women) marathon performances: 1970–99*

Year	Male	Female	Year	Male	Female
1970	170	0	1985	996	894
1971	140	2	1986	1024	1003
1972	156	0	1987	1026	1092
1973	165	2	1988	980	1202
1974	209	9	1989	943	1031
1975	234	18	1990	954	1121
1976	260	39	1991	1070	1268
1977	286	45	1992	1048	1201
1978	448	91	1993	1097	1126
1979	580	209	1994	1145	1203
1980	754	310	1995	1034	1219
1981	731	448	1996	1040	1337
1982	834	694	1997	1037	1246
1983	1134	1038	1998	1033	1278
1984	1101	1203	1999	1081	1348

performance time limit. Peronnet and Thibault used data available up to 1987[12], and projected the best men and women's marathon performances for 2000 as 2:05:23 and 2:18:43, respectively. The men's predicted time has been reached, at least within the error of estimation, with Khannouchi's 2:05:42. For women, the rate of performance improvement since 1987 has slowed more than was predicted. Similar regression analysis techniques applied to the data in Figure 1 provide trend lines that suggest men will break the two-hour barrier in the marathon in 2015, and women will break the two-hour and 20 minutes barrier sometime during spring 2002.

Table 2 summarizes the increasing number of top-level marathon performances each year from 1970 to 1999 using 2:20:00 for men and 2:55:00 for women as lower limits. During the 1970s, breaking these time barriers was an achievement synonymous with world-class status in the marathon. Today, these standards have quickened to sub-2:10:00 and sub-2:30:00 for men and women respectively. There was an exponential rise in the numbers of top-class performances between 1978 and 1982. The number of such performances has stabilized from 1983 to 1999, averaging 1,044 under the 2:20:00 mark delivered each year by men and 1,165 by women faster than 2:55:00.

Within individual countries, several different patterns of top athlete achievement exist, shown for men in Table 3. The national passion for marathon racing in Japan produces large numbers of sub-2:20:00 performances every year. In Great Britain and the US, however, a substantial reduction has occurred in the number of their top-level athletes participating in the marathon[12]. One suggested explanation for this decline in the US has been that, with such stiff competition for only three Olympic marathon team spots, athletes have opted to focus on other events, such as shorter-

Table 3   *Changing patterns in the number of sub-2:20:00 marathon performances by men: 1983–99*

Nation	1983	1984	1985	1986	1987	1988	1989	1990	1991	1992	1993	1994	1995	1996	1997	1998	1999
KEN	4	11	17	18	22	16	21	18	19	32	43	79	86	110	163	216	254
ETH	9	10	18	20	13	22	24	26	32	24	44	53	49	56	75	62	50
USA	267	165	100	114	96	65	63	75	93	64	57	57	59	40	27	36	48
GBR	137	116	96	73	66	62	52	38	46	37	40	34	19	17	20	17	8
JPN	88	102	100	103	116	90	83	104	122	113	124	128	123	137	123	152	143

distance road racing and track events. However, for reasons not entirely clear, the quality of performance standard by the US and British athletes even in these other events has decreased substantially.

Table 3 also shows the rapid increase in numbers of top-level marathon performances by two African countries — Kenya and Ethiopia. Kenya's athletes in particular have recently become enamoured with racing marathons to an extent almost never seen in other countries. In 1999, 156 Kenyan men delivered a total of 254 sub-2:20:00 performances (up from 216 in 1998) — more than any other nation in history except for the 268 performances achieved by the much larger US during its peak of activity in 1983. Kenyan men won 51 major world marathons in 1999, compared to nine for second-best Russia and a tie for third-best with eight performances each by Ethiopia and Japan.

Are Kenyan distance runners uniquely gifted for achieving performance excellence with such apparent dominance, or is it simply a fortuitous combination of their lifestyle, altitude residence and training? Recent scientific studies published on elite-level Kenyan distance runners[13] when compared to Scandinavian runners suggest that Kenyan athletes may have a higher maximal oxygen uptake, better running economy, and lower lactate threshold than their European counterparts. This difference is likely not due as much to genetic influences as it is to lifestyle and training effects[14]. The dominance of the Kenyans as runners is discussed in detail in Professor Lambert's and Professor Noakes' chapter.

Conclusions

The marathon foot race began 105 years ago as a competitive event of the highest calibre, oriented around the Olympic games. It has since been transformed into a social movement of its own. Training to complete a marathon at whatever pace is a challenge demanding a focused lifestyle towards improved fitness that will, hopefully, occur without injury. Hundreds of thousands of people around the world have completed anywhere from one marathon to hundreds of marathons. Back in the pack, everything from marriages occurring along the route to heart transplant patients completing the journey makes the event a microcosm of society itself. At the front of the pack remain those vying for the title of Marathon Champion and, if their dreams come true, the coveted title of Olympic gold medallist in this celebrated sporting event.

References

1 Milvy P. *Ann N Y Acad Sci* 1977; **301**: 1–1090.

2 Godolphin FRB. *The Greek historians. The complete and unabridged historical works of Herodotus.* Translated by George Rawlinson. New York: Random House; 1942.

3 White J, ed. *Lives of Miltiades, Cimon, Pausanias, Aristidis.* London: Longmans, Green & Co, 1886.

4 Martyn SG. Book review. *Olympika* 1997; **6**: 129–36.

5 Browning R. *The complete poetical works.* Boston: Houghton Mifflin, 1895.

6 Kyle D. The ancient world. In: Magill FN, ed. *Dictionary of world biography.* Hackensack: Salem Press, 1998.

7 Ioannides I. The true course run by the marathon messenger. *Olympic Review* 1976; **109–110**: 599–602.

8 Wallechinsky D. *The complete book of the summer Olympics.* New York: Little Brown & Co, 1996.

9 Anonymous. Handbook: International Amateur Athletic Federation 1912–21.

10 Senn AE. *Power, politics, and the Olympic Games.* Champaign (IL): Human Kinetics, 1999.

11 Martin DE, Gynn RWH. *The Olympic marathon.* Champaign (IL): Human Kinetics, 2000.

12 Peronnet F, Thibault G. Mathematical analysis of running performance and world running records. *J Appl Physiol* 1989; **67**: 453–65.

13 Saltin B, Larsen H, Terrados N *et al.* Aerobic exercise capacity at sea level and at altitude in Kenyan boys, junior and senior runners compared with Scandinavian runners. *Scand J Med Sci Sports* 1995; **5**: 209–21.

14 O'Connell C. Environmental conditions, training systems and performance development of Kenyan runners. *New Studies in Athletics* 1996; **11**: 25–36.

Ageing and the marathon

PROFESSOR CRAIG SHARP

PROFESSOR OF SPORT SCIENCE, DEPARTMENT OF SPORT SCIENCES,
BRUNEL UNIVERSITY, WEST LONDON
AND HONORARY RESEARCH FELLOW, UNIVERSITY OF STIRLING, UK

'And so, from hour to hour, we ripe and ripe,
And then from hour to hour, we rot and rot;
And thereby hangs a tale.'

(Shakespeare; *As you like it*: II; vii 26)

'You will never live to my age without you keep yourselves in breath with exercise,
and in heart with joyfulness.'

(Sir Philip Sidney; *Old Age*, 1580)

Ageing, leading to death, has been an evolutionary development and a necessary corollary to sexual reproduction. Sexual reproduction arose from gene-mixing, possibly due to an early form of phagocytosis among primitive eukaryotic life-forms where phagocytosed nuclei may not have been completely digested, leading to their nucleic acid fusing with host genetic material. This mixing of genes may have conferred survival advantage in an unstable environment. However, such increase in variety would have had little advantage if population numbers were kept high by older members living too long — hence, perhaps, the evolutionary need for an ageing process leading to death. Death may, thus, be viewed as the price to be paid for sex, in that asexual reproduction involves the parent living on as part of the offspring.

In sexual reproduction, the force of natural selection declines with age, and beyond reproductive age there is no transmissible genetic benefit except, perhaps, the prospective ability to look after one's young to create better chances for survival. This may be why some primates, especially homo sapiens, live well beyond reproductive age. In this context, it is worth noting that middle-aged mothers may live longer than younger mothers. Perls *et al* compared two groups of women born in 1896 (78 centenarians and 54 who died in 1969) and noted that those who reached 100 years were four times more likely to have had children in their 40s than the women who lived to 73 years[1]. They concluded that 'evolutionary pressure to extend lifespan is closely linked to prolonging the time during which a woman can bear children'[1].

Longevity in general

The oldest (authenticated) person in the world was Madame Jeanne Louise Calment who was born in 1875, lived in Arles, France, and once sold pencils to Van Gogh from her father's shop. She was 122 years and seven months when she died in August 1997. The oldest Briton, Lucy Askew of Buckhurst Hill, Essex, was reported to be 115 years, and the oldest man, David Henderson of Laurencekirk, Aberdeenshire, was six years younger, in 1999.

In 1900, people were considered old when they reached their 40s. Even 40 years ago, people were deemed old when they approached 60, but today many do not feel their age when they reach 80 — this is a feature known as 'youth creep'. There is no common experience in the ageing process. For instance, a 50-year-old orchestral conductor may feel to be a mere youngster, while a 20-year-old rhythmic gymnast can feel hopelessly middle-aged. Marathon runners are more immune to such strictures.

Older marathon and other sports performers

The oldest Olympic medallist was Swedish rifleman Oscar Swahn, who obtained the silver at the age of 72 in 1920 having won gold in 1912. He was chosen for the 1924 Paris Games but had to withdraw due to injury. The oldest British sports competitor was dressager Hilda Johnstone who, at the age of 70 years, performed at the Munich Olympics. At least six Olympians have spanned 40 years: three in yachting, two in fencing and one equestrian.

In 1995, Spirduso wrote in her book[2]:

> *'With so much negative news about one's aging physical ability, an analysis of the great athletic performances of some of our septuagenarians and octogenarians is inspiring and uplifting. I believe that almost all professionals underestimate the physical abilities and potentials of the elderly. At a time in their lives when so many people are telling the elderly that they can't, we professionals at least should be telling them that they can.'*

She ended her landmark text with: 'They (master's athletes) reveal the limits of human physical potential in all adult age categories. They inspire an upward look, provide a standard, and give hope, and that is the note on which any book about the physical dimensions of aging should conclude'.

In 1994, Eamon Coughlan ran the mile in three minutes and 58.15 seconds (3:58.15) at the age of 41. Yekaterina Podkopayeva, at 42 years, beat 38-year-old Mary Decker in the 1997 world indoor 1,500 m final by running 3:59.10. In the marathon, Carlos Lopez won the Los Angeles event in an Olympic record of two hours, nine minutes and 21 seconds (2:09:21) at the age of 38, having broken the world 10,000 m record at 37 years, running 27:17.48. A 79-year-old man has run the marathon in 3:49:0 (8:44.1/mile), and a 76-year-old woman has registered 4:31:0 (10:20.2/mile) (Table 1). At 80 years, men and women have been found to be able to run 10 km in <45 and 59 minutes respectively, and in all track distances, from 100 m to 10,000 m, the Master's records reveal that the general decline with age in trained men and women is linear and gradual until the eighth decade, when the times become less consistent[3].

Table 1 US single-age marathon records

Age (years)	Male	Female	Age (years)	Male	Female
4	6:03:0	—	49	2:33:0	2:51:0
5	5:25:0	4:56:30	50	2:25:42	2:50:0
6	4:07:0	4:00:30	51	2:29:0	2:52:0
7	4:04:0	3:52:0	52	2:25:0	3:01:0
8	3:37:0	3:13:30	53	2:31:0	3:00
9	3:07:0	3:11:0	54	2:32:0	2:52:0
10	3:02:0	3:07:0	55	2:34:0	2:52:0
11	2:47:0	3:04:0	56	2:39:0	3:07:0
12	2:46:30	2:58:0	57	2:38:0	3:13:0
13	2:43:0	2:53:0	58	2:38:0	3:21:0
14	2:41:30	2:51:0	59	2:48:0	3:24:0
15	2:29:0	2:46:30	60	2:47:0	3:15:0
16	2:23:0	2:34:0	61	2:43:0	3:28:0
17	2:24:0	2:47:0	62	2:49:0	3:31:0
18	2:17:0	2:42:0	63	2:48:0	3:30:0
19	2:15:0	2:34:42	64	2:43:0	3:39:0
20	2:13:0	2:30:18	65	2:51:0	3:37:0
23	2:08:0	2:30:10	66	2:43:0	3:49:0
25	2:09:18	2:26:0	67	2:55:0	4:02:0
26	2:11:0	2:29:0	68	2:52:0	4:03:0
27	2:08:40	2:28:0	69	3:01:0	4:01:0
28	2:10:40	2:21:0	70	3:01:0	4:09:0
29	2:10:0	2:31:0	71	3:01:0	4:25:0
30	2:10:0	2:28:0	72	3:09:0	4:38:0
31	2:09:30	2:30:0	73	3:13:0	4:57:0
32	2:11:30	2:30:0	74	3:37:0	4:48:0
33	2:11:30	2:28:0	75	3:18:0	4:32:0
34	2:13:12	2:30:0	76	3:35:0	4:31:0
35	2:12:0	2:32:0	77	3:33:0	5:13:0
36	2:15:30	2:36:0	78	3:37:0	5:01:0
37	2:12:42	2:28:0	79	3:49:0	5:04:0
38	2:17:18	2:27:0	80	4:28:0	5:10:0
39	2:14:18	2:31:0	81	4:50:0	5:51:0
40	2:17:0	2:40:30	82	4:38:0	6:14:0
41	2:19:18	2:38:0	83	5:20:0	6:33:0
42	2:20:0	2:42:0	84	4:18:0	6:02:0
43	2:23:0	2:40:0	85	5:22:0	6:54:0
44	2:25:0	2:35:0	86	5:40:0	7:57:0
45	2:26:0	2:45:0	87	6:49:0	7:09:0
46	2:26:0	2:53:0	88	6:52:0	8:03:0
47	2:27:0	2:52:0	89	6:36:0	8:09:0
48	2:31:0	2:51:0	90	7:53:0	10:13:0

Thus, there does not appear to be a particular age threshold at which performance suddenly deteriorates. Hardly any deterioration in marathon performance is seen between the ages of 20 and the mid- or late 30s; however, between 40 and 80 years

Table 2 *Total and annual percentage increases in marathon times in the UK, US and whole world from ages 40 to 80. These data are open to marked secular influences but are nevertheless appended for interest*

Age (years)	World		UK		US	
	Male	Female	Male	Female	Male	Female
40	2:11:04	2:26:51	2:15:46	2:34:35	2:17:0	2:40:30
80	3:43:27	5:10:04	3:47:04	5:47:19	4:28:02	5:10:10
% increase	70	111	67	125	96	93
Annual % increase	1.8	2.8	1.7	3.1	2.4	2.3

% time increments were calculated as [(time at age 80 – time at age 40/time at age 40) x 100] = % increase in time. Time is expressed as being more appropriate for runners than velocity

the rate of slowing is about 1.7–3.1% per year (Table 2). In power events, such as the throws, the rate of decline in the Master's performances is about 2% annually, although the rate is also still relatively linear until the eighth decade after which the trend becomes less regular[4].

It is important to note that most data are cross-sectional, and marked secular trends have been observed in the physique, training methods and racial mix in athletic populations over the past 30–40 years. Successive age cohorts have been exposed to different nutritional, motivational, psychological, social, training and exemplar influences at varying stages of sporting lives. The data presented are non-stationary and are not derived from a homogeneous population; the calculated decrements are of low validity. In the original New York Academy of Sciences 1976 marathon conference, Rose and Cohen expressed much caution about secular variables, referring to '… a nagging problem haunted the original data analysis, the secular contamination of the data …'[5]. Nevertheless, the raw data in Tables 1 and 2 (and the partially derived data in Tables 3 and 4), even if mostly cross-sectional, are of interest in terms of indicating approximate magnitudes. They also currently represent much of the data available. Rose and Cohen quote Keys who noted that '… insistence on scientific purism … can lead to a degree of conservatism in which nothing is done.'[5]. These tables provide much incentive and enjoyment for runners, and at least a guide for those who study them.

Young marathon performers

Outstanding performances at the lower end of the age scales have also been recorded. Among earlier publications, the 1981 'Big-M' Australian marathon was documented with 190 entrants aged between seven and 17 years, 56 of whom were under 15[6]. Of these, a seven-year-old ran 3:31:10, while the 11- and 12-year-old age categories were won by girls completing the race in 3:31:30 and 3:13:12, respectively. A 13-year-old boy ran the marathon in 2:55:24. However, these data are shaded by the current American marathon age-best tables (Table 1) which show a four-year-old boy completing the distance in 6:03:0, and a six-year-old boy and girl in 4:07:0 and 4:00:30 respectively. Girls were also faster in the next two age categories of seven and eight years, with 3:52:0 and 3:13:30 compared with the boys' 4:04:0 and 3:37:0; however, completion times appeared to level out at 10 years. The 11-year-old winner was a boy with a time of 2:47:0, and the first girl under three hours was a 12-year-old with 2:58:0.

Age-graded tables

The compilation of age-graded tables by the World Association of Veteran Athletes (WAVA) has produced an extensive and comprehensive series of 'age standards' and 'age factors' for both genders and all ages from eight to 100 years, for all track and field events[7]. For the marathon, the 'age standard' is an idealized list of current or predicted world best times (Table 3). By calculating a given marathon runner's time as a percentage of the 'age standard', it is possible to compare, for example, the marathon time of a 20-year-old man with that of his 50-year-old mother. If the 50-year-old mother ran 3:15:30 and her son ran 2:48:40, her 'performance related percentage' would be 79% and his 75%; she could, therefore, claim to be the relatively better marathon runner. The table's function is comparable to the scoring tables for the decathlon or heptathlon, or the handicap system in golf. The 'age factor' is a correction factor that can be applied to the marathon time; the time could be normalized to allow comparison with the time of other runners in the race (Table 4). For example, if a 14-year-old girl ran the marathon in 2:36:56, her 'marathon factor' would be 0.9254 and her run would represent a potential of 2:25:14. Similarly, a finishing time of 2:42:00

Table 3 *Marathon 'age standards', where the given age standard should be divided by the actual marathon time, and the result expressed, if required, as a percentage. Between 20 and 37 years for men, and 20 and 36 years for women, no allowance is made for increasing age; women's 'open-age' standard (20–37) is faster than the current world record*

Age (years)	Male	Female	Age (years)	Male	Female
10	2:31:56	2:50:42	65	2:39:2	3:01:16
15	2:14:11	2:27:12	70	2:48.:1	3:13:21
20–37	2:06:50		75	2:59:24	3:28:20
20–36		2:18:51	80	3:13:37	3:47:35
40	2:08:58	2:22:29	85	3:32:40	4:13:53
45	2:13:42	2:28:29	90	4:01:02	4:54:03
50	2:18:55	2:35:08	95	4:53:48	6:12:03
55	2:24:44	2:42:38	100	7:14:37	10:52:29
60	2:31:21	2:51:13			

Table 4 *Marathon 'age factors' used to compare a marathon runner's performance with what he or she could have achieved at their best. The factor expresses a calculated rate of decline (or improvement) based on observed world best times with age. The actual marathon time is multiplied by the 'age factor'*

Age (years)	Male	Female	Age (years)	Male	Female
8	0.7565	0.7258	40	0.9835	0.9745
9	0.8020	0.7727	45	0.9486	0.9351
10	0.8348	0.8134	50	0.9130	0.8950
11	0.8634	0.8485	55	0.8763	0.8538
12	0.8884	0.8785	60	0.8380	0.8110
13	0.9101	0.9040	65	0.7975	0.7660
14	0.9289	0.9254	70	0.7541	0.7181
15	0.9452	0.9432	75	0.7070	0.6665
16	0.9591	0.9579	80	0.6551	0.6101
17	0.9710	0.9699	85	0.5964	0.5469
18	0.9810	0.9794	90	0.5262	0.4722
19	0.9894	0.9870	95	0.4317	0.3732
20–37	1.0000		100	0.2758	0.2128
20–36		1.0000			

in a 40-year-old woman with a factor of 0.9745 would represent a completion time of 2:37:52 in her prime. Also, a man of 65 years who ran 3:39:0 would represent 2:54:39 in his prime with a factor of 0.7975. Such tables are compiled from track and field data by an appointed committee of the WAVA. It is difficult to truly validate these tables, in the same way that it is not easy to validate decathlon tables. However, acting as a normalizing mechanism, they have added much to the enjoyment and motivation regarding performances of individuals, clubs, groups and families competing in the marathon, and in track and field athletics in general. Their accuracy will improve with time and following the accumulation of longitudinal data.

Physiological aspects of ageing and endurance running performance

Anthropometry

Body fat composition is about 16–8% at the age of eight. However, this changes to 12–6% and 23–8% in 20-year-old men and women, respectively, then rises steadily to 19–26% and 28–38% or more by the ages of 60 to 70; lean body mass declines both relatively and absolutely. Height tends to decrease by about 1cm per decade after 40 years.

Effect on skin

The rete pegs, which anchor the dermis to epidermis, shorten with age — this leads to increased susceptibility of older (especially novice) runners to blister formation and greater tendency to skin trauma, as on the removal of adhesive tape. Melanocytes diminish at an approximate rate of 2% annually when people reach their 40s; the cutaneous inflammatory response also diminishes. Hence, older, and especially novice, runners are more susceptible to sunburn but do not show visible evidence of its acute pathology as markedly as seen in the young.

Cardiorespiratory effects

Forced vital capacity decreases by about 250 ml/decade. The elasticity of pulmonary support structures declines and the alveolar size increases, which collectively can increase the work of breathing to approximately 20% of the energy cost of exercise in the over-60s age group, compared with 10% in those in their 20s. Reduction in the number of pulmonary capillaries, as well as perfusion quality, is observed; there is an increased sensitivity with age of the respiratory centre to given blood levels of carbon dioxide, as in pregnancy. Thus, ventilation increases disproportionately to oxygen intake in older subjects, leading novice runners in particular to presume that they are less fit than they actually are, as non-athletes often subjectively gauge their 'fitness' by their ventilation response to effort. Maximum heart rate declines with age by about 40 beats/min between 20 and 60 years. This is partly due to decreased sympathetic stimulation of the sinoatrial node (which loses β-adrenergic sensitivity) and a loss of up to 50% in the number of sinoatrial node cells, and possibly due to a decreased sarcoplasmic reticulum take-up of calcium in the myocardium as a result of slowing of calcium-pump kinetics.

The Framingham and other studies have shown, somewhat paradoxically, that age-related myocardial hypertrophy leads to a diminishing stroke volume by decreasing ventricular chamber size[8]; between the ages of 25 and 80, left ventricular wall thickness increases by 30%. These cardiorespiratory changes contribute to a decline in maximal volume uptake (VO_{2max}) of about 5 ml/kg/min per decade, from an approximate initial value of 50 ml/kg/min for untrained men in their 20s and about 5 ml lower in women[9]. This downward trend is also present in those who remain in training, but their VO_{2max} may still stay consistently higher than the untrained, eg by 20 ml/kg/min at the age of 40 and by 10 ml/kg/min at 70. Nevertheless, untrained elderly subjects may increase their work capacity by 80% over three months, with up to 15% improvement in VO_{2max} and corresponding increases in the 'anaerobic threshold' (onset of blood lactate accumulation) after training[10].

Muscle endurance

Skeletal muscle capillarization has been found to be as high in older runners (388±93 capillaries/mm^2) as in young runners (367±60/mm^2) of equivalent performance[11]. Ageing muscle has been shown by some workers to tend towards higher percentages of type 1 fibres, demonstrating on histology whole fascicles consisting entirely of slow fibres — this indicates re-innervation with type-1 nerve following possible type-2 denervation as an age change[12], although the evidence is equivocal. This may be of potential benefit to older marathon runners. Myosin adenosine triphosphatase (ATP-ase) decreases with age and the size and number of mitochondria seem to diminish, although much less so if relative habitual activity remains constant. This decrease may be due to disuse atrophy, often called 'detraining' by athletes.

Muscle strength and power

Progressive muscle atrophy occurs with ageing. Between 65 and 90 years, muscle power is lost more rapidly than strength — a decline rate of 3.5%/year for power and 1.8%/year for strength has been observed[13]. Concentric force development is also lost more rapidly than eccentric. There is little fall-off in strength in both sexes until about the mid-40s, which then drops by about 25% by the mid-60s. In women, there may be an accelerated postmenopausal fall-off in power and strength. Muscle power can translate into speed over the ground. Lundgren-Lindquist et al found in their study of traffic crossings in Gothenburg that, after the crossing signal was extinguished, pedestrians had to walk at a rate of 1.4 m/s to cross safely. Of the pedestrians >70 years, 28% and 68% of untrained men and women respectively were unable to attain this velocity[14].

These force parameter losses appear to be reversible to some extent[15]. This was demonstrated when 56–70-year-old men produced marked improvements in local muscle endurance following eight weeks of strength training[16]. Muscle strength training, even of nonagenarians, may produce a doubling of force development by the quadriceps[17]. Apart from benefits such as an improved ability to get out of a chair or off the toilet, these increases in leg muscle function in the aged may improve balance capability, leading to both increased mobility and reduction in the number of falls. However, the exercise regimen must be maintained if improvement is to be sustained. Leg strength as a fitness parameter for endurance runners could be important in elderly competitors, although much less so for the young.

Reaction times

Regular exercise appears to be accompanied by a slowing in the rate of decline in movement/reaction times in the elderly; this could help minimize falls on stumbling, especially during the later stages of endurance runs or races. Simple and complex movement times have been shown to be faster in 'old active' subjects (145 ms and 190 ms, respectively) than in both 'old non-active' (240 ms and 250 ms) and 'young non-active' (170 ms and 200 ms) subjects[18]. 'Young active' runners scored 120 ms and 180 ms respectively on testing. Such speed indicates a general response mechanism of the central nervous system and, with age, the simple reaction time slows by the order of 0.6 ms/year. Limb tremor, especially of the hands, changes with age such that its frequency diminishes, but the velocity and amplitude increase resulting in fewer but larger tremors[19]; this probably relates more to hand/arm actions than to running.

Collagen and the series elastic component

A well-used tendon retains much of its elastic properties. It does not necessarily show a decrease in collagen molecular cross-bonding, but a lower degree of stabilization may occur in the bonds already in place. Collagen turn-over is increased with exercise; thus cross-bonding is less stable, and elasticity and elastic storage of energy may be greater. Not only will this assist small proprioceptive stabilizing movements, but it may also decrease the work of running by allowing greater elastic energy storage in tendon and ligament, which may contribute up to 50% of the work of walking or running at marathon pace[20]. Thus, improved running economy could be maintained through greater turnover of collagen.

Osteoporosis, thermal control and immunity

Regular physical exercise, especially weight-bearing exercise such as walking, running, racket sports, aerobics and country dance, has been widely shown to decrease the rate of bone demineralization, although it is reasonably specific to the body segments exercised[2]. Exercise is also thought to improve thermal control, helping the elderly to resist hypothermia in the cold and to remain cooler in hot weather or during activity. There is increasing evidence that moderate exercise, perhaps particularly in the elderly, may enhance some immune responses and lead to a lowered incidence of, for example, respiratory disease, and to fewer days in hospital with respiratory and other infections[21].

Detraining

It is reasonable to suppose that a substantial percentage of the physiological deterioration due to ageing is not necessarily a genetically programmed response to time, but is in fact due to a detraining effect of reduced exercise that is often coupled with increased body (fat) mass. The athletes' motto: 'If you don't use it, you lose it!' applies equally, if not more, to the ageing population. The extraordinary marathon performances of elderly trained runners appear to confirm this, although their genetics may also play a disproportionate role[22].

Psychology

In addition to socialization factors, well-documented beneficial psychological effects on mood and morale[23,24], and possible cognitive advantages, exercise such as distance running has much to offer older members of society in terms of being a distinctly beneficial and benign form of therapy against the depressing nature of the ageing process. WB Yeats cautiously assessed this:

> 'I thought no more was needed / Youth to prolong
> Than dumb-bell and foil / To keep the body young.
> O who could have foretold / That the heart grows old?'

(Yeats WB; *A song*)

Conclusions

An important question to ask senior citizens, or those nearing seniority, is how old they would think they were if they did not know their age. The disparity between theory and fact in the answer could indicate the activity and exercise levels of the individual. The exercise and fitness decrements of ageing are, to some extent, a reversible or at least a decelerative process of bodily detraining and disuse within the confines of injury, disease, and genetic and social programming.

Marathon runners >40 years continue to produce extraordinary running times, although the inevitable slow-down with age may be countered, at least psychologically, by the use of various normative tables. Improving or maintaining physical function, eg via running, may also affect mental aspects, especially in terms of mood-state. As time gradually turns us all into history, this provides some grounds for optimism.

Acknowledgements

Special thanks for their ready help to: Steve Seaton, Editor of *Runner's World*, Rodale Press Ltd, London; and Nicola Cockarill, librarian of the National Sports Medicine Institute, London. Also, to Niobe Jonilla Menendez of the University of Limerick and especially the World Association of Veteran Athletes for generously encouraging the reproduction of their tables and data.

References

1 Perls TP, Alpert L, Fretts RC. Middle-aged mothers live longer. *Nature* 1997; **389**: 133.

2 Spirduso WW. *Physical dimensions of aging*. Champaign Ill: Human Kinetics, 1995.

3 Burton D. British and world veteran's track and field records 1996. *Veteran's Athletics* 1996; Autumn issue: 17–8.

4 Mundle P, Dietderich S, Harvey R. *Masters age records 1999*. California: National Masters News, 1999.

5 Rose CL, Cohen ML. Relative importance of physical activity for longevity. In: The marathon: physiological, medical, epidemiological and psychological studies. Conference proceedings: *Ann N Y Acad Sci* 1977; **301**: 671–702.

6 Roberts R. Marathon running and children. In: Russo P, Gass G, eds. *Children and exercise*. Cumberland, Australia: NSW Sport Sciences Research Centre, 1982: 51–5.

7 World Association of Veteran Athletes. *Age-graded tables for track and field athletics 1998*. California: National Masters News, 1998.

8 Savage DD, Abbott RD, Padgett S *et al.* Epidemiologic features of left ventricular hypertrophy in normotensive and hypertensive subjects: recent Framingham data. *J Cardiovasc Ultrasonography* 1985; **4**: 3–16.

9 Quiron A, de Careful D, Laurencelle L *et al.* The physiological response to exercise with special reference to age. *J Sports Med Physical Fitness* 1987; **27**: 143–50.

10 Blumenthal JA, Emery CF, Madden DJ *et al.* Effects of exercise training on cardiorespiratory function in men and women over 60 years of age. *Am J Cardiol* 1991; **67**: 633–9.

11 Coggan AR, Spina RJ, Rogers MA *et al.* Histochemical and enzymatic characteristics of skeletal muscle in master athletes. *J Appl Physiol* 1990; **68**: 1896–901.

12 Jones DA, Round JM. *Skeletal muscle in health and disease: a textbook of muscle physiology*. Manchester: Manchester University Press, 1990.

13 Skelton DA, Greig CA, Young A *et al.* Strength, power and related functional ability of healthy people aged 65–89 years. *Age and ageing* 1994; **23**: 371–7.

14 Lundgren-Lindquist B, Aniansson A, Rundgren A. functional studies in 79-year-olds. III. Walking perform-ance and climbing capacity. *Scand J Rehabil Med* 1983; **15**: 125–31.

15 Klitgaard H, Mantoni M, Schiaffino S *et al*. Function, morphology and protein expression of ageing skeletal muscle: a cross-sectional study of elderly men with different training backgrounds. *Acta Physiol Scand* 1990; **140**: 41–54.

16 Suominen H, Heikkinen E, Liesen H *et al*. Effects of 8 weeks' endurance training on skeletal muscle metabolism in 56–70-year-old sedentary men. *Eur J Appl Physiol* 1977; **37**: 173–80.

17 Fiatarone MA, Marks EC, Ryan ND *et al*. High intensity strength training in nonagenarians. *JAMA* 1990; **263**: 3029–34.

18 Spirduso WW. Reaction and movement time as a function of age and physical activity level. *J Gerontol* 1975; **30**: 435–40.

19 Lakie M. Is essential tremor physiological? *J Neurol Neurosurg Psychiat* 1986; **49**: 660–76.

20 Alexander RM. *The human machine*. London: Natural History Publications, 1992: 76–80.

21 Sharp NCC, Parry-Billings M. Can sport damage your health? *New Sci* 1992; **32**: 33–7.

22 Williams AG, Rayson M, Montgomery HE *et al*. The ACE gene and muscle performance. *Nature* 2000; **403**: 614–5.

23 Steinberg H. School of Psychology, University of Middlesex, Enfield, EN3 4SF; personal communication, 1999.

24 Steinberg H, Sykes E. Mood enhancement through physical exercise. In: Schroder, ed. *Health psychology, potential in diversity*. Regensberg: S Roderer Verlag, 1993: 171–209.

Further reading

Bortz WM. *Dare to be 100*. New York: Simon and Schuster, 1996.

Gosden R. *Cheating time: science, sex and ageing*. London: McMillan, 1996.

Medina JJ. *The clock of ages*. Cambridge: Cambridge University Press, 1996.

McPherson BD. *Sport and aging*. Champaign Ill: Human Kinetics, 1986.

Spirduso W. *Physical dimensions of aging*. Champaign Ill: Human Kinetics, 1995.

WAVA. *Age-graded tables*. Van Nuys CA: National masters News PO Box 2372, 1999.

DISCUSSION

Dr Roger Wolman: Do you think that the degree of fall-off in performance that you showed to occur in women around the age of 50 is related to postmenopausal changes in bone and muscle?

Professor Craig Sharp: You may well be right. Because of secular influences on cross-sectional data, we need to obtain good longitudinal data to see if there is a particular negative inflection in the performance graph around the menopause. As you indicate, after the menopause musculo-skeletal function may decline more sharply, although if women do maintain reasonable levels of exercise through the postmenopausal few years they may slow the rate of deterioration. The effect of peri-menopause is certainly something that should be looked at in performance terms.

Dominance of the Africans in distance running

PROFESSOR MIKE LAMBERT & PROFESSOR TIMOTHY NOAKES

MRC/UCT BIOENERGETICS OF EXERCISE RESEARCH UNIT, FACULTY OF HEALTH SCIENCES,
UNIVERSITY OF CAPE TOWN, SPORT SCIENCE INSTITUTE OF SOUTH AFRICA, NEWLANDS,
SOUTH AFRICA

In 1960, Abebe Bikila of Ethiopia won the marathon at the Rome Olympics in a world record time of two hours, 15 minutes and 16 seconds (2:15:16). This was the first time that an African had won a high-profile long-distance running event. There was some mystique attached to his victory as he was relatively unknown before the race, he ran barefoot and did callisthenics in the stadium after the race. A few years later, Professor Ernst Jokl noted that 'Africa harbours a great athletic reserve army which has not yet been fully mobilized for the Olympic contests. Athletes from African nations are bound to play an increasingly important role in the Olympic Games in the future'[1]. Jokl compared black and white athletes and concluded that black men were 'athletically most efficient', and suggested that black athletes have superior genetic endowment for sprinting and middle-distance running[1].

Four decades later, African runners are clearly dominant in the running events in track, cross-country and the marathon. Kenyan runners in particular have dominated the lucrative American road races to such an extent that attempts have been made to limit their participation in these events[2].

The dominance of the sport of running by Africans raises interesting questions. For example, what factors explain their superior running ability? Do these factors have an environmental, socio-economic or physiological basis? Are any of these factors heritable? In an attempt to answer these questions, this chapter will investigate the records of running performance to establish the extent to which Africans, or sub-groups within Africa, dominate different events. The physiological studies that have been conducted on distance runners from Africa will be discussed, and a hypothesis for a physiological explanation for their superior running ability will be proposed.

Analysis of running performance records

The 50 best marathon runners of all-time represent 17 countries (Table 1). Twenty-seven of these runners are from African origin, mostly from a relatively small geographical region in eastern and southern Africa (Figure 1, October 2000). Five countries have four or more marathon runners in the 50 fastest marathon times. Kenya heads the list with 14 runners, followed by Japan (*n*=6), Spain (*n*=5), Ethiopia (*n*=5) and South Africa (*n*=4).

Table 1 *The 50 fastest marathon runners of all-time divided into the countries and continents they represent (October 2000)*

Country	Continent	Number of runners
Kenya	Africa	14
Japan	Asia	6
Spain	Europe	5
Ethiopia	Africa	5
South Africa	Africa	4
Portugal	Europe	3
Morocco	Africa	2
Korea	Asia	2
Australia	Australasia	1
Belgium	Europe	1
Brazil	South America	1
Djibouti	Africa	1
France	Europe	1
Great Britain	Europe	1
Italy	Europe	1
Mexico	North America	1
Tanzania	Africa	1

If athletic ability was distributed purely in proportion to differences in population numbers, then Asia, which is home to 61% of the world population, should produce an equivalent proportion of the top 50 marathon runners in the world whereas Africa,

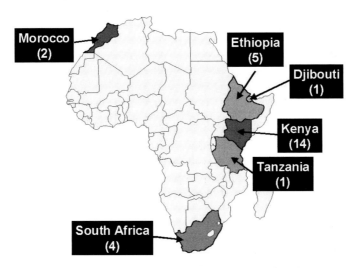

Figure 1

The 27 runners from Africa rated in the top 50 marathon runners of all-time (October 2000). The number of runners from each country is shown in brackets

with 13% of the world population, should produce only seven medals, not 27 (54%) of these runners. Africa, especially the east and southern regions, clearly produces a disproportionately large number of elite marathon runners.

Ethnic differences within Africa

Even within regions in Africa, there are differences in running ability between the ethnic groups. For example, although black athletes in South Africa comprise only 20% of the competitive running population, they fill at least 90% of the top positions in the major races over distances of 8 to 56 km[3].

Kenya has a reputation as the strongest cross-country nation, having won the world team championships for the past 15 years. Their superiority is so great that on five occasions (in 1988, 1991, 1993, 1994 and 1996), the Kenyans' points tally in the world cross-country championships was good enough to beat a team chosen from the best finishers from the rest of the world. Further examination shows that most of Kenya's world-class runners come from an area about the same size as Wales, with a population of approximately three million — this represents about 10% of Kenya's total population[4]. Runners from the Kalenjin ethnic group, one of about 40 groups in Kenya, have won 40% of all major international honours in distance runners in the past 10 years. Bale and Sang calculated that a geographical region of about 60% of Kenya has not produced any elite runners[5]. Within the Kalenjin-speaking groups, the Nandi tribe has contributed the greatest proportion of elite runners.

The dominance of the Kenyans, in particular the Kalenjin-Kenyans, has been shown by calculating the countries of origin of all medal winners at the Olympic Games from 1964 to 2000 for men track runners (800 m to 10,000 m)[4]. The Kenyans, considered as a group, won more than three times the total number of medals for the

Table 2 *Medals at the Olympic Games from 1964 to 2000 for men track runners (800 m to 10,000 m) (excluding the Olympic Games of 1976 and 1980 as these were boycotted by many countries[4])*

Country	Number of gold medals	Total number of medals
Kenya (Kalenjins)	10	32
US	3	10
Morocco	3	9
Ethiopia	3	8
Britain	1	8
Kenya (non-Kalenjins)	4	7
Germany (East and West)	2	7
Finland	3	4
New Zealand	2	4
Tunisia	1	4
Algeria	2	2

second country (the US). However, the results of the Kalenjin-Kenyans are even more remarkable because, as a smaller subgroup within Kenya, they have won more than twice the number of medals than did athletes representing the US (Table 2).

The numerical probability of the success of the Kenyans in the 1988 Olympic games has been calculated as one in 1.6 billion[6]. At this event, Kenyan runners won gold medals in the 800 m, 1,500 m, 3,000 m steeple-chase and the 5,000 m. This probability is calculated using the whole Kenyan population and is, thus, a further underestimation of the true probability of this happening, as the elite runners originate from such a small proportion of the total Kenyan population[4].

Is superior running ability inherited or acquired?

The discussion on whether or not superior running ability can be inherited is dominated by emotive rhetoric as the arguments are currently not supported by scientific data. However, in the analysis of running performances within the African ethnic groups, there is no doubt that the west Africans outclass the east Africans in the 100 m and 200 m events. The performances overlap at the 400 m distance, but above 800 m the east Africans are clearly dominant[7]. Within the group of east Africans, the Kenyans and their Ethiopian neighbours are the dominant athletes. Although this provides a strong case for running ability being inherited, it does not confirm the point and an environmental and socio-economic basis for success cannot be excluded. However, a case-control study of school children in Kenya provides some evidence for a familial-linked basis for running success (Nurok and Noakes, unpublished data). In this study, 18 of 25 competitive runners at a high school had a first-degree relative who had run competitively. In contrast, only 2 of 25 non-competitive runners at the same school had a relative who had run competitively. This study clearly reveals the strong family influence on running performance and begs the question of an inherited trait that determines superior running ability.

Environmental and socio-economic factors and running proficiency

A rather simple interpretation of Kenya's success in distance running is that many areas in Kenya are above an altitude of 2,000 m. It has been assumed that Kenya's high altitude and its apparent ability to produce an above average number of elite runners are causally related. This argument, however, is countered by the fact that other parts of the world (ie Nepal and Peru) are also located at high altitudes but do not have an abundance of world class long-distance runners. Thus, factors other than living at a high altitude need to be considered.

The influence of prevailing socio-economic factors and the environment on performance capacity cannot be ignored. Josiah Thugwane — the 1996 Olympic marathon gold medallist (2:12:36) — is an example of a world-class athlete who began training as an adult. He was raised in a humble environment and it was only while working in

South Africa as a coal miner that his exceptional talent was noticed. Thugwane's coach, Jacque Malan, believes the social circumstances that prevailed in Thugwane's life caused an insatiable hunger and desire for him to succeed in long-distance running. His Olympic gold medal earned him immediate fame and fortune, and elevated him and his family into an upper income group. He was illiterate; however, after obtaining his Olympic gold medal, he learnt to conduct interviews with the media from around the world, speaking confidently in English, his second language. Such examples provide a convincing argument that socio-economic conditions act as a catalyst in developing athletic talent to its full potential, but they do not diminish the argument that a specific physiological talent must first be present for it to be developed.

A popular explanation for the Kenyans' dominance in distance running is that it results from a combination of living at altitude, a simple diet, a lifestyle without a motor car, and children who cover as much as 30 km daily to and from school. Paul Tergat — five times winner of the world cross-country championships, third all-time best for 5,000 m, second all-time best for 10,000 m, and current world record holder for 21.1 km — does not agree with this theory, and has stated: 'That's what people say, but it is a myth about young children running many kilometres to school. In my case, home to school was just 800 m. In fact I did not like running at school and was not particularly good at it. It was only when I went to the armed forces and I was made to run that I discovered I had a talent for it.'[8].

The Kenyans were already a dominant force in running much before any lucrative scholarships at American Universities, race appearance fees and prize money were received. The foundation for national excellence in distance running was laid when Mike Kosgei became Kenya's national coach in mid-1985; his disciplined training and the positive influence of world cross-country champion John Ngugi were the combined factors associated with Kenya's rise to dominate the rest of the world[9]. Success on the track, which followed the disciplined hard training, was accompanied by financial success — this converted the runners into heroes and role models.

Although environmental and socio-economic factors may contribute to success in distance running (see Dr Martin's chapter), they are not the main factors and it stands to reason that they will only influence the outcome if the runner has the physiological profile for success in this field.

Studies on the physiological basis for success in African distance runners

Although the physiological and biochemical adaptations induced by endurance training are well described[10,11], the link between these adaptations and endurance performance is not very well understood. Similarly, cellular changes associated with fatigue after endurance exercise are well described[12], but how changes in these variables explain endurance performance is not yet completely established. Both deficiencies in explaining how variables influence endurance performance can be attributed to the fact that sports performance in the laboratory is difficult to measure. Even under the most ideal conditions, it is difficult to distinguish performance differences of <5%. However, in competition, the differences in performance between the medal winners and the other runners in the field may be a fraction of 1%. Therefore, research studies explaining the functional significance of the physiological and biochemical adaptations to training, or the fatigue mechanisms during exercise, are lacking. This makes it difficult to provide strong scientific evidence explaining the dominance of the Africans in distance running.

It is highly unlikely that under all conditions the superior running ability can be explained by a single physiological, biochemical or fatigue mechanism. Instead, it is more logical to assume that there are many factors which manifest under different conditions and which may affect running performance[13].

Maximal oxygen consumption

The superior running performance of Kenyan runners cannot be explained using the conventional cardiovascular anaerobic model of exercise physiology and athletic performance[13,14]. This model is based on the concept that endurance performance is determined by the capacity of the heart to pump blood and oxygen to the muscles, thereby allowing the muscles to work harder before developing anaerobiosis[13-5].

The maximal oxygen (O_2) uptake (VO_{2max}) of elite African runners has been measured, revealing high but unremarkable values that cannot explain the superior running performance of these athletes[16,17]. This is not surprising as VO_{2max} is a poor predictor of endurance performance in an homogenous group of athletes[13-5]. This confirms that the VO_{2max} test does not measure all the physiological variables determining success during prolonged exercise.

An observation has been made that hard-training Scandinavian boys may have a VO_{2max} of 70 ml O_2/kg/min[18] while physically active Kenyan boys are in the range of 60–70 ml O_2/kg/min (measured at altitude), which compares to a value of around 80 ml O_2/kg/min measured at sea level[16]. This suggests that there is a large pool of young Kenyans with a high aerobic capacity suited for long-distance running.

Running economy and fatigue resistance

Running economy, measured as O_2 consumption at a submaximal running speed, was superior in two world-class Kenyan runners[16], but was not different between elite black South African runners and the white middle-distance runners who acted as controls[17]. In the latter study, however, the elite black South African runners were able to sustain a higher percentage of their VO_{2max} values for longer than the middle-distance control runners, suggesting that they had an enhanced ability to resist fatigue. The ability to sustain a high percentage of VO_{2max} has been a recognized predictor of endurance performance for several years[19].

The enhanced fatigue resistance was also measured in the skeletal muscle of elite black South African runners after repetitive isometric contractions[17], and was identified in non-elite black athletes compared to Caucasian athletes matched for running performance[3,20].

The mechanism causing this increased resistance to fatigue is not clear and may originate in the central nervous system or in the peripheral skeletal muscle[17].

Muscle fibres

It is logical to assume that differences in muscle characteristics may explain the superior ability of elite South African runners to resist fatigue. It is widely appreciated that type 2 (fast twitch) muscle fibres fatigue at a faster rate than type 1 (slow twitch) fibres. Young sedentary west African boys were shown to have a dominance of fast twitch fibres[21], which is not surprising as this population has produced many world-class sprinters. In contrast, successful distance runners had a higher proportion of slow twitch fibres[23]. Despite the superior fatigue resistance of the elite black South African runners, their proportion of skeletal muscle type 1 fibres was not as high (approximately 50%) as expected[17]. Also, Scandinavian and Kenyan runners have similar muscle fibre compositions, fibre size, level of capillarization and oxidative capacity[23]. Kenyan runners had a higher 3-hydroxyl-acyl coenzyme A dehydrogenase (3-HAD) activity and lactate dehydrogenase activity than Scandinavians. Black South African runners also had a higher 3-HAD activity than white runners matched for VO_{2max} and 10 km running performance[20]. These changes may have caused a lower blood lactate concentration and increased lipid oxidation in the Kenyan and black South African runners, although these effects would have been fairly subtle and of unknown physiological significance[20,23].

Body composition

For many years, it has been thought that body composition is directly associated with distance running performance. In general, Kenyan runners are smaller than Scandinavian runners[16]. In a study carried out by Coetzer et al, elite black South African runners were found to be shorter, weigh less and have less body fat and muscle than the white control group of middle-distance runners matched for running performance over distances up to 3 km[17]. The body compositions of nine black South African runners (61.15 ± 0.33 min for 21.1 km (Lambert, unpublished data)) were compared with the body composition measurements of 20 elite long-distance runners from the US (Table 3)[24]. Although the race times of the US runners were not published, the group included several Olympians and represented the best US runners at that time (1976). The US athletes were heavier and taller than the South African runners and both groups had similar body fat content. The muscle girths, and by implication the muscle mass, of the US runners were also greater but the nature of this benefit has yet to be established[25].

Table 3   *The body composition of elite black South African runners (n=9) with an average 21.1 km race time of 61.15 ± 0.33 min (Lambert, unpublished) compared to elite American runners (n=20)[25]*

Variable	Elite black South African runners (*n*=9)	Elite US runners (*n*=20)[25]
Age (years)	27.1±3.4	–
Mass (kg)	53.9±3.7	63.1±4.8*
Stature (cm)	168.3±4.2	177.1±6.0*
Skinfolds (mm):		
Triceps	4.7±1.3	5.0±1.1
Subscapular	6.5±1.1	6.4±0.9
Abdomen	5.4±0.9	7.1±2.1
Suprailiac	4.0±0.7	4.6±1.0
Thigh	5.6±2.0	6.1±1.8
Girth measurements (cm):		
Thigh	46.8±1.8	51.9±2.3*
Calf	32.6±1.6	35.4±1.3 *
Arm	23.3±1.5	28.2±1.0 *
Forearm	22.8±1.1	26.4±0.9*
Diameters (cm):		
Femur	8.5±0.3	9.5±0.4*

* $P<0.05$

This reveals that African distance runners are generally smaller than Caucasian runners. It has been observed for more than a century that a smaller size is beneficial for distance running.

Muscle mass and heat loss

The small size and small muscle mass of African distance runners may be a partial explanation for their ability to resist fatigue during sustained exercise of long duration, particularly when exercising in the heat. Each athlete can store a critical amount of heat before being forced to reduce exercise intensity[26]. A smaller muscle mass reduces the amount of heat produced when running at any speed. When environmental conditions limit the capacity for heat loss, smaller runners have an advantage[25]. It is, therefore, not surprising that Josiah Thugwane was the smallest (43 kg) athlete in the field of the 1996 Olympic marathon that was held in warm conditions.

The mechanism of fatigue associated with exercise in the heat is not related to high levels of skeletal muscle anaerobiosis or energy depletion in the active muscles[26]. Instead, there is evidence to suggest that heat-induced fatigue is associated with a reduced drive of the central nervous system resulting in a lowered skeletal muscle recruitment. In essence, this causes the muscle activity and power output to decrease. It has been argued that this reduced central nervous system recruitment of skeletal muscle is a mechanism designed to prevent organ damage[14].

It is therefore tempting to speculate that the superior long-distance runners accumulate less heat as a result of their smaller muscle mass. Consequently in these runners the point is delayed at which the body temperature exceeds a certain critical temperature causing a reduced muscle recruitment. In other words, the superior long-distance runners can sustain a high exercise intensity for longer before fatigue develops than can runners of lesser ability. This theory supports the finding that superior runners have an improved ability to resist fatigue and needs to be evaluated in further laboratory trials.

Future areas of research

Noakes has described a series of physiological models to help understand the physiology of training for enhanced endurance performance[13]. Three additional research models need to be applied to explain superior running performance: the muscle power model of exercise physiology, the biomechanical model, and the central fatigue model (teleoanticipation).

Muscle power model

This suggests that muscle contractile capacity, or the ability to generate force per unit of muscle, is greater in athletes with superior performance. The model is accepted by cardiac physiologists, who would argue that delivery of calcium ions (Ca^{2+}) to the myofibres and the activity of the enzyme involved in adenosine triphosphate (ATP) hydrolysis — myosin ATPase — determine the contractile state of the myocardium in both health and disease[27]. It seems logical to assume that the same applies to skeletal muscle.

The only study that has examined the contractility of skeletal muscle, isolated from athletes, revealed measurable changes in maximal shortening speed of the muscle fibres and significant changes in the relationship between the Ca^{2+} and fibre force relationship after 10 days of intensive swimming training[28]. These results confirm that this is an area of research that offers great potential for explaining the superior fatigue resistant of elite athletes.

Biomechanical model

Roberts *et al* showed that locomotor muscles hold the 'springs' (tendons) rigid during horizontal running to allow them to store energy with each step[29]. This concept is central to the biomechanical model[13] of endurance exercise, which predicts that the greater the muscles' capacity to act as springs, the less torque they must produce and hence the more efficient they are. This will offer some advantage during running and is compatible with an increased ability to resist fatigue.

There are structural and neural components regulating the 'springiness' of muscle. The structural proteins in skeletal muscle (eg desmin, titin and nebulin) comprise the cytoskeleton and maintain the structural integrity of the myofibrillar lattice[30]. A significant amount of desmin was lost in 2.5% of rabbit muscle recruited during five minutes of eccentric contractions[31]. Disruption of the desmin network in skeletal muscle affects muscle function as these proteins form intermediate filaments that link adjacent Z discs and maintain structural cross-sectional integrity of muscle fibres[32]. Perhaps a loss of desmin in the skeletal muscle during exercise comprises the integrity of the sarcomere and coincides with the onset of fatigue? Perhaps elite runners have a more robust desmin network which protects the structural integrity of the myofibrillar lattice and delays the onset of fatigue?

Titin is a large structural protein with a chain length of approximately 27,000 amino acids and a molecular weight of about three million[33]. It is designed to act as a spring in the muscle by connecting the thick filaments and the Z discs, preventing movement of the thick filaments from the centre of the sarcomere. Titin's unique structure allows it to accommodate physiological stretch by first straightening without unfolding, and then unfolding a portion of the molecule called the PEVK domain[34]. The unfolding of the PEVK portion increases the capacity of the muscle to stretch further. The length of the PEVK sequence varies depending on the type of muscle and determines the stiffness of the muscle tissue. For example, a higher titin:actin ratio is seen in fast twitch fibres with more elasticity than the less elastic slow twitch fibres[35]. The significance of how the structural proteins influence muscle function has been underestimated[36]. Although speculative, the explanation for the enhanced ability to resist fatigue of elite African runners may be found in the titin composition of the skeletal muscles. This hypothesis needs further analysis.

The neural component to the 'springiness' of muscle also plays an important role[37]. The ability of muscle to store and use elastic energy depends on the muscle's activity before the foot lands[38], which is programmed from the higher centres of the central nervous system[39]. The reflex potentiation after the impact of the foot plays a major role by increasing stiffness in muscles, leading to a more rapid transition from the braking to the propulsion phase[38]. Fatigue of this stretch-shortening cycle so developed results in a reduced tolerance to muscle stretch and a delayed transfer from muscle stretch to muscle shortening as well as a loss in the recoil characteristics of the muscles[40]. As a result, the duration of both the braking and push-off phases of the running stride is increased. This leads to mechanical changes in the stride with landing occurring on a more extended leg but with greater knee flexion. These neuromuscular changes, which occur during running[41], will decrease the efficiency of movement and reduce the ability to resist fatigue. This suggests that the neural control of muscle force production and the capability to store and use elastic energy may have an important role in explaining distance running performance.

Central fatigue model (teleoanticipation)

Recent studies in this unit (St Clair Gibson et al, unpublished data) indicate that fatigue during prolonged exercise has a subconscious central (brain) component. This leads to the concept of a 'teleoanticipation', in which the brain regulates skeletal muscle recruitment patterns during exercise, perhaps to prevent body damage.

Reduced muscle damage during exercise in elite black distance runners as a result of enhanced 'springiness' of the muscles, or a robust cytoskeleton for example, could influence 'teleoanticipation' during exercise, maintaining higher levels of muscle recruitment during exercise and delaying fatigue. This interesting theory requires further investigation.

Conclusions

There is strong evidence that the elite runners represent geographically distinct regions. Although environmental and socio-economic factors may have encouraged them to develop their running potential, these are unlikely to be the only factors explaining the success of the African runners.

The few scientific studies of elite African runners have shown that they have an enhanced capacity to resist fatigue. An explanation for this characteristic of fatigue resistance has not been forthcoming from traditional measurements of O_2 consumption according to the cardiovascular anaerobic model of exercise physiology and athletic performance. Skeletal muscle consists of various structural proteins and is designed to protect the integrity of the sarcomere during contractions. Titin is one such protein that has elastic properties. It is tempting to speculate that elite runners with an enhanced ability to resist fatigue can be identified by the composition of the titin in their muscles.

The muscle power and biomechanical models suggest a strong theoretical basis that the enhanced fatigue resistance of elite African runners originates in the neuromuscular mechanisms, which regulate the stretch-shortening cycle with each stride while running. The elite distance runners may have a refined 'teleoanticipation' mechanism which may explain their ability to resist fatigue.

Acknowledgements

The author's research is funded by the University of Cape Town, the Medical Research Council and the Founding Donors of the Sports Science Institute of South Africa.

References

1 Jokl E. *Physiology of exercise*. Springfield, IL: Thomas 1964.

2 Maselli G. *Denver Post* 1998 May 23: D-01.

3 Bosch AN, Goslin BR, Noakes TD, Dennis SC. Physiological differences between black and white runners during a treadmill marathon. *Eur J Appl Physiol* 1990; **61**: 68 72.

4 Manners JH. Kenya's running tribe. *The Sports Historian* 1997; **17**: 14–27.

5 Bale J, Sang J. *Kenyan running*. London: Frank Cass, 1996.

6 Noakes TD. Why do Africans run so swiftly? A research challenge for African scientists. *SA J Science* 1998; **94**: 531–5.

7 Sailer S, Seiler S. Track & battlefield. *National Review* 1997 Dec 31: 44–7.

8 MacKay D. Out of Africa. *Runners World* (South African edition) 1997 Aug: 35–7.

9 Manners JH. Baker's Dozen. *Runners World* (South African edition) 1998 May: 40–6.

10 Saltin B, Gollnick PD. Skeletal muscle adaptability: significance for metabolism and performance. In: Peachey LD, Adrian RH, Geiger SR, eds. *Handbook of physiology; section 10: Skeletal muscle*. Bethesda, Maryland: American Physiological Society, 1983.

11 Holloszy JO, Coyle EF. Adaptations of skeletal muscle to endurance exercise and the metabolic consequences. *J Appl Physiol* 1984; **56**: 831–8.

12 Fitts RH. Cellular mechanisms of muscle fatigue. *Physiol Rev* 1994; **74**: 49–94.

13 Noakes TD. Physiological models to understand exercise fatigue and the adaptations that predict or enhance athletic performance. *Scand J Med Sci Sports* 2000; **10**: 123–45.

14 Noakes TD. Challenging beliefs: ex Africa semper aliquid novi. *Med Sci Sports Exerc* 1997; **29**: 571–90.

15 Noakes TD. Maximal oxygen uptake: 'classical versus 'contemporary' viewpoints'. A rebuttal. *Med Sci Sports Exerc* 1998; **30**: 1381–98.

16 Saltin B, Larsen H, Terrados N *et al*. Aerobic exercise capacity at sea level and at altitude in Kenyan boys, junior and senior runners compared with Scandinavian runners. *Scand J Med Sci Sports* 1995; **5**: 209–21.

17 Coetzer P, Noakes TD, Sanders B *et al*. Superior fatigue resistance of elite black South African distance runners. *J Appl Physiol* 1993; **75**: 1822–7.

18 Andersen LB, Henckel P, Saltin B. Maximal oxygen uptake in Danish adolescents 16–19 years of age. *Eur J Appl Physiol* 1987; **56**: 74–82.

19 Costill DL, Thomason H, Roberts E. Fractional utilization of the aerobic capacity during distance running. *Med Sci Sports Exerc* 1973; **5**: 248–52.

20 Weston AR, Karamizrak O, Smith A *et al*. African runners exhibit greater fatigue resistance, lower lactate accumulation, and higher oxidative enzyme activity. *J Appl Physiol* 1999; **86**: 915–23.

21 Ama PFM, Simoneau JA, Boulay MR *et al*. Skeletal muscle characteristics in sedentary Black and Caucasian males. *J Appl Physiol* 1986; **61**: 1758–61.

22 Costill DL, Fink Wl, Pollock M. Muscle fiber composition and enzyme activities of elite distance runners. *Med Sci Sports Exerc* 1976; **8**: 96–100.

23 Saltin B, Kim CK, Terrados N *et al*. Morphology, enzyme activities and buffer capacity in leg muscles of Kenyan and Scandinavian runners. *Scand J Med Sci Sports* 1995; **5**: 222–30.

24 Pollock ML, Gettman LR, Jackson A *et al*. Body composition of elite class distance runners. *Ann N Y Acad Sci* 1977; **301**: 361–70.

25 Dennis SD, Noakes TD. Advantages of smaller body mass for distance running performances in warm, humid conditions. *Eur J Appl Physiol* 1999; **79**: 280–4.

26 Nielsen B, Strange S, Christensen NJ *et al*. Acute and adaptive responses in humans to exercise in a warm, humid environment. *Plügers Arch* 1997; **434**: 49–56.

27 Opie LH. *The heart: physiology from cell to circulation*. 3rd ed. New York: Lipincott-Raven, 1998: 1–637.

28 Fitts RH, Costill DL, Gardetto PR. Effect of swim exercise training on human muscle fiber function. *J Appl Physiol* 1989; **66**: 465–75.

29 Roberts TJ, Marsh RL, Weyand PG, Taylor CR. Muscular force in running turkeys: the economy of mini-mising work. *Science* 1997; **275**: 1113–5.

30 Patel TJ, Lieber RL. Force transmission in skeletal muscle: from actomyosin to external tendons. *Ex Sports Sci Rev* 1997; **25**: 322–63.

31 Lieber RL, Thornell L-E, Fridén J. Muscle cytoskeletal disruption occurs within the first 15 min of cyclic eccentric contraction. *J Appl Physiol* 1996; **80**: 278–84.

32 McComas J. *Skeletal muscle — form and function*. Champaign, IL: Human Kinetics, 1996.

33 Baringa M. Titanic protein gives muscles structure and bounce. *Science* 1995; **270**: 236.

34 Erickson HP. Stretching single protein molecules: titin is a weird spring. *Science* 1997; **276**: 1090–2.

35 Askter HA, Granzier HlM, Focant B. Differences in the I band structure, sarcomere extensibility, and electrophoresis of titin between two muscle types of the perch (Percafluviatilis l). *J Ultrastruct Mol Struct Res* 1989; **102**: 109–21.

36 Waterman-Storer CM. The cytoskeleton of skeletal muscle: is it affected by exercise? A brief review. *Med Sci Sports Exerc* 1991; **23**: 1240–9.

37 Aura O, Komi PV. Effects of prestretch intensity on mechanical efficiency of positive work and on elastic behaviour of skeletal muscle in stretch-shortening cycle exercise. *Int J Sports Med* 1986; **7**: 137–43.

38 Dietz V, Schmidtbleicher D, Noth J. Neuronal mechanisms of human locomotion. *J Neurophysiol* 1979; **42**: 1212–22.

39 Moritani T, Oddson L, Thorstensson A. Electromyographic evidence of selective fatigue during the eccentric phase of stretch/shortening cycles in man. *Eur J Appl Physiol* 1990; **60**: 425–9.

40 Nicol C, Komi PV, Marconnet P. Fatigue effects of marathon running on neuromuscular performances. I. Changes in muscle force and stiffness characteristics. *Scand J Med Sci Sports* 1991; **1**: 10–7.

41 Paavolainen LM, Nummela AT, Rusko HK. Neuromuscular characteristics and muscle power as determinants of 5-km running performance. *Med Sci Sports Exerc* 1999; **31**: 124–30.

DISCUSSION

*'There is nothing special about me.
There will soon be many Kenyans as good as me'*

Kipchoge (Kip) Keino of Kenya
WR Holder 3,000 m and 5,000 m
Olympic Champion 1,500 m 1968, Steeplechase 1972
Olympic Silver medal 5,000 m 1968, 1,500 m 1972

Mr Christopher Brasher: There is an incredible concentration of Olympic medallists in one area of Kenya. There is a precedent for this which I remember researching some time ago: between the two wars at the Olympic games (ie between 1920 and 1936 inclusive) in the 1,500 m, 3,000 m steeple chase, 5,000 m and 10,000 m, 50% of the medallists came from one small nation and the other half from the rest of the world — that nation was Finland and this was entirely due to the Finnish culture. Competitors at that time were almost restricted to Anglo Saxons. There were very few Africans except from South Africa, and hardly any Asians except from Japan, but now there is a huge change. Competitors in the Olympic games today are truly worldwide; yet, in the same events, there is an incredible concentration from a very small area of Africa. The dividing line between the explosive and stamina events is the middle of Africa — colour is not related to this.

Attendee: Is the African in north-east Africa more active than the white European?

Professor Mike Lambert: There is a lot of subsistence living in north-east African areas, so the inhabitants do have to be physical in their day-to-day activity from an early age.

Sir Roger Bannister: It would seem on first principles that if someone were running a great deal during the phase of body growth in youth, the adaptation of the heart and the lung might become more efficient. Are you suggesting this is irrelevant?

Professor Mike Lambert: I think there are several predisposing factors that collectively produce a champion; having the physiological attributes is probably the basis on which all of them depend. Altitude is important but not the only factor; if it was, then countries such as Peru and Tibet would also have an abundance of elite runners, but we do not see many top runners from these regions. If lifestyle including exercise from a young age were the only factor, then you could find many less-developed countries in which children work from an early age producing many elite runners. These factors probably contribute, but without the physiological framework the runners cannot develop fully into top-class athletes.

Professor Eric Newsholme: During each stride, the Achilles tendon stores some kinetic energy as elastic energy, which is released in the next stride[1]. This increases the efficiency in running from 25% to 40%. How far is it possible to measure the elasticity of these tendons in athletes and, thus, the precise efficiency?

Professor Mike Lambert: This is difficult to measure. When oxygen consumption became a parameter of interest years ago, it became relatively easy to measure. However, parameters which have been more difficult to measure have lagged behind. There are laboratories, particularly in Finland, which have been focusing on muscle elasticity for a while but the concept has not been fully accepted.

Professor Craig Sharp: Some time ago, one of my PhD students based part of his research on the elastic component of muscle. His external examiner was Professor McNeill Alexander who has calculated that elastic return possibly contributes up to 50% of the energy of each running stride in the marathon. However, we do not know how to measure it in vivo. We do not know how to train it (although I think that pliometrics may help) — even if we did, as we cannot measure it, we cannot quantify any training effect except through measures of running economy, and possibly simplistically through some form of rebound vertical jump. Regarding the former, Professor Carlton Cooke, who was the postgraduate in question, did find that elite distance runners used of the order of 5 ml/kg/min less oxygen at the same pace compared to good club and recreational marathoners (the latter two being much the same). Carlton asked his subjects to run over a force platform, filmed them and biomechanically analysed their techniques, but felt that the difference did not lie in their running action. We speculated whether or not there might be differences in elastic energy storage and recovery[2].

Dr Dan Tunstall Pedoe: While we are discussing muscle and tendon elasticity, I would like to mention an American television documentary film about the differences between white and black athletes, which caused consternation in the US and was accused of being racist. A basketball coach and sports scientist claimed that with athletes jumping on a force platform, you could tell from the shape of the curve whether or not it was a white or a black person who had jumped because there was such a big difference. I wonder whether anyone has biomechanical evidence on this or whether or not it was a very selective study.

Professor Mike Lambert: I saw the same documentary. I remember the scientist standing next to the force platform and dictating 'this is white', 'this is black', and everyone in the audience laughed, as the way in which he was doing this did seem a little far-fetched. I am not sure if it can be measured to the degree of confidence that he was implying.

Attendee: Why do some elite marathon runners experience only one or two years of world-class performance while others stay at their peak for some years?

Professor Mike Lambert: We have come across runners who can run fairly competitively for up to 30 years and are still competitive in their age group; on the other hand, there are runners who seem to succumb to the stresses of training and racing after about five years. An explanation may be related to differences in muscle structure, or perhaps the antioxidant systems.

Mr Christopher Brasher: I carried out some research in the 1980s relating to the powers of recuperation and ability to stay at the top of great marathon runners such as Salazar, Rogers and Steve Jones. They each had about four to five good marathon runs but at the same time Ingrid Kristiansen and Greta Waitz were at the top of the women's rankings and remained there. They had 14 or 15 world class runs. Both are Norwegian and female, but that cannot be the only explanation.

Attendee: Have the Kenyan runners been studied by sports psychologists?

Professor Craig Sharp: I know a little about the Kenyan athletes, as they have a main training camp based near my work place, and my PhD student, Brian Moore, works with them. I do not believe they have any major sports psychological input in their training.

Professor Norman Myers: I have resided in Kenya for 24 years. I thoroughly agree that the 'Rift Valley' athletes of Kenya have established a formidable record, winning medals galore. I would like to add to what several speakers have said. First, there is no such thing as the Kalenjin tribe. Rather, it is an ethnic grouping that includes the Nandi, the Kipsigis (both of whom have produced a lengthy list of champions), and several other tribes. They live on the plateau to the west of the Rift Valley, not in the Valley itself, and at altitudes 5,500–8,500 feet (1,800–2,900 m). These other tribes live in the same plateau region. In cultural, sociological and anthropological senses, these tribes have much in common; I guess one could postulate the same physiologically. Tribes other than Nandi and Kipsigis have produced few runners, and nobody to my knowledge has a credible explanation.

Second, other tribes in Kenya possess exceptional running talent but have not produced many champions, eg the Maasai. While spending a year coaching so-called Rift Valley tribes, I repeatedly found that the Maasai appeared to possess the most natural ability. Boys who had not yet reached their teens could cover 50 miles in a single night on a cattle-raiding exercise. What the Maasai did not possess, and still apparently do not, was much interest in developing their in-born talent. Apart from Konchellah and a handful of others, they have been far from prominent on the international scene.

Third, other tribes have displayed remarkable capacity; for instance, the Kisii, who live at 6,000–8,000 feet (2,000–2,700 m) above Lake Victoria and, as a Bantu tribe, are as ethnically distinct from the Kalenjin as the British (Anglo Saxons) are from the Eskimos (Inuit). In the late 1950s, I coached a number of Kisii athletes who, after a few months of three or four moderate-intensity training sessions per week could run under 30 minutes for 10,000 m in Nairobi (altitude 1,700 m). Two runners chose to perform more training in terms of both quantity and quality for six months, and responded rapidly to coaching, gaining a gold and a silver at the Commonwealth Games of 1962. Another Bantu runner, although a Kikuyu, is Wakihuru, who won the London marathon a few years ago. He is not only non-Kalenjin but has spent most of his life on the Kenya coast, ie with no altitude benefit (unless it had been genetically encoded in his parents who had lived their lives at 2,000 m). Note, too, the feats of runners from Somalia and

Djibouti, who come from territories where people have long lived at low altitude. The same applies to certain runners from Tanzania.

During the 1960s and early 1970s, Kenyans began to emerge on the international running scene, capturing sizable numbers of medals at world level. Yet their training was often not a patch on their counterparts' regimens. It was not that Kenyan runners were idle in training; quite the opposite. But their coaching regimens were not nearly so informed and organized. Their success appeared to be due in major measure to a natural talent. It was not until the 1980s that they started to undergo training of a quantity and quality to match those of non-Africans. Once the runners were in the hands of coaches with sufficient experience, Kenyan stars started to become not only super stars but appear in large numbers (as witness their record in the steeplechase). Judging by what I have seen of them while visiting Kenya in recent years, they train with a commitment, indeed a ferocity that I rarely find elsewhere. Perhaps they can sustain training of extraordinary volume and quality because they have remarkable genes for recovery between training sessions. They may have other built-in physiological attributes. But I suspect a further factor lies with their cultural background, which often places a premium on capacity to withstand physical discomfort (as befits people living in difficult environments). A problem for these tribes for generations if not centuries has been lock-jaw (Tetanus) disease. In an apparent attempt to counter this threat, boys have had their two lower front teeth (incisors) knocked out at an early age, so that if necessary they can still be fed protein-rich liquids, such as cow's blood and milk, through the gap. This tradition is still practiced today: note the facial features of several of the current Kenyan runners. Boys are required to undergo the "operation" without any anaesthetic or any slight sign of pain. The same applies to certain other traditional tribal rites (such as ritual circumcision) which mark the transition to manhood, with extreme emphasis on readiness to be indifferent to pain. Young men take great pride in outdoing each other in feats of pain tolerance. This, I believe, is why they can sustain extremely demanding training regimes. Of course the physiological factors are probably most important of all. Kenyans can run fast, not only after many years of training but even as soon as their late teens.

Attendee: I am intrigued by so many male marathon runners, especially Kenyans dipping below two hours and 10 minutes in the past few years. Is there a logical explanation for why many are suddenly running fast?

Mr Christopher Brasher: Yes there is. The IAAF ratified payments for races! Shall I give you one date and one place? Athens, 1982 . What happened there? The time that payments became open and legal was the dividing line between amateurs and professional. What is the difference between Herb Elliot and Seb Coe, two of the greatest middle distance runners, who was the greatest? One — the professional Coe — did two Olympics, one — the amateur Elliott — did only one because he had a wife and two kids to support and had to go back to work whereas Coe did not. Since 1982, running has become a career.

Professor Craig Sharp: I think that our silence is meaningful in that this increase in the number of 2:10 marathon runners is probably a sociological phenomenon, possibly in terms of 'hungry runners' like the hungry boxers of the 30s and 50s, and outwith our orbit of competence.

Dr David Martin: I could offer that this is an 'agent-induced phenomenon'. By that I mean simply that the Kenyan athletes do not have either the worldly savvy or the political ease to know that certain marathon races around the world have more lucrative prize money than others.

They also do not know how to secure an entry, and how to obtain the necessary papers to leave their country. However, they do know that the home purchasing power of the prize purses provided is immense, so they are willing to train arduously to prepare themselves. Agents based in Kenya — primarily Europeans — similarly realize that there is an enormous potential profit in 'managing' such details for these excellent athletes, taking a percentage of their prize winnings in return. As the number of world marathons with prize money increases, and as the depth of those finishers receiving such money increases, so the number of travelling athletes to these various events increases. Given ideal racing conditions, highly fit runners racing for huge sums, and the excellent negotiating skills of Kenyan athlete agents ensuring that a generous assortment of Kenyan runners toe the start line, the end result is the unprecedented number of fast Kenyan times. The runners (and their agents) become very wealthy, their athlete compatriots back home see this as a desirable way to make a living, and the agents are there to recruit these additional athletes into the process. In earlier years, before such prize money was offered, there was little need for Kenyan or other runners to leave their country to compete except for major international competitions, which did not have prize money offerings.

Professor Peter Radford: It is not only money; it is also about self-respect. From my generation and Sir Roger Bannister's and Mr Chris Brasher's, there were many people when we were competing who thought that we were wasting our time. Why weren't we doing the more important things of life? That is a mind set, however hard you work to get rid of it. We inherited a sporting culture in the West which says that sport was trivial and a young man's fling until he got down to the serious business of life. There are some cultures where it is now possible, with money and the rewards that go with it, to believe that running is *the* serious thing in life, and I think that changes everything.

Mr Christopher Brasher: It is so much about respect and social status. For example, British Boxing World Champions in the 1920s and 1930s came from the slums of Cardiff and Glasgow. I will tell you one story to end this; I was talking to Jimmy Reid, at one time a Communist, and one of the two union leaders who led the 'work-in' at Fairfield Ship Yard in Glasgow. He told me that at one stage during the negotiations between management and the union in a cinema full of 600 workers, there was a short recess. He asked the men, 'How many of you have ever been on a track, put up your hand?' Not one. 'How many of you have ever worn spikes?' … not one. He poked me in the ribs and said, There probably, was the first four minute miler and not you Oxford and Cambridge men.

Sir Roger Bannister: I know my parents said, 'We are very worried about you spending so much time on running. The main thing is for you to pass your exams and become a doctor'. They were lovable and nice people, but that was their attitude, let alone the attitude of those in Oxford. I remember I got back from a race in Philadelphia, one of the 'miles of the century' and I was asked by a don from my college, 'Have you just been in America?'. He said 'Weren't you running in a Benjamin Franklin mile?' He then said, 'Tell me how far is a Benjamin Franklin mile?'

Reference

1 Kram R, Taylor CR. Energetics of running: a new perspective. *Nature* 1990; **346**: 265–7.

2 Cooke CB. *Running efficiency: a biomechanical and physiological evaluation of normal and loaded horizontal running*. Birmingham: University of Birmingham, 1989. PhD thesis.

Muscle metabolic factors decisive for marathon running

DR JØRN HELGE, DR GERRIT VAN HALL
& PROFESSOR BENGT SALTIN

THE COPENHAGEN MUSCLE RESEARCH CENTRE, RIGSHOSPITALET (UNIVERSITY HOSPITAL),
COPENHAGEN, DENMARK

There are three biological prerequisites for a marathon runner to be successful: high aerobic power, the ability to use a high fraction of it for long periods (ie hours), and a good running economy (ie low energy costs at marathon pace throughout the race) (Figure 1). Before the Munich Olympic games in 1972, the demand of a high maximal oxygen uptake (VO_{2max}) for optimal marathon performance had been the point of focus. However, Frank Shorter's performance in 1972 indicated that other factors were also influential. Shorter was the winner of the marathon whose VO_{2max} was 71.4 ml/kg/min compared with 80 ml/kg/min of some of the other competitors. His advantages were a good running economy, an oxygen uptake of only 53–4 ml/kg/min when running at 19.4 km/h (not competitive speed) on the flat, and use of 92% VO_{2max} at com-

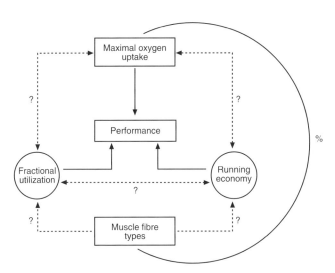

Figure 1

Schematic view of the main physiological variables influencing marathon performance. Solid arrows indicate that the interrelation is well demonstrated, whereas dotted arrows show a potential relationship although the causality remains to be demonstrated or refuted

petitive running speed as opposed to 85–7% in other top-class marathon runners. The magnitude of difference in these two variables between Shorter and his rivals was pronounced; his running economy in particular is among the lowest reported energy cost for a marathon runner and equals that of the best Kenyan cross-country or road race runners. Thus, a high VO_{2max} alone does not make the winner in a marathon race; the

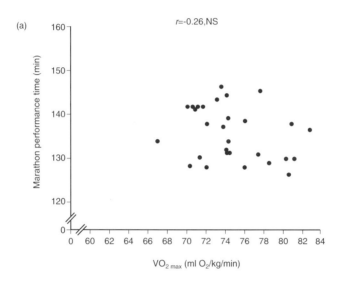

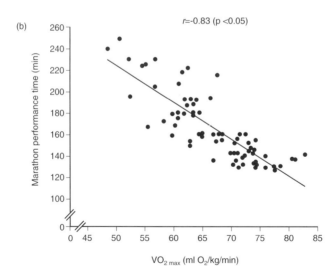

Figure 2

Marathon performance expressed as a function of VO_{2max} representing: (a) data on elite athletes performing better than two hours and 30 minutes (b) a wide range of performance times

Redrawn and adapted from[1,2,49].

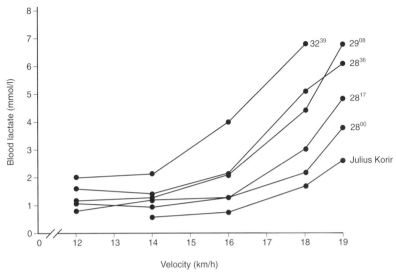

Figure 3

Blood lactate expressed as a function of running velocity at a 2.8% incline to mimic air resistance and ground friction. The data represent Kenyan elite male runners (n=5) and a well trained Danish runner (n=1, 32[39]), and the numbers are the 10 km road race times (minutes) achieved in a race that took place three days earlier

Redrawn from[7].

finding that the fastest runners have a poor correlation between VO_{2max} and the marathon running time, therefore, comes as no surprise[1]. If the entire crowd of marathon runners ranging from the fastest to the slowest is studied, the correlation between performance and VO_{2max} is very good (Figure 2)[1]. This is explained by the fact that aerobic power can vary with a factor of two between the 'untrained' and the most well-trained marathon runner, whereas running economy and relative exercise intensity may only vary by 10–5% each, when comparing the two hours and 10 minutes runners with the three or four hour runners. There is already ample literature on the different running variables and their statistical coupling to performance[1-3]. This chapter will discuss various aspects of skeletal muscle plasticity and factors related to a good running economy. It will also explain why certain features of skeletal muscle metabolism are important in marathon running and why the blood lactate response when running has such a high predictive value for performance (Figure 3).

Skeletal muscle fibre types

Our knowledge on human skeletal muscle fibre types, their characteristics and the degree of adaptability has greatly improved over the past few years. For example, we now know that the human muscle fibre type IIb does not have the same characteristics

Table 1 *Variables characterizing different types of runners*

	VO$_{2max}$ (ml/kg/min)	Fibre types (%)			Capillaries/ fibre	Enzyme activity (mmol/kg/min)	
		I	IIa	IIx		CS	HAD
Track runners	74.6	58	37	5	2.2	15.9	12.6
800–1,500 m)	70–78	52–63	24–42	1–7	2.0–2.4	13.0–18.4	9.9–14.1
(n=7)							
3,000–10,000 m	79.9	64	33	3	2.6	18.6	19.0
(n=10)	76–84	58–76	12–41	0–5	2.3–2.9	16.0–21.4	16.0–23.1
Road/cross-country	80.1	73	27	0	2.9	22.2	21.6
(n=9)	75–85	57–89	11–43	0–3	2.6–3.3	18.8–24.6	18.9–22.0
Sedentary	48	52	36	12	1.1	6.0	5.1
Controls	39–55	36–70	18–48	6–18	0.9–1.3	4.8–8.9	3.9–6.0
(n=12)							

Fibre type I=slow twitch; Fibre type IIa=fast twitch a; Fibre type IIx=fast twitch x; CS=citrate synthase; HAD=B-hydroxy-acyl CoA dehydrogenase. All runners are either European or world-class elite runners. Kenyan runners are represented in the group of long-distance and road cross-country runners. Data are mean and range[6,7]

as that found in muscles from rats and other smaller vertebrates. The human type IIb fibre has slower contractile characteristics and is similar to the type IIx fibre of the rat — it has, therefore, been renamed type IIx. It is also less glycolytic with a sizable oxidative capacity. Equally important is the fact that, with regular use, the type IIx fibre can quickly be transferred to type IIa[4,5]. Hence, only very few or no type IIx fibres can be found in muscles of well-trained endurance athletes (Table 1)[5].

Muscle fibre types are not easily changed from type II to type I with training[5]. Electrophoretic methods have been used to identify the myosin heavy chain isoform pattern (I, IIa and IIx), but there has been no longitudinal training study in humans that has demonstrated a complete transformation of type IIa to type I fibres. The relative amount of major histocompatibility complex (MHC)-I may, however, be enlarged. This means that more type IIa fibres co-express MHC-I and MHC-IIa, which may not be easily detectable when using the histochemical adenosine triphosphate (ATP)-ase staining to identify muscle fibre types. Early studies by Komi and Karlsson on mono- and dizygotic twins indicated that genetic endowment may be critical for muscle fibre type composition[8]. Although this finding has been challenged by Bouchard *et al*[9], the most recent studies on monozygotic twins lend further support to a strong hereditary factor in the occurrence of type I or II muscles fibres in humans. Another example of genetic endowment is the difference in east and west Africans in regard to muscle fibre types. In vastus lateralis, Nigerian boys had an average of 30% type I fibres in their muscles whereas active east African boys had a mean of 62%. It cannot be stated conclusively that this difference is solely due to heredity as recent, more detailed studies of east African boys revealed a lower percentage of type I fibres in the more sedentary boys[10]. A large variation in fibre type composition was also observed, opening up for selection to be a contributing factor. Although this may be the case, it does not change the conclusion that there is a high threshold for type IIa fibres to transform into type I fibres with endurance training, whereas there is no or a very low threshold for converting IIx into IIa fibres.

Skeletal muscles have three to four times greater mitochondrial enzyme activity after extreme endurance training compared to those seen in sedentary people, giving type I and IIa fibres a similar mitochondrial respiratory capacity[11]. In this light, it could be anticipated that muscle fibre types would not matter much in regard to the metabolic response to prolonged exercise and endurance performance. Coyle *et al* have studied this particular problem with intriguing results[12]. In cyclists with a VO_{2max} of 67 ml/kg/min, the blood lactate response to submaximal exercise was used to divide well-trained cyclists into either low or high lactate responders to cycle exercise. Endurance performance was markedly different in the two groups. The high lactate responders could only cycle half the time at 88% VO_{2max} compared to the low lactate responders. Leg muscles were studied for mitochondrial marker enzymes, fibre types and their sizes as well as capillaries, and no difference was found between groups with regard to mitochondrial enzyme activity and capillaries/muscle fibre. Thus, neither the lactate response nor the performance could be related to these indices of muscle adaptation. Both variables are easily affected by changes in physical activity level and are proposed as a link to a more efficient muscle metabolism[13]. Two other muscle indices differed: those with a poor performance and a lower lactate threshold had less type I muscle fibres (47% vs 67%) than the good performers, and had a 15% larger mean muscle fibre size. These results do not relate to running. In the same study, the subjects performed uphill running at a steep incline (10%) to ensure a heavy load on the vastus lateralis of the knee extensors (the muscle portion from which the biopsy was taken)[12]. There was no difference in lactate threshold, which was high (>80%

Table 2 *Comparison of the vastus lateralis portion of quadriceps femoris and gastrocnemius (lateral head) with regards to two mitochondrial enzymes (citrate synthase (CS) and β-hydroxy-acyl CoA dehydrogenase (HAD)) and capillaries per fibre*

	Track runners, distance ≥3,000 m (n=14) Enzymes (mmol/kg/min ww)			Road runners, cross-country (n= 7) Enzymes (mmol/kg/min) ww		
	CS	HAD	Cap/fibre	CS	HAD	Cap/fibre
Vastus lateralis	17.2	15.6	2.2	20.2	19.6	2.6
Gastrocnemius (lateral head)	24.8	20.1	2.7	23.0	22.2	2.7

All subjects were world-class runners and included Kenyans and Scandinavians. Muscle fibre types were similar in the two muscles with a trend for more ST fibres in vastus lateralis (about 5%)[6,7]

VO_{2max}) regardless of fibre type composition. This finding supports the notion that capillaries and enzyme activity have a major role in the muscle metabolic response to exercise regardless of fibre type composition, however it renders no explanation for the differences observed in cycling by Coyle *et al*[12]. It is worth mentioning that, although all leg muscles are engaged in running, the load on the various muscle groups or portions of them may vary depending on the type of run, ie whether or not it is on the flat, uphill, on track, road or cross-country. A reflection of this is the fact that capillarization and enzyme profile of various leg muscles can be quite different when comparing various types of runners, although fibre type compositions are similar (Table 2).

Running economy

It is easy and precise to measure mechanical efficiency or energy costs in cycling, but difficult or even impossible in other forms of exercise such as running. For direct efficiency estimations in running, uphill walking has provided values between 15–20% for net mechanical efficiency which is slightly lower than in cycling. When running on the flat at submaximal speeds, the energy cost is a good measure of running economy. There are, however, two important factors to consider when extrapolating this estimate to represent competitive speed conditions for the marathon. First, whether or not energy costs increase linearly with velocity of running — this is presently unknown. Second, the anaerobic contribution to the energy yield at high exercise intensities. For all running distances except the marathon, these limitations make it impossible to provide an exact measure of the energy costs when running with competitive speed, because VO_{2max} is used in all distances up to 10,000 m. Top speed in competitive marathon running is 19–20 km/h and, although the top runner may use 90% VO_{2max}, the ATP resynthesis from anaerobic glycolysis is minor (discussed below). Thus, the oxygen uptake at a competitive running speed in a marathon should provide a fair estimate of the running economy. As mentioned above, there is a multitude of such measures which provide the same result. A large variation in oxygen consumption is seen at the marathon speeds. At a running speed of 19 km/h, the most efficient runners have a VO_2 of 54–5 ml/kg/min as compared to 60 ml/kg/min and 65 ml/kg/min for a good and the least efficient runner respectively, a maximum difference that approaches 20% (Figure 4). In this example, body weight differences were normalized for kilogrammes only but should strictly be (body weight)$^{0.75}$ kg[7].

What is the explanation for this variation in energy costs when running? The answer is that there is a lack of knowledge to provide anything else than suggestions! The biomechanical aspects relate to elevation of the centre of gravity, movement of the legs, and elastic recoil. Data are emerging on the first two factors, as they are measurable. A running style with pronounced elevation in the vertical direction with each step is costly and can explain a fair fraction of the observed variation[14]. Similarly, increased leg mass is associated with a higher oxygen uptake at a given running speed.

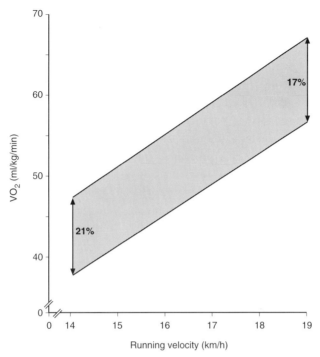

Figure 4

VO$_{2max}$ expressed as a function of marathon running velocity. The grey band indicates the observed variation possible in these parameters

Redrawn from[1].

The size of the foot, the lower leg and the thigh also have a peripheral role, but the more the weight/volume, the higher the energy costs. If a single factor was to be selected as being important for a good running economy in a marathon, the length and shape of the leg combined with its size would most probably be chosen (Henrik Larsen, personal communication). Among other factors suggested, the role of muscle fibre composition has been studied in cycling. It has been hypothesized that the relative activation of type I fibres in exercise that does not demand a high fraction of VO$_{2max}$ is larger than in exercise that does require a high fraction of VO$_{2max}$ and thus, the mechanical efficiency is higher. The reasoning is that type I fibres are recruited with a frequency that makes them metabolically efficient. The experimental data support this notion, although only weakly[15]. Moreover, when cycling for several hours, both type IIa and IIx fibres are recruited to produce the force without a more marked elevation in VO$_2$. This argues against the fast muscle fibres being energetically ineffective when recruited in rhythmic concentric exercise requiring low force.

An important and overlooked aspect of running efficiency is that, in contrast to cycling, where efficiency is reasonably maintained, a marked deterioration is seen with time in running. Furthermore, it appears that for the better runners a more moderate drift

in oxygen uptake is occurring during running. There are two obvious conditions causing a drift in VO_2 at constant exercise intensity: the gradual switch to more fat being
used as substrate for oxidative metabolism and the slight increase in ventilation. In
cycling, these changes can to a large extent explain the drift in VO_2. In running, the
elevation in VO_2 is much greater and even in well-trained athletes amounts to 0.3–
0.5 l/min. A major difference between cycling and running is that there is no eccentric component in the former, but even when running on the flat the eccentric impact
on the muscle is noticeable. Thus, one possibility for the mentioned difference could
be that elastic recoil vanishes in prolonged running due to the eccentric component
that causes mechanical wear and tear. In the process of fatigue, structural alterations
may also occur at the molecular level thereby changing the elastic recoil capacity, which
may lead to a less efficient stride. The magnitude of increase over a two to three-hour
run is in the order of 0.3–0.5 l/min or about 10%. In more extreme situations such as
in a 100 km race, a given speed costs 1 l/min more oxygen at the end of the race than
at the start — this represents an elevation in energy cost of 30–40%[2]. It is worth
noting that the reduction in running pace is not due to a lower fractional use of VO_{2max},
which is kept quite constant; instead, there is an inverse relationship between the
increased metabolic costs and running speed.

Training induced shifts to lipids

The coupling between fractional use and performance for the marathon distance is
clear (Figure 1). However, maintaining a high fractional use despite the drift in oxygen uptake (0.3–0.5 l/min) and the concurrent decrease in muscle glycogen requires
an optimal partitioning of substrates. The importance and partitioning of lipid as a
substrate during exercise, and the mechanism regulating this will be discussed below.

Endurance training has profound effects on the capacity to transport and oxidize
substrates, which induces a greater capacity for total substrate flux and in some circumstances leads to an increased contribution of fat as a substrate during submaximal
exercise. Most studies have demonstrated an increased combustion of fat when exercising on the same absolute intensity as before training. This may be due to the concurrent decrease in relative exercise intensity, allowing for a higher fat oxidation at
the lower relative exercise intensity[16,17]. At the same relative exercise intensity, the
presence of a shift in substrate use towards a higher fat use is less clear. In a recent
series of cross-sectional[18] and longitudinal[19] studies, it was demonstrated that during submaximal exercise the respiratory exchange ratio (RER) was not lowered with
training in men at the same relative exercise intensity. A decrease, although small in
RER at the same relative exercise intensity, has also been demonstrated[20]. These
findings are to some extent confirmed by data available in the literature that failed or
only found a significant change in RER measured at the same relative exercise load at
one point after three hours of submaximal exercise. A confounder of this issue is clearly

the efficacy of diet as a potent moderator of substrate flux during exercise. As such the lack of a training induced increase in fat use after four[21] and seven[22] weeks aerobic training and a carbohydrate-rich diet suggests that the interaction of training and macronutrient intake play an important role when the effect of training on substrate utilization is evaluated.

Does training induce a shift in substrate use across the exercising leg muscle at the same relative load? This point has been addressed applying different exercise and training models and in all but one, leg RQ during exercise was unchanged after training. The difference, found in one study[23], was measured during two-legged cycle exercise after training of one leg. Although a difference was present in blood flow, the normal training effect on hormonal and arterial substrate concentration was absent — caution should, therefore, be exercised when interpreting this finding! It was suggested in a recent study that substrate use was shifted towards fat oxidation in inactive tissues[19], but during exercise at higher workloads the inactive tissue receives a small fraction (10–5%) of the cardiac output and as such is not of great importance for athletes.

In a controversial paper, Whipp et al predicted that female athletes were on the move to surpass male performance in long-distance running[24] (see Dr Tunstall Pedoe's chapter on *Marathon myths and marathon medicine*)! Although it is generally believed that females have a higher fat oxidation during submaximal exercise which would render them less prone to fatigue, there are indications that this difference is attenuated in well-trained female athletes. Thus, based on the development in running world records over recent years and the gender difference in percent body fat and haemoglobin, the gender difference remains status quo.

Training induced shifts in lipid sources (blood and muscle)

The advent of stable isotope tracer methodology and the significantly refined analytical capacity of mass spectrometers have stimulated studies of the regulation and partition of fat recruited for oxidation, originating from the circulation and/or from triacylglycerol stored within the muscle. Romijn et al demonstrated that the contribution of plasma derived fatty acids (FA) tended to decrease with increasing workload[25]. After endurance training in male subjects at the same relative workload, 65% VO_{2max} fat oxidation was unchanged. Although the rate of appearance (RaFA) was increased[26]. In a follow-up study, Bergman and colleagues applied a similar training and exercise protocol and showed that RQ measured over the leg remained unchanged at the same relative load after training.

Although remarkably high (1.01), the net FA uptake increased and the muscle triglyceride (TG) lipolysis decreased[19]. These results indicate that substrate partitioning remains unchanged after training when measured at the same relative workload. To our knowledge, solid data are lacking for higher workloads and, as a result, it is difficult to evaluate the training effect on fuel partitioning at higher workloads.

From a training perspective, it may be worth focusing on studies based on electron microscopy. These demonstrated that endurance training[27], even when comparing animals of similar size and markedly different aerobic capacity[28], caused a significant increase in muscle triacylglycerol storage around the mitochondria. Based on a phylogenetic rationale and recent data demonstrating a significant muscle triacylglycerol breakdown during post-exercise recovery, and no breakdown during exercise[29], it is tempting to suggest that an important role for muscle triacylglycerol might also be delivery of substrate during exercise recovery. However, the observed increased storage of triacylglycerol surrounding the mitochondria in well-trained athletes might suggest that this fuel source could be important during more intense exercise, when glycolytic flux is high and the transport of substrates, particularly FA, across the sarcolemma reaches 'saturation'[30]. Specifically in the case of marathon performance sports drinks are consumed; this inevitably triggers an insulin-induced attenuation of lipolysis and subsequent FA delivery, thus adding to the importance of intracellularly stored lipid for maintaining lipid oxidation and avoiding carbohydrate depletion and the resulting fatigue.

In addition to understanding the effect of training on fat oxidation, it is necessary to consider whether or not training changes the recruitment of glucose from intra- or extramuscular depots during whole body exercise at the same relative exercise load. It is well known that glycogen breakdown is dependent on the relative exercise intensity across a wide degree of training status, and maintenance of carbohydrate oxidation at a given relative exercise load must therefore imply that the contribution from plasma derived glucose remains unchanged. Such a contention is supported by findings of similar plasma derived glucose contributions applying both cross-sectional and longitudinal experimental designs[31].

Unfortunately, data are sparse on the direct measurement of substrate use and partitioning in elite marathon runners during a race; however, based on training studies and pre-competition measurements, RER values should reside in the broad range of 0.85–0.95 (even close to 1.0). When oxygen use is 60–7 ml O_2/kg/min during a competition in elite marathon runners, the RER values can only be sustained if intramuscular triacylglycerol contributes heavily to the lipid oxidation. Although the literature on the importance of mTG breakdown during exercise is controversial, some data are available to support this notion[32].

Limits to lipid oxidation in trained athletes

Galbo[33] and later Romijn et al[25] demonstrated that fat oxidation in absolute terms is highest at about 55–65% VO_{2max}, but it is still not clear which factors limit fat oxidation and whether or not training alters this limitation. In an elegant series of papers, Dick Taylor and colleagues compared the Labrador retriever dog with the pygmy goat, animals of similar size but different aerobic capacities (3,026 and

6,517 μmol O_2/kg/min, respectively). They found that, at comparable exercise intensities, the dog and the goat supplied the same fraction of their maximum aerobic capacity from fat oxidation. Thus the relative capacity for fat oxidation does not seem to be higher in the more aerobic animal dog compared to the less aerobic animal goat. This finding supports the lack of evidence for training induced increases in fat use at the same relative workload mentioned previously[19]. This clearly implies that fat oxidation is limited by the maximal flux rate of the aerobic system and/or the amount of available oxygen at a given point in time during exercise.

Several theories have sought to explain the mechanism that regulates the proportional oxidation of fat and carbohydrate. The glucose-FA cycle was suggested >35 years ago but, although many attempts have been made, there is still unsatisfactory evidence that this cycle is operational during exercise in man. Sidossis and colleagues[34] suggested that flux through the glycogenolytic pathway and an increased production of acetyl-coenzyme A (CoA), leading to formation of malonyl-CoA with subsequent allosteric inhibition of long-chain fatty acyl-CoA transport into the mitochondria, could be the regulatory mechanism. This substrate cycle was termed the reverse glucose FA cycle and, although one experiment demonstrated that glucose ingestion during exercise limited long-chain FA recruitment and oxidation, the available evidence supporting the operation of this cycle is sparse.

Recent interest has focused on the role of adenosine 5′-monophosphate (AMP)-activated protein kinase (AMPK) in skeletal muscle as a 'metabolic master switch' which, by phosphorylation of key proteins, has a dual role increasing muscle glucose uptake and decreasing malonyl-CoA and subsequently enhancing FFA-oxidation[35]. Ruderman and colleagues suggested that since the glucose-derived increase in cytosolic citrate (which stimulates acetyl-CoA-carboxylase-β (ACCβ)-activity) and concurrent exercise-induced increase in 5′-AMP with a subsequent increase in AMPK-activity (which inhibits ACCβ-activity) both affect ACCβ activity and the malonyl-CoA regulatory mechanism, this provides a link to Randle's glucose FA cycle[36]. The increased glucose availability and subsequent increase of malonyl-CoA would just as nicely support the presence of the reverse glucose FA cycle in function. It follows that, although AMPK activation is undoubtedly involved in the regulation of substrate selection, there are still major unresolved issues.

What is the role of training in the regulation of substrate selection? Implicitly there is still the possibility that substrate availability via mass action could potentially be influential to substrate use, through the partitioning of substrate delivery from glycogen and muscle triacylglycerol stores, and the FA and glucose from the bloodstream. It has consistently been described that long-term training increases both the number of intramuscular substrate stores and the transport capacity for both glucose and fat. It could simply be speculated that training exerts its influence on substrate selection via an enhanced substrate delivery and storage capacity and an overall increase in the total oxidative flux capacity. This would imply that dietary habits, timing of intake and diet composition are important in the partitioning of substrates during exercise.

How is the adaptive training response regulated?

Advanced methodological techniques have profoundly increased our knowledge on the mechanisms involved in induction of adaptive training response. Early findings by Issemann and Green introduced the peroxisome proliferator-activated receptors (PPARs)[37], which are ligand-activated transcription factors belonging to the nuclear hormone receptor superfamily, and evidence has since accumulated that these could play a major role for the coordinate transcriptional regulation of nuclear genes involved in the cellular FA oxidation[38]. PPARs are expressed in a variety of tissues: α-PPARs predominantly in tissues with a high rate of β-oxidation, such as liver, kidney, heart and muscle; γ-PPARs predominantly in adipose tissue; and δ-PPARs exhibiting less tissue specificity[39]. PPARs are activated by a number of substances, but physiological ligands include dietary long-chain FA, eicosanoids and heat shock proteins (HSPs)[38]. α-PPAR is considered to be a major regulator of intra- and extracellular lipid metabolism up-regulating the expression of enzymes and proteins involved in the transport of FA into the cell, transport into the mitochondria, and in mitochondrial and peroxisomal FA oxidation[39]. The HSP72 has been linked to the PPARs, and it has been proposed that it plays a role in the signalling pathway of PPAR. In line with this there is evidence that a gene encoding medium-chain acyl-CoA dehydrogenase (MCAD), a mitochondrial β-oxidative enzyme, was regulated in a pattern that paralleled the skeletal muscle fibre type-specific energy use. Furthermore, there is emerging evidence that α-PPAR is also affected by glucocorticoids and insulin and that this occurs via upstream response elements, although at present the insulin response element is not characterized[40]. The later convergence of the hormonal and metabolic transcriptional pathways in conjunction with inclusion of an HSP stress response indicates this system could potentially emphasize the major effectors known to alter lipid metabolism (Figure 5).

Although the flux rate of the lipid metabolising system is important to the limitation of the system, the absolute flux rate also depends on the oxygen delivery capacity and specifically mitochondrial function. In 1997, two new uncoupling proteins (UCPs), UCP2 and UCP3, were discovered; UCP3 is abundantly expressed in muscle[41]. The levels of UCP3 and UCP2 messenger ribonucleic acid (mRNA) were shown to be significantly reduced after eight weeks endurance training in rat soleus and tibialis[41]; a similar finding in man was recently reported when trained and untrained subjects were compared[42]. This indicates that metabolic efficiency is improved with training. As more oxygen is needed to maintain the same ATP-synthesis with fat compared to carbohydrate as substrate during exercise, a sparing of proton 'leakage' by a decreased mitochondrial UCP expression will allow, although small, somewhat higher fat oxidation even when the oxidative system is at its upper limit.

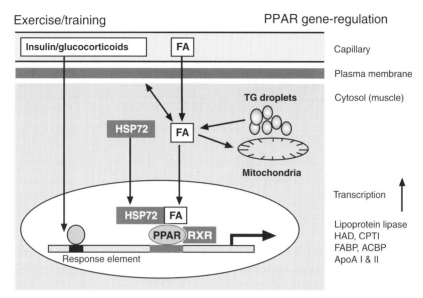

Figure 5

Simplified diagram of the convergence of three pathways within skeletal muscle which, by generation of FA, HSP72 and insulin/glucocorticoids respectively, produce agonists (response element for hormones) that are potential activators of genes coding for transport proteins and enzymes involved in the metabolism of fat via the PPAR system

Lactate metabolism

In marathon running, even experts would consider anaerobic glycolysis to be insignificant. The running pace is even and most courses quite flat, which combined with two or more hours of running time would imply a complete aerobic energy yield with lipid contributing as substrate rather than only carbohydrate and, if so, a very high rate of glycolysis. Moreover, the close link between a high lactate threshold and success in marathon running has underscored the belief that there is no or very little muscle lactate production when running the marathon. Nothing could be more wrong. Lactate is continuously produced, released to the blood, but cleared as well[43]. This uptake of lactate by the tissues particularly includes the active leg muscle, where the largest fraction of lactate clearance of the leg occurs. Lactate is converted to pyruvate and fully oxidized in the contracting muscles[43]. The ability to run at a high speed without accumulating lactate is not only due to keeping lactate production low but also a high capacity for lactate clearance. Thus, the two questions to be dealt with relate to why lactate is formed and the extent to which lactate is cleared from the blood and oxidized by active muscles.

A high fat utilization by the leg muscles is decisive for successful marathon running as it conserves the limited muscle glycogen stores. This does not preclude a high rate of glycolysis in active muscles. RER values observed when running at marathon pace range from 0.85 to close to 1.0. In prolonged exercise, the RER may gradually become reduced with time but at a relative exercise capacity above 80% VO_{2max} — such a reduction is small or non-existent (Figure 5[44]). This means that ≥ 2.5 g/min carbohydrate is used by active skeletal muscles, and from this follows a high rate of glycolysis and a high rate of pyruvate production. In prolonged exercise the elevation in muscle pyruvate is in absolute values quite small but in relative terms there is a doubling or more, which increases with time, reflecting an ongoing high rate of pyruvate production as well as use in prolonged exercise. As shown by Huckabee et al in the 1950s, lactate formation is closely related to rate of pyruvate formation rather than lack of oxygen[45]. In this light, the role of the maintained or even slightly elevated lipid oxidation when exercising at a high VO_{2max} is to reduce the dependence on glycolysis. Even the smallest elevation in lipid combustion will have an impact on the rate of glycolysis which will be lowered. In turn this means that less lactate is being produced. Thus, one of the main reasons for the right shift in the blood lactate response to increasing running speed is its effect on the capacity of the trained muscles to use lipids. The higher this fraction is of the total substrate turnover, the lower the relative rate of glycolysis and the amount of pyruvate and lactate produced.

Several longitudinal endurance-training studies support this notion. The most conclusive data come from studies where only one leg or muscle group was trained, and both legs were tested for their substrate metabolism simultaneously. Henriksson was the first to demonstrate that a difference in lipid combustion, of 18% vs 31% total energy turnover of an untrained and trained leg respectively, was accompanied by no net release of lactate from the trained leg after the initial 10 minutes of exercise, whereas the untrained leg on average released close to 2 mmol/min during the one-hour exercise period[23]. Interestingly, systemic blood lactate concentration was constant (around 4 mmol/l) throughout the exercise period. Moreover, muscle lactate was essentially the same in the thigh muscles of the two legs, measuring about 6.5 mmol/kg (wet weight) at the end of the exercise. This indicates a continuous production of lactate during exercise in both legs but less so in the trained leg. Although the lactate efflux from the trained skeletal muscle was smaller than from the untrained leg, it is of note that the trained leg in Henriksson's study exhibited a no net release of lactate. This can only be explained by an equal magnitude of lactate uptake and efflux in the trained leg.

Within a muscle bundle, lactate can potentially be produced in one fibre and consumed in the other when these are in relative close proximity to each other. In 1930, Owles suggested 'lactate may be produced in some muscles and subsequently oxidised in others, or even adjacent fibres of the same muscle'[46]. To date, the focus has been on type II fibres producing lactate and type I fibres consuming lactate. However, type I and II fibres have similar enzymatic machinery and transport systems available to produce and handle lactate, although in different activities and quantities. Therefore, it seems unlikely that lactate is exclusively produced in type II fibres and in part consumed in type I fibres, or that lactate taken up from the circulation is exclusively consumed by type I fibres. However, the described phenomenon of one fibre producing and another potentially consuming the produced lactate may occur if not all fibres are recruited during exercise. The significance of such a mechanism would be minor as the metabolic rate is important for the rate by which lactate can be metabolised in the cell. Synthesis of glycogen from lactate occurs, but it is a rather slow process.

Lactate transport and lactate dehydrogenase in human skeletal muscles

In humans an increase in physical activity can improve the lactate transport capacity of skeletal muscle and is associated with a rise in sarcolemmal monocarboxylate transporters (MCT) (and a relative increase in MCT1) (Figure 6)[47]. It is interesting that the type II fibres, which seem to produce more lactate, possess a lower lactate transport capacity. It has been estimated that a muscle with only type II fibres can be expected to have one-half of the lactate transport capacity of a muscle composed of entirely type I fibres. This seems to be contradictory, but it has been suggested that MCT1 expression in muscle fibres may reflect the extent to which transport of lactate into the cell is required for its oxidation as a respiratory fuel. In contrast, MCT4 expression may be more important for lactate efflux from the muscles that rely more on glycolytic metabolism[47].

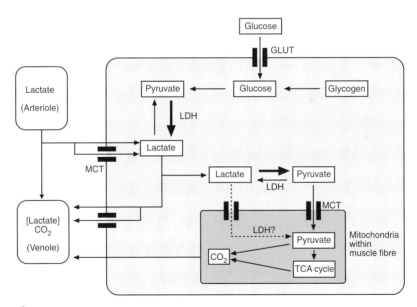

Figure 6

A schematic diagram showing the pathways of lactate (pyruvate) into and within the muscle cell. Arrows represent the transport and metabolic pathways of lactate from the arterial microcirculation to the mitochondria and subsequently to the venoles as lactate or carbon dioxide. The broken arrow into the mitochondria represents the possible transport of lactate into the mitochondria[43]

Skeletal muscles possess all isozymes of lactate dehydrogenase (LDH); the total LDH activity in type I fibres is roughly one-half compared to type II fibres. However, the relative contribution of heart-specific $LDH_{1,2}$ to total LDH activity is higher in the type I than the type II fibres. Endurance runners have a higher percentage of type I fibres, a lower total LDH activity and a higher relative contribution of the heart-specific $LDH_{1,2}$ than untrained runners. In parallel with these findings, endurance training causes a decrease in total LDH activity and an increase in relative activity of $LDH_{1,2}$; similarly, sprint training causes an increase in total LDH activity and a decrease in relative activity of heart-specific $LDH_{1,2}$. However, the relatively higher $LDH_{1,2}$ content in type I fibres and in skeletal muscle of endurance athletes should be interpreted with care, since the absolute specific activity of $LDH_{1,2}$ hardly changes. This implies that the changes in total LDH activity are mainly in the muscle type LDH. Illustrative is the negative correlation observed in top athletes between $LDH_{4,5}$ activity and running distance (Figure 7)[7]. The differences in $LDH_{1,2}$ were minimal (42–53 μmol/min/g muscle) although it seemed positively correlated with running distance.

The picture that emerges is of a fairly complex muscle metabolic scheme. At a high relative exercise intensity (>80% VO_{2max} and up to about 90% in some of the best runners) as in running the marathon, there is a mandatory carbohydrate use at a high rate with a concomitant rate of pyruvate formation. This leads to an overflow of pyruvate to lactate by simple mass action in the LDH reaction. The mechanism by which use of fat can retard glycolysis is via elevated mitochondrial citrate production, which

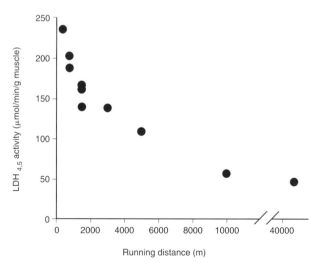

Figure 7

The activity of the $LDH_{4,5}$ expressed as a function of the runner's optimum performance distance. The data represent Swedish male international elite runners (n=10)

Redrawn from[7].

in turn causes the cytosolic concentration to increase and inhibits the activation of phosphofructose kinase. However, lactate production is unavoidable even in the most well-trained skeletal muscles when the metabolic rate is high. Lactate is metabolised in order to minimize its accumulation in the body. In an ordinary situation, liver, heart and inactive muscles are sufficient to clear the lactate. However, this is not sufficient when running a fast marathon, in which case the active skeletal muscle contributes most. In addition to lactate production being limited due to a lowering of the total LDH activity, the fact that LDH_{1-2} activity is maintained and the MCT capacity elevated will enlarge the clearance of lactate from the blood by the active skeletal muscle.

Conclusions

VO_{2max}, fractional use of VO_{2max} and running economy play a major role in determining marathon performance. Joyner predicted in his 1992 article that one hour and 58 minutes was an achievable running time, which is 6–8% better than that achieved today[48]. This appears to be a plausible prediction. With the best possible running economy, maintained throughout the race, the oxygen requirement is about 65 ml/kg/min at 2 l/km/h (a more average running economy demands about 70 ml/kg/min). A VO_{2max} of 80 ml/kg/min, of which 87% is used, provides a VO_2 of 69.6 ml/kg/min. On the mechanistic side, the cardiorespiratory fitness sets the limit for VO_{2max} while skeletal muscle variables such as capillaries, transport proteins and mitochondrial enzymes and mitochondrial 'location' are crucial for a high fractional use of VO_{2max}. Low body weight and long, slender legs are important for running economy, but muscle fibre types may also play a role. Proper training can improve VO_{2max} and the muscle metabolic potential, but there is a conflict as high-intensity exercise is most likely to improve VO_{2max} while prolonged running at around or just below competitive speed is better for obtaining an adequate muscle adaptation. Body size and leg length relative to body height are hardly trainable.

Acknowledgement

The original studies by the authors cited in the present article were made possible by a grant from the Danish National Research Foundation (#504-14).

References

1   Svedenhag J, Sjodin B. Maximal and submaximal oxygen uptakes and blood lactate levels in elite male middle- and long-distance runners. *Int J Sports Med* 1984; **5**: 255–61.

2   Noakes TD. *Lore of running*. Champaign: Leisure press, 1991.

3   Joyner MJ. Physiological limiting factors and distance running: influence of gender and age on record performance. In: Holloszy JO, ed. *Exercise and sports sciences reviews*. Baltimore: Williams and Wilkins, 1993: 103–33.

4   Andersen P, Henriksson J. Training induced changes in the subgroups of human type II skeletal muscle fibres. *Acta Physiol Scand* 1977; **99**: 123–5.

5 Harridge SDR. The muscle contractile system and its adaptation to training. In: Marconnet P, Saltin B, Komi P, Poortmans J, eds. *Human muscular function during dynamic exercise*. Basel: S Karger, 1996: 82–94.

6 Rolf C, Andersson G, Westblad P, Saltin B. Aerobic and anaerobic work capacities and leg muscle characteristics in elite orienteers. *Scand J Med Sci Sports* 1997; **7**: 20–4.

7 Saltin B, Kim CK, Terrados N *et al.* Morphology, enzyme activities and buffer capacity in leg muscles of Kenyan and Scandinavian runners. *Scand J Med Sci Sports* 1995; **5**: 222–30.

8 Komi PV, Karlsson J. Physical performance, skeletal muscle enzyme activities, and fibre types in monozygous and dizygous twins of both sexes. *Acta Physiol Scand Suppl* 1979; **462**: 1–28.

9 Bouchard C, Simoneau JA, Lortie G *et al.* Genetic effects in human skeletal muscle fiber type distribution and enzyme activities. *Can J Physiol Pharmacol* 1986; **64**: 1245–51.

10 Larsen HB *et al.* Trainability of Kenyan village boys compared with Kenyan town boys. *J Physiol (London)* 2000; 528P, 42P.

11 Jansson E, Kaijser L. Muscle adaptation to extreme endurance training in man. *Acta Physiol Scand* 1977; **100**: 315–24.

12 Coyle EF, Coggan A, Hopper M, Walters T. Determinants of endurance in well-trained cyclista. *J Appl Physiol* 1988; **64**: 2622–30.

13 Gollnick PD, Saltin B. Significance of skeletal muscle oxidative enzyme enhancement with endurance training. *Clin Physiol* 1982; **2**: 1–12.

14 Cavagna GA. Mechanical work in running. *J Appl Physiol* 1964; **19**: 249–56.

15 Coyle EF, Sidossis LS, Horowitz JF, Beltz JD. Cycling efficiency is related to the percentage of type I muscle fibers. *Med Sci Sports Exerc* 1992; **24**: 782–8.

16 Gollnick PD, Saltin B. In: Horton ES, Terjung RL, eds. *Exercise, nutrition and energy metabolism*. New York: Macmillan, 1988: 72–88.

17 Brooks GA, Mercier J. Balance of carbohydrate and lipid utilization during exercise: the 'crossover' concept. *J Appl Physiol* 1994; **76**: 2253–61.

18 Bergman BC, Brooks GA. Respiratory gas-exchange ratios during graded exercise in fed and fasted trained and untrained men. *J Appl Physiol* 1999; **86**: 479–87.

19 Bergman BC, Butterfield GE, Wolfel EE *et al.* Evaluation of exercise and training on muscle lipid metabolism. *Am J Physiol* 1999; **276**: E106–17.

20 Koivisto V, Hendler R, Nadel E, Felig P. Influence of physical training on the fuel-hormone response to prolonged low intensity exercise. *Metabolism* 1982; **31**: 192–7.

21 Helge JW, Wulff B, Kiens B. Impact of a fat rich diet on endurance in man: role of the dietary period. *Med Sci Sports Exerc* 1998; **30**: 456–61.

22 Helge JW, Richter EA, Kiens B. Interaction of training and diet on metabolism and endurance during exercise in man. *J Physiol (Lond)* 1996; **292**: 293–306.

23 Henriksson J. Training induced adaptations of skeletal muscle and metabolism during submaximal exercise. *J Physiol (Lond)* 1977; **270**: 661–75.

24 Whipp BJ, Ward SA. Will women soon outrun men? [letter] [see comments]. *Nature* 1992; **355**: 25.

25 Romijn JA, Coyle Ef, Sidossis LS *et al.* Regulation of endogenous fat and carbohydrate metabolism in relation to exercise intensity and duration. *Am J Physiol* 1993; **265**: E380–91.

26 Friedlander AL, Casazza GA, Horning MA *et al.* Endurance training increases fatty acid turnover, but not fat oxidation, in young men. *J Appl Physiol* 1999; **86**: 2097–105.

27 Hoppeler H. Exercise-induced ultrastructural changes in skeletal muscle. *Int J Sport Nutr* 1986; **7**: 187–204.

28 Vock R, Hoppeler H, Claassen H *et al.* Design of the oxygen and substrate pathways VI. Structural basis of intracellular substrate supply to mitochondria in muscle cells. *J Exp Biol* 1996; **199**: 1689–97.

29 Kiens B, Richter EA. Utilization of skeletal muscle triacylglycerol during postexercise recovery in humans. *Am J Physiol Endocrinol* 1998; **38**: E332–7.

30 Hoppeler H, Weibel ER. Limits for oxygen and substrate transport in mammals. *J Exp Biol* 1998; **201**: 1051–64.

31 Bergman BC, Butterfield GE, Wolfel EE *et al.* Muscle net glucose uptake and glucose kinetics after endurance training in men. *Am J Physiol* 1999; **277**: E81–92.

32 Staron RS, Hikida RS, Murray TF *et al.* Lipid depletion and repletion in skeletal muscle following a marathon. *J Neurol Sci* 1989; **94**: 29–40.

33 Galbo H. Hormonal and metabolic adaptation to exercise. New York: Georg Thieme, 1983.

34 Sidossis LS, Stuart CA, Schuman GI *et al.* Glucose plus insulin regulate fat oxidation by controlling the rate of fatty acid entry into the mitochondrion. *J Clin Invest* 1996; **98**: 2244–50.

35 Ruderman NB, Saha AK, Vavvas D, Witters LA. Malonyl-CoA, fuel sensing, and insulin resistance. *Am J Physiol* 1999; **276**: E1–18.

36 Vavvas D, Apazidis A, Saha AK *et al.* Contraction-induced changes in acetyl-CoA carboxylase and 5′-AMP-activated kinase in skeletal muscle. *J Biol Chem* 1997; **272**: 13255–61.

37 Issemann I, Green S. Activation of a member of the steroid hormone receptor superfamily by peroxisome proliferators. *Nature* 1990; **347**: 645–50.

38 Bishop-Bailey D. Peroxisome proliferator-activated receptors in the cardiovascular system. *Br J Pharmacol* 2000; **129**: 823–34.

39 Gervois P, Torra IP, Fruchart JC, Staels B. Regulation of lipid and lipoprotein metabolism by PPAR activators. *Clin Chem Lab Med* 2000; **38**: 3–11.

40 Steineger HH, Arntsen BM, Spydevold O, Sorensen HN. Retinoid X receptor (RXR alpha) gene expression is regulated by fatty acids and dexamethasone in hepatic cells. *Biochimie* 1997; **79**: 107–10.

41 Boss O, Samec S, Desplanches D *et al.* Effect of endurance training on mRNA expression of uncoupling proteins 1, 2, and 3 in the rat. *FASEB J* 1998; **12**: 335–9.

42 Schrauwen P, Troost FJ, Xia J *et al.* Skeletal muscle UCP2 and UCP3 expression in trained and untrained male subjects. *Int J Obes Relat Metab Disord* 1999; **23**: 966–72.

43 van Hall G. Lactate as a fuel for mitochondrial respiration. *Acta Physiol Scand* 2000; **168**: 643–56.

44 Saltin B, Gollnick PD. In: Horton ES, Terjung RL, eds. Exercise, nutrition and energy metabolism. New York: Macmillian Publishing,1988: 45–71.

45 HuckabeeWE. Relationships of pyruvate and lactate during anaerobic metabolism II. Exercise and formation of O_2-debt. *J Clin Invest* 1958; **37**: 255–63.

46 Owles WH. Alterations in lactate acid content of the blood as a result of light exercise, and associated changes in CO_2-combining power of the blood and the alveolar CO_2 pressure. *J Physiol (Lond)* 1930; **69**: 214–37.

47 Juel C, Halestrap AP. Lactate transport in skeletal muscle — role and regulation of the monocarboxylate transporter. *J Physiol (Lond)* 1999; **517**: 633–42.

48 Joyner MJ. Modeling: optimal marathon performance on the basis of physiological factors. *J Appl Physiol* 1991; **70**: 683–7.

49 Foster C, Daniels JT, Yarbrough RA. Physiological and training correlates of marathon running performance. *Aust J Sports Med* 1977; **9**: 58–61.

Genetics and maximal oxygen uptake

PROFESSOR CLAUDE BOUCHARD

EXECUTIVE DIRECTOR, PENNINGTON BIOMEDICAL RESEARCH CENTER,
HUMAN GENOMICS LABORATORY, BATON ROUGE, LOUISIANA, USA

Endurance performance depends on several factors, including the physical, biomechanical, physiological, metabolic, behavioural, psychological and social characteristics of the individual. Although some of these determinants are probably little influenced by genetic heterogeneity, most are affected to a significant extent. A comprehensive review of evidence for the contribution of genetic variation to all these determinants is beyond the scope of this paper. This chapter will focus on maximal oxygen uptake (VO_{2max}) as a surrogate for cardiorespiratory endurance. It is commonly accepted that VO_{2max} — determined by a combination of central factors (eg cardiac output) and peripheral factors (eg muscle capillary density) — is one of the factors limiting endurance performance. Evidence, based on the genetic epidemiology literature, for a role of genetic factors in VO_{2max} in the sedentary state and its response to exercise training will be discussed in this chapter. Results from candidate gene studies and other molecular markers will also be summarized.

Quantitative genetic studies

Much research had been carried out to determine whether or not VO_{2max} is influenced by genetic factors. This has enabled us to address the following questions: is there a familial concentration for VO_{2max} in the sedentary state and its response to training? What is the relative contribution of the estimated genetic effect (heritability) to the total population variation? Is there evidence for a stronger maternal or paternal influence in the transmission pattern?

Sedentary state

One approach to assessing the importance of familial resemblance in relevant phenotypes is to compare the variance between families or sibships with that observed within nuclear families or sibships. In order to obtain meaningful results, relevant concomitant variables such as age, gender, body mass and body composition must be controlled.

Several studies have suggested that VO_{2max} is characterized by a significant familial resemblance[1–3]. The HERITAGE Family Study, for example, determined an F ratio of 2.72 from the comparison of the between-family and within-family variance for VO_{2max} (adjusted for age, sex, body mass and body composition) in the sedentary state. The intraclass coefficient for the familial resemblance was 0.41[4].

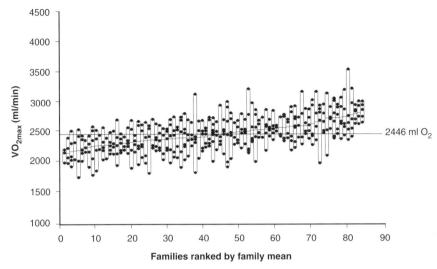

Figure 1

VO_{2max} (adjusted for age, body weight, fat mass and fat-free mass) plotted by family rank in the HERITAGE Family Study. Each family is enclosed in a box, with individual data points plotted as dots and each family mean as a dash; the horizontal reference line is the group mean

Redrawn and reproduced with permission[4].

The heritability of VO_{2max} has been estimated from three family studies[1,5,6] and seven studies on twins[7,8]. The most comprehensive is the HERITAGE Family Study, which involved two cycle ergometer VO_{2max} tests performed in sedentary families of Caucasian descent[4]. Based on structural modelling of the data, the maximal heritability of the age, sex, body mass and body composition-adjusted VO_{2max} was shown to be about 50%. Figure 1 illustrates the concept of family lines with low and high VO_{2max} phenotypes in the sedentary state.

Results of the seven studies conducted with pairs of monozygous (MZ) and dizygous (DZ) twins have also been reviewed. The intraclass correlations for MZ twins ranged from 0.6 to 0.9, while that for DZ twins, with one exception, was between 0.3 and 0.5[7]. The largest twin study was derived from a population-based twin panel of conscripts[8]. The data were based on predicted VO_{2max} values that were subsequently transformed to categorical scores, from low to high maximal aerobic power — the intraclass correlations for these scores were similar to those found in other twin studies. In our own study, carried out at the Laval University, Quebec City, Canada, and which involved 27 pairs of brothers, 33 pairs of DZ twins and 53 pairs of MZ twins, the heritability was about 40% for VO_{2max}/kg body mass[6].

Statistical modelling analytical strategies have been applied to estimate genetic and environmental sources of variation in VO_{2max}. For example, Fagard *et al* performed a path analysis of VO_{2max} in 28 MZ and 19 DZ twin pairs[9]; when data were adjusted for body mass, skinfold thickness and sports participation, heritability was estimated as 66%. In 1996, Maes and colleagues applied structural equation modelling to data on 105 10-year-old twin pairs and their parents (97 mothers and 84 fathers) from the Leuven Longitudinal Twin Study[10]. They quantified genetic and environmental sources of variation in several fitness components, including VO_{2max} measured during a maximal treadmill test, and observed strong assortive mating for absolute VO_{2max} (l/min) with a husband–wife correlation of 0.42 (n=79 pairs), markedly higher than in the HERITAGE Family Study[4]. The results did not provide a straightforward indication as to which model best explained the data. However, there was clear evidence for a strong genetic component to absolute VO_{2max}, but the genetic influence was reduced when VO_{2max}/kg body mass was considered.

One of our early familial studies suggested the likelihood of a specific maternal effect for VO_{2max}/kg mass or VO_{2max}/kg fat-free mass[1]. This hypothesis was prompted by the observation that correlations reached ≥0.20 in mother–child pairs, but were zero in father–child pairs. More recently, the HERITAGE Family Study has provided strong evidence for a substantial maternal heritability in VO_{2max} adjusted for age, sex, body mass and body composition[4]. About one-half of the maximal heritability of VO_{2max} observed in the sedentary state was compatible with a maternal, and possibly a mitochondrial, transmission.

Response to training

There are many inter-individual differences of VO_{2max} in response to exercise training. Among young adults, for example, some individuals exhibit a large response, whereas others show no or minimal response; a broad range of response phenotypes lies between these extremes. Figure 2 depicts the individuality of response in terms of gain in VO_{2max} with a standardized 20-week endurance training programme across the four clinical centres involved in the HERITAGE Family Study[11]. The mean gain in VO_{2max} was about 400 ml oxygen (O_2)/min but the range extended from no gain to 1 l O_2/min. The same range of changes with exercise-training had been observed in some earlier training studies with sedentary subjects[7].

What is the main cause of the heterogeneity in response to training? We believe that it is largely related to genetic characteristics that have yet to be determined. In order to test this hypothesis, training studies with pairs of monozygotic twins were performed, with the rationale that the response pattern will vary for individuals having the same genotype (within pairs) compared to subjects with differing genetic characteristics (between pairs). The results showed that individuality in trainability of VO_{2max} is highly familial and primarily genetically determined. Indeed, studies performed with pairs of MZ twins revealed that VO_{2max} response to standardized training was six to nine times more variant between genotypes (ie between pairs of twins) than within genotypes (ie within pairs of twins)[12]. Figure 3 illustrates the similarity of training response among members of the same MZ twin pairs in one of these experiments.

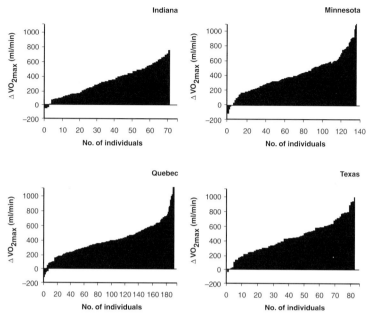

Figure 2

Individual values for the increase in VO$_{2max}$ among whites across the four clinical centres of the HERITAGE Family Study in response to a 20-week endurance training programme

Redrawn and reproduced with permission[11].

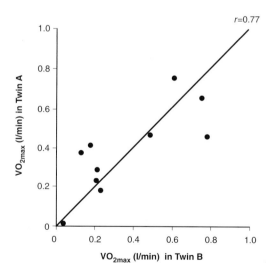

Figure 3

Intrapair resemblance (intraclass coefficients) in 10 monozygotic twin pairs for training changes in VO$_{2max}$ (l O$_2$/min) after 20 weeks of endurance training

Reproduced with permission[12].

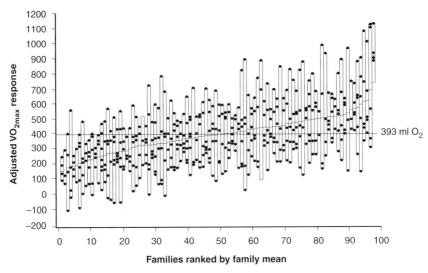

Figure 4

VO$_{2max}$ response to a 20-week endurance training programme in the white families of the HERIT-AGE Family Study. Each family is enclosed in a box, with individual data points plotted as dots and each family mean as a dash; the horizontal reference line is the group mean

Reproduced with permission[11].

Gains in absolute VO$_{2max}$ showed almost eight times more variance between than within pairs of twins[12,13].

The most convincing evidence for the presence of family lines in the trainability of VO$_{2max}$, however, is provided by the HERITAGE Family Study. The increase in VO$_{2max}$ in 481 individuals from 98 two-generation families of Caucasian descent was adjusted for age, sex and baseline VO$_{2max}$. The adjusted VO$_{2max}$ response showed 2.6 times more variance between families than within families, and the model-fitting analytical procedure yielded a maximal heritability estimate of 47% (Figure 4)[11].

Molecular markers

Genetic epidemiology studies provide justification to search for genes and mutations associated with VO$_{2max}$ in the sedentary state and its responsiveness to training. The genetic dissection of VO$_{2max}$ will clearly require a wide array of designs and technologies, eg case and control studies, family studies, association studies, linkage studies from genomic scans or with candidate genes, transmission disequilibrium tests, rodent transgenic models, crossbreeding studies with informative mouse or rat strains, knockout models, conditional knockout models, ambitious sequencing projects, and sophisticated bioinformatics. Most available reports have focused on candidate genes encoded in nuclear deoxyribonucleic acid (DNA) and on a few mitochondrial DNA (mtDNA) sequences. Recently, a first genomic scan for VO_{2max} was published[14]. But first, let us review the evidence for a role of selected candidate genes and mtDNA on VO_{2max}. It seems unlikely that a single gene or a few loci will be sufficient to define the genetic component of endurance performance and its determinants, and the ability to train. The investigation of the molecular basis of human variation in performance and in trainability is still in its infancy. However, the databases necessary to undertake such studies have been or are currently being established, and it is hoped that a wealth of new data will be available in the near future.

Angiotensin-converting enzyme gene

Over the past few years, studies have reported significant associations between an angiotensin-converting enzyme (ACE) insertion/deletion (I/D) polymorphism and performance-related phenotypes. In a case-control study of 64 Australian Olympic level rowers and 114 non-athlete controls, higher frequencies of the I allele and the I/I genotype were observed in athletes (0.57 and 0.30, respectively) than in controls (0.43 and 0.18, respectively)[15]. Similarly, in 25 British male mountaineers with a history of ascending >7,000 m without using supplementary O_2, the I allele was more common than in a cohort of 1,906 British males free from clinical cardiovascular disease[16]. The relationship between ACE I/D polymorphism and VO_{2max} was also investigated in three groups of postmenopausal women with low (sedentary, n=19), moderate (physically active, n=19) or high (athletes, n=20) levels of habitual physical activity[17]. In all physical activity subgroups, women with the I/I genotype were shown to have the highest VO_{2max} value and, in the pooled data, differences between genotypes were statistically significant. However, both genotype and allele frequencies were similar across the physical activity subgroups.

Although these results seem to support the hypothesis of an association between high cardiorespiratory fitness and the I allele of the ACE I/D polymorphism, the small number of subjects and the study designs have become a cause of concern. As a result, a DNA bank of >350 Caucasian male endurance athletes with VO_{2max} reaching at least 75 ml/kg/min along with sedentary control subjects with VO_{2max} <50 ml/kg/min (the GENATHLETE cohort) has been established in collaboration with laboratories in Canada (Quebec), Germany (Freiburg), Finland (Kuopio), the US, and other countries — this has been used to investigate the hypothesis. One report, based on data from 192 athletes and 189 controls, revealed no difference in distribution of the ACE I/D genotypes between the two groups[18]. Further classification of the athletes based on measured VO_{2max} did not provide evidence for an excess of the I allele or the I/I genotype among athletes with high VO_{2max} levels (>85 ml/kg/min). Similarly, in 476 Caucasian and 248 black subjects from the HERITAGE Family Study cohort, no associations were observed between cardiorespiratory fitness phenotypes measured in the sedentary state and the ACE I/D polymorphism[18].

A series of reports based on a cohort of young British male military recruits noted significant associations between the ACE I/D polymorphism and training responses of cardiac phenotypes and muscular endurance performance[16,19]. Following a 10-week military training period, the homozygotes for the D allele of the ACE polymorphism showed significant increases in cardiac septal and posterior wall thickness and in the left ventricular mass, whereas no changes were evident in the I/I homozygotes[19]. It was later reported that the increase in the number of repetitive elbow flexions with a 15-kg barbell was 11-fold greater in the I/I homozygotes than in the D/D homozygotes[16]. Considering the physiological role of ACE, results on the responses of cardiac dimensions seem biologically plausible. However, the lack of a reasonable mechanism for the latter association with skeletal muscle performance raises doubts over these results.

In the HERITAGE Family Study cohort, the associations between the ACE I/D polymorphism and the training responses of fitness-related phenotypes (O_2 consumption, power output, heart rate, cardiac output, stroke volume, minute ventilation, tidal volume, blood lactate level) at maximal and submaximal exercise were tested in 476 Caucasian and 248 black subjects[20]. No evidence was found for a greater training response in the subjects with the I/I genotype. Of the 216 association tests performed on 54 phenotypes in four subject groups, only 11 showed significant p-values. In contrast to previous studies, the D/D homozygotes in Caucasian offspring showed the greatest increases in VO_2 and power output phenotypes, and decreases in heart rate at submaximal exercise at a constant power output (50 W). No associations were evident in Caucasian parents or in black parents or offspring.

Considering the negative findings from the larger studies and the lack of a plausible physiological explanation for an association between cardiorespiratory fitness phenotypes and ACE polymorphism, it is unlikely that DNA sequence variation in the ACE gene is a determinant of VO_{2max} and cardiorespiratory endurance in humans.

Skeletal muscle-specific creatine kinase gene

Skeletal muscle-specific creatine kinase (CKMM) is an enzyme involved in skeletal muscle energy metabolism — it catalyzes the formation of adenosine triphosphate (ATP) from phosphocreatine and adenosine diphosphate (ADP). CKMM is more abundant in type II than type I skeletal muscle fibres, and low levels are typically observed in the skeletal muscles of endurance athletes. In CKMM knockout mice, the initial isometric maximal twitch force and the twitch time to peak tension did not differ from those of the wild-type controls[21]. However, the muscle force induced by continuous electrical stimulation (1 Hz and 5 Hz) in the mutant animals showed a rapid drop at the onset of the stimulation but was regained as the stimulation continued. After 225 s, force production was greater than in the wild-type animals. This suggests that the muscles of the mice lacking CKMM were more resistant to fatigue[21].

The association between CKMM polymorphisms and fitness-related phenotypes in humans has been investigated in three studies. An early study indicated that a CKMM protein charge variant was weakly associated with the ability to perform a 90-minute endurance test[22]. More recently, both association and sib-pair linkage analyses supported the hypothesis of a role of the CKMM gene locus on VO_{2max} in the Caucasian subjects of the HERITAGE Family Study cohort[23,24]. In the sedentary state, the parents who were homozygotes for the rare allele of the CKMM NcoI marker had a lower VO_{2max} than the other two genotypes[23]. Moreover, both in parents and in offspring, the same genotype was associated with a lower VO_{2max} training response. However, in the GENATHLETE cohort, both the allele and the genotype frequencies were similar in endurance athletes and in sedentary controls[25]. This may indicate that the variation in the CKMM gene locus modifies the trainability of VO_{2max} in sedentary subjects but is not a key determinant of the elite endurance athlete status, that is, when VO_{2max} is at or near its maximum potential.

Mitochondrial DNA

Due to the apparent maternal effect on VO_{2max}[4,7], mtDNA is of particular interest as it is inherited solely from the maternal oocyte. Human mtDNA is a 16,569 base pairs (bp) circular duplex molecule that does not recombine and is self-replicative. It codes for 13 of the 67 polypeptides involved in the respiratory chain and oxidative phosphorylation, plus two ribosomal and 22 transfer ribonucleic acids (tRNAs). The displacement-loop (D-loop) region is a non-coding segment that contains the promoters for transcription of heavy and light mtDNA strands, the origin of replication of the heavy strand, and conserved sequences essential for mtDNA expression[26,27]. The mtDNA concentration is about 1.5-fold higher in endurance-trained athletes than in sedentary controls[28].

It has been found that carriers of three mtDNA morphs — one due to a base change for threonine in the tRNA and two others caused by base substitutions in subunit 5 of the reduced nicotinamide adenine dinucleotide (NADH) dehydrogenase (MTND5) gene — had a body mass-adjusted VO_{2max} in the untrained state that was significantly higher than that found in non-carriers[29]. A low response of VO_{2max} to endurance training was also observed for three carriers of a variant in MTND5 in the same study.

A MTND5-NciI polymorphism at bp 13,364, a BamHI marker at bp 13,470 and a D-loop KpnI variant at bp 16,133 were assessed in 125 endurance athletes from the GENATHLETE cohort and in a group of matched controls[30]. The MTND5-NciI variant was found in 12.9% of athletes and 14% of controls, and the MTND5-BamHI variant was observed in 12.8% of endurance athletes and 12.3% of sedentary controls. The D-loop KpnI mutation was found in 5.8% of athletes and in 1.6% of controls. It was concluded from this study that the three mtDNA polymorphisms were not more prevalent in either of the two subject groups. However, it cannot be excluded that some mtDNA variants may have functional implications in sedentary subjects and are not important in elite endurance athletes.

Na,K-ATPase α2

The maintenance of a membrane potential is a prerequisite for excitability and contraction of skeletal muscle cells. Both in vitro and in vivo studies have shown that the sarcolemmal sodium (Na), potassium (K)-ATPase plays a central role in the regulation of membrane potential, and during acute exercise its activity increases markedly to re-establish the K^+ and Na^+ gradients across cell membrane and to facilitate the generation of new action potentials and muscle contractions[31]. The Na,K-ATPase concentration in skeletal muscle has been shown to increase in response to exercise training in humans[32], whereas the inhibition of the enzyme has significantly decreased skeletal muscle contractile endurance in animal models[31].

In the HERITAGE Family Study cohort, we investigated the associations between two Na,K-ATPase α2 gene markers (an isoform expressed mainly in skeletal muscle) and VO_{2max} and maximal power output (W_{max}) in the sedentary state and their responses to 20 weeks of endurance training[33]. Sib-pair linkage analysis revealed a suggestive linkage between the Na,K-ATPase α2 gene locus and the training responses of VO_{2max} ($p=0.054$) and W_{max} ($p=0.003$) in 309 Caucasian sib-pairs. In the association analyses, the homozygotes for the rare allele of the exon 1 marker showed a 48% lower VO_{2max} training response than the homozygotes for the common allele, with the heterozygotes exhibiting an intermediate response. Moreover, a second marker located at the 3' end of the gene revealed a significant association with the VO_{2max} training response in the offspring. The rare allele homozygotes had 39% and 29% greater increase in VO_{2max} with training than the common allele homozygotes and the heterozygotes, respectively. These results suggest that DNA sequence variation at the Na,K-ATPase α2 locus, or a locus nearby, is associated with the responsiveness of VO_{2max} to endurance training in previously sedentary Caucasian adults.

Heritage genomic scan

Another approach to identify genes pertaining to cardiorespiratory endurance is the detection of quantitative trait loci (QTL) by a genomic scan. A genomic scan based on crossbreeding studies with information strains of mice or rats has not been reported to date.

The first paper on a genomic scan for VO_{2max} in the sedentary state and its response to endurance training was published recently[14]. The scan was based on 289 polymorphic markers covering all 22 pairs of autosomes with a mean spacing of 11 cM. A total of 99 Caucasian nuclear families and 415 pairs of siblings of the HERITAGE Family Study were available for the study. For the sedentary state VO_{2max} (adjusted for age, sex, body mass and body composition), the results indicated suggestive linkage ($p<0.01$) with markers on chromosomes 4q12, 8q24, 11p15 and 14q21, whereas markers on 1p11, 2p16, 4q26, 6p21 and 11p14 yielded positive signals for the VO_{2max} training response (also adjusted for age, sex and baseline VO_{2max}).

Although these observed linkages were not very strong in accordance with the polygenic nature of the VO_{2max} phenotypes, the results suggest that selected chromosomal regions should be investigated further for potential candidate genes or expressed sequences.

Conclusions

There is increasing evidence that genes play a role in performance determinants in the sedentary population — this is based on the methods of genetic epidemiology, considering one phenotype at a time, including VO_{2max}. Data are available for a variety of these performance phenotypes, and the heritability is generally low ($\leqslant 25\%$) and rarely exceeds 50%[12]. The genetic effect seems to be polygenic, although this has not yet been thoroughly investigated. There is also evidence that individuals have different abilities to adapt to and benefit from exercise training. Those with the same genotype have a similar response to training than those with differing genotypes. Thus, the genotype appears to be a very important determinant of the trainability of VO_{2max}.

The search for genetic markers of trainability status will probably be more productive than that of the performance phenotype in the untrained state. Many candidate genes have been investigated in the GENATHLETE case-control study, including erythropoietin, angiogenin, carnitine palmityl transferase, fatty acid binding proteins, hormone-sensitive lipase, lipoprotein lipase, insulin-like growth factors and their related binding proteins, transforming growth factors, heat-shock proteins, nitric oxide synthase, tumour necrosis factors and others[34]. However, a single gene with a clear and strong effect has not yet been determined.

Candidate gene studies and genomic scans for the identification and localization of QTL contributing to endurance performance phenotypes will produce useful information, but this will not be sufficient. There is a need for crossbreeding studies of informative rodent strains to provide evidence of QTL and to delineate the mechanisms associated with these genetic signals. This will provide a foundation for investigation of the relevant human syntenic chromosomal regions. The between-strain differences among inbred rat strains strongly suggest that there are genes affecting endurance performance[35]. A variety of transgenic and knockout rodent models will also be needed if we are to have a better understanding of the role of genes and mutations evidenced in human studies. These rodent models will, undoubtedly, foster new and innovative human molecular studies.

Although much remains to be investigated, the exercise science and sports medicine research domains are not well funded and this has resulted in slow progress. Therefore, it is not surprising that the genetic and molecular foundations of human endurance performance is still rudimentary.

Acknowledgements

The research on genetics and exercise is supported by the National Institutes of Health (HL-45670) and the Pennington Biomedical Research Center. It was also supported in the recent past by NSERC (Canada) (OPG 0042791) and FCAR (Quebec) (ER-2449).

References

1 Lesage R, Simoneau JA, Jobin J et al. Familial resemblance in maximal heart rate, blood lactate and aerobic power. *Hum Hered* 1985; **35**: 182–9.

2 Lortie G, Bouchard C, Leblanc C et al. Familial similarity in aerobic power. *Hum Biol* 1982; **54**: 801–12.

3 Montoye HJ, Gayle R. Familial relationships in maximal oxygen uptake. *Hum Biol* 1978; **50**: 241–9.

4 Bouchard C, Daw EW, Rice T et al. Familial resemblance for VO_{2max} in the sedentary state: The HERIT-AGE Family Study. *Med Sci Sports Exerc* 1998; **30**: 252–8.

5 Bouchard C, Boulay MR, Simoneau JA et al. Heredity and trainability of aerobic and anaerobic perform-ances. *Sports Med* 1988; **5**: 69–73.

6 Bouchard C, Lesage R, Lortie G et al. Aerobic performance in brothers, dizygotic and monozygotic twins. *Med Sci Sports Exerc* 1986; **18**: 639–46.

7 Bouchard C, Malina RM, Pérusse L, eds. *Genetics of fitness and physical performance.* Champaign, Illinois: Human Kinetics Publishers, 1997.

8 Sundet JM, Magnus P, Tambs K. The heritability of maximal aerobic power: a study of Norwegian twins. *Scand J Med Sci Sports* 1994; 181–5.

9 Fagard R, Bielen E, Amery A. Heritability of aerobic power and anaerobic energy generation during exer-cise. *J Appl Physiol* 1991; **70**: 352–62.

10 Maes HH, Beunen GP, Vlietinck RF et al. Inheritance of physical fitness in 10-yr-old twins and their parents. *Med Sci Sports Exerc* 1996; **28**: 14479–91.

11 Bouchard C, An P, Rice T et al. Familial aggregation of $VO_{(2max)}$ response to exercise training: results from the HERITAGE Family Study. *J Appl Physiol* 1999; **87**: 1003–8.

12 Bouchard C, Dionne FT, Simoneau JA, Boulay MR. Genetics of aerobic and anaerobic performances. *Exerc Sport Sci* Rev 1992; **20**: 27–58.

13 Prud'homme D, Bouchard C, Leblanc C et al. Sensitivity of maximal aerobic power to training is genotype-dependent. *Med Sci Sports* Exerc 1984; **16**: 489–93.

14 Bouchard C, Rankinen T, Chagnon YC et al. Genomic scan for maximal oxygen uptake and its response to training in the HERITAGE Family Study. *J Appl Physiol* 2000; **88**: 551–9.

15 Gayagay G, Yu B, Hambly B et al. Elite endurance athletes and the ACE I allele — the role of genes in athletic performance. *Hum Genet* 1998; **103**: 48–50.

16 Montgomery HE, Marshall R, Hemingway H et al. Human gene for physical performance. *Nature* 1998; **393**: 221–2.

17 Hagberg JM, Ferrell RE, McCole SD et al. VO_2max is associated with ACE genotype in postmenopausal women. *J Appl Physiol* 1998; **85**: 1842–6.

18 Rankinen T, Wolfarth B, Simoneau JA et al. No association between the angiotensin-converting enzyme I/D polymorphism and elite endurance athlete status. *J Appl Physiol* 2000; **88**: 1571–5.

19 Montgomery H, Clarkson P, Dollery CM et al. Association of angiotensin-converting enzyme gene I/D polymorphism with change in left ventricular mass in response to physical training. *Circulation* 1997; **96**: 741–7.

20 Rankinen T, Pérusse L, Gagnon J et al. Angiotensin-converting enzyme ID polymorphism and fitness pheno-types in the HERITAGE Family Study. *J Appl Physiol* 2000; **88**: 1029–35.

21 van Deursen J, Heerschap A, Oerlemans F et al. Skeletal muscles of mice deficient in muscle creatine kinase lack burst activity. *Cell* 1993; **74**: 621–31.

22 Bouchard C, Chagnon M, Thibault MC *et al*. Muscle genetic variants and relationship with performance and trainability. *Med Sci Sports Exerc* 1989; **21**: 71–7.

23 Rivera MA, Dionne FT, Simoneau JA *et al*. Muscle-specific creatine kinase gene polymorphism and VO₂max in the HERITAGE Family Study. *Med Sci Sports Exerc* 1997; **29**: 1311–7.

24 Rivera MA, Pérusse L, Simoneau JA *et al*. Linkage between a muscle-specific CK gene marker and VO₂max in the HERITAGE Family Study. *Med Sci Sports Exerc* 1999; **31**: 698–701.

25 Rivera MA, Dionne FT, Wolfarth B *et al*. Muscle-specific creatine kinase gene polymorphisms in elite endurance athletes and sedentary controls. *Med Sci Sports Exerc* 1997; **29**: 1444–7.

26 Clayton DA. Replication of animal mitochondrial DNA. *Cell* 1982; **28**: 693–705.

27 Greenberg BD, Newbold JE, Sugino A. Intraspecific nucleotide sequence variability surrounding the origin of replication in human mitochondrial DNA. *Gene* 1983; **21**: 33–49.

28 Puntschart A, Claassen H, Jostarndt K *et al*. mRNAs of enzymes involved in energy metabolism and mtDNA are increased in endurance-trained athletes. *Am J Physiol* 1995; **269**: C619–25.

29 Dionne FT, Turcotte L, Thibault MC *et al*. Mitochondrial DNA sequence polymorphism, VO₂ max and response to endurance training. *Med Sci Sports Exerc* 1991; **23**: 177–85.

30 Rivera MA, Wolfarth B, Dionne FT *et al*. Three mitochondrial DNA restriction polymorphisms in elite endurance athletes and sedentary controls. *Med Sci Sports Exerc* 1998; **30**: 687–90.

31 Nielsen OB, Harrison AP. The regulation of the Na⁺,K⁺ pump in contracting skeletal muscle. *Acta Physiol Scand* 1998; **162**: 191–200.

32 McKenna MJ, Harmer AR, Fraser SF, Li JL. Effects of training on potassium, calcium and hydrogen ion regulation in skeletal muscle and blood during exercise. *Acta Physiol Scand* 1996; **156**: 335–46.

33 Rankinen T, Pérusse L, Borecki IB *et al*. The Na,K-ATPase α2 gene and trainability of cardiorespiratory endurance: The HERITAGE Family Study. *J Appl Physiol* 2000; **88**: 346–51.

34 Bouchard C, Wolfarth B, Rivera MA *et al*. Genetic Determinants of Endurance Performance. In: Shepherd RJ (ed). *Endurance in sport*. Oxford: Blackwell Science, in press.

35 Barbato JI, Koch LG, Darvish A *et al*. Spectrum of aerobic endurance running performance in eleven inbred strains of rats. *J Appl Physiol* 1998; **85**: 530–6.

Cellular fatigue, muscle stiffness and free radicals

DR ALAN DONNELLY

SENIOR LECTURER, DEPARTMENT OF PHYSICAL EDUCATION AND SPORTS SCIENCE,
UNIVERSITY OF LIMERICK, LIMERICK, IRELAND

Exercise including eccentric muscle contractions, where the muscle lengthens as it produces force, is associated with delayed onset muscle soreness (DOMS) or muscle stiffness. Running, particularly downhill, is a common cause of DOMS. Anecdotal evidence suggests that most runners experience this stiffness at some point during their training, usually at the beginning of a season or when training volume increases. This chapter will focus on the causes and effects of DOMS, and will discuss the evidence for the involvement of free radical-mediated processes in the aetiology of contraction-induced muscle damage.

Unaccustomed exercise

Temporary muscle soreness can occur during the final stages of high-intensity exercise bouts, probably as a result of metabolite accumulation; this recedes on cessation of exercise. In contrast, DOMS is characterized by its late onset, most commonly one day after unaccustomed exercise and with maximum soreness occurring two or three days after exercise[1,2]. Muscle soreness is felt when the limb is moved or on palpation, and declines completely between five and nine days after exercise[1]. The precise mechanism by which muscle soreness arises is not clear, although monocyte-derived prostaglandins and tissue oedema have been proposed as causative factors[3].

Range of muscle motion

Unaccustomed exercise restricts the range of muscle movement. This was demonstrated by Clarkson *et al* who studied damaged human biceps and reported that the angle to which the affected arm could be flexed was reduced immediately after exercise and for several days thereafter, while the relaxed arm angle decreased, restricting the range of motion of the muscle[1]. These changes could reflect muscle contracture or swelling of the affected muscle.

Muscle force production

The ability of a muscle to produce force is reduced in both voluntary and stimulated contractions following unaccustomed exercise[1,2]. Force loss can be ⩾50% of pre-exercise values immediately after cessation of exercise, with no change in force or a subsequent small loss one day post-exercise; this is followed by gradual recovery, which may not be complete until ⩾10 days after the initial bout. Some authors report a biphasic pattern to force loss in humans where immediate loss may be partially due to metabolic fatigue resulting in a slight temporary recovery, followed by a greater force loss one or more days after the initial bout[4]. This pattern is also observed in animal studies[5].

Exercise-induced muscle damage is associated with a characteristic change in the force-frequency relationship of the affected muscle[6]. Low frequency fatigue, where a disproportionate force loss occurs at low frequencies of stimulation, can be detected at

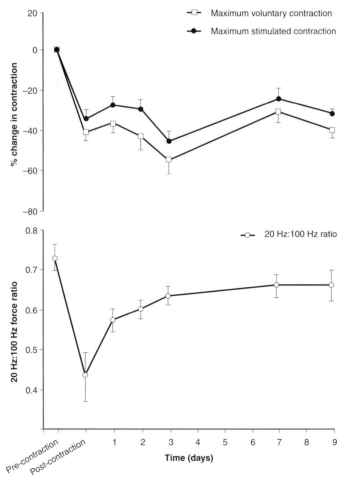

Figure 1

Results of voluntary and stimulated eccentric contractions to induce temporary muscle damage in nine volunteers showing % change and decline in 20 Hz:100 Hz stimulated force ratio

Redrawn and reproduced with permission[4].

20 Hz, 50 Hz and 100 Hz stimulation — 20 Hz shows greatest force loss. Further-more, damaged human muscle appears to respond more slowly to stimulation and has an increased excitation-contraction coupling time after eccentric contractions[5].

Results from a study in which eccentric muscle contractions were stimulated to induce temporary muscle damage to the knee extensors of nine volunteers are shown in Figure 1[4]. The stimulated contractions produced more reproducible results than the voluntary contractions, with consistent levels of muscle damage in all volunteers. Voluntary force declined by >50% with peak force loss occurring three days after the exercise bout; this suggested that secondary processes lead to further force loss after eccentric contractions. Although stimulated force loss was significantly less than voluntary force loss, the same pattern of force decline was observed. The sharp decline in the stimulated 20 Hz:100 Hz force ratio indicates low frequency fatigue. The more rapid recovery of 20 Hz:100 Hz force ratio in this study is representative of the normal pattern after eccentric contractions; recovery from low frequency fatigue occurs more rapidly than that for muscle force as a whole, and low frequency fatigue does not seem to show the secondary decline observed for maximal voluntary and stimulated force. This example of damage-induced force loss presents a typical pattern that might be observed after unaccustomed eccentric contractions.

Evidence of muscle damage

Exercise that induces DOMS often results in elevated circulating levels of muscle-derived proteins. For ease of measurement, serum or plasma creatine kinase (CK) activity has been used most frequently as a marker of muscle damage[1,7,8]. Running, particularly marathon running, has been shown to increase levels of both CK iso-enzymes — CK MM and CK MB[9]. Studies on participants following marathon running reveal that CK MB is derived from skeletal muscle and not from the heart, reflecting its increased synthesis in aerobically trained muscle[10]. As a result of changes in CK levels, other enzymes (eg lactate dehydrogenase) and muscle-derived proteins (eg myoglobin and myosin light chain) increase in the blood. Together, these changes suggest that exercise-related muscle damage results in a loss of muscle sarcolemmal integrity.

Histological examination of damaged muscle reveals disturbances to many important muscle components, mainly the myofibrils, with A band disruption and disorganization of the Z discs reported immediately after exercise[11]. Damage to cytoskeletal proteins has also been noted, with desmin staining being reduced 15 minutes after eccentric contractions[12]. These damage-related changes are observed in the muscles of runners after a marathon, with Z line disruption, phagocyte infiltration and contracture knots recorded during three days after running[13]. Interestingly, this study revealed that eight of the 10 volunteers showed evidence of muscle damage before the marathon, possibly indicative of training induced damage[13].

Effects of DOMS on exercise performance and training

The effects of muscle damage and muscle soreness encountered by athletes and other sports people during a training programme have received very little direct study. We know that DOMS and its associated effects result in decreased efficiency when further exercise is undertaken, with greater heart rate and rate of perceived exertion reported during exercise using damaged muscle[14]. This, along with muscle weakness, limits the ability to train effectively; the associated muscle weakness may increase the risk of injury during training.

Another prolonged effect of eccentric contractions and muscle damage is impaired muscle glycogen resynthesis[15]. This may partly be due to effects on the concentration of GLUT-4 — a glucose transporter protein — in damaged muscle, which has been shown to be significantly reduced in eccentrically exercised vastus lateralis muscle after contraction of the knee extensors in humans[16]. Glycogen concentration within the muscle was also decreased at these times. Asp *et al* suggested that membrane damage due to eccentric contractions might make it difficult for the insertion of GLUT-4 into the plasma membrane which would result in defective translocation or more rapid degradation of the protein. GLUT-4 is normally translocated to the cell surface in response to insulin binding; however, damaged muscle may be less sensitive to insulin. Failure of glycogen repletion following eccentric contractions may prove a limiting factor in training and exercise performance.

Initiation of DOMS

Sarcomere overstretch

Not all contraction types are damaging. It is well established that eccentric contractions are more damaging than isometric or concentric contractions[11]. Eccentric contractions are energetically less costly than the other contraction types, which indicates that metabolic processes do not initiate the damage process. Moreover, it seems likely that eccentric contractions performed at long muscle lengths are the most damaging[7,17], supporting a mechanical rather than a metabolic initiation of the damage process.

The susceptibility of muscle to eccentric contractions may result from random inhomogeneity in sarcomere length, ie the shorter, weaker sarcomeres are stretched more than adjacent longer sarcomeres during muscle lengthening. This causes the weaker sarcomeres to move away from the peak tension and reduce force output[18]. The initiating events in muscle damage may be overextension of these weaker sarcomeres during continued eccentric contractions, resulting in instabilities within the adjacent myofibril regions and subsequent production of focal regions of overstretched sarcomeres[19]. Such lesions are commonly reported in damaged muscle[11].

Supporting evidence for sarcomere overstretch is provided by examination of the muscle length-tension relationship immediately after eccentric contractions. The optimal length for muscle contraction increases significantly in toad muscle[19] and in human muscle[19,20], suggesting an immediate increase in length of the muscle resulting from eccentric contractions — this could be attributed to overextension of sarcomeres. As the overextended sarcomeres cannot contribute to force production, they may account for part of the decrease in force production recorded immediately after eccentric contractions.

Failure of excitation-contraction coupling

The failure of excitation-contraction coupling may also play a role in reducing muscle force. Ingalls *et al* studied the effects of eccentric contractions in mice and concluded that 57–75% of the observed decline in maximal force could be accounted for by a defect in excitation-contraction coupling[21]. We know the sarcolemma is not the site of excitation-contraction coupling failure as the resting membrane potential remains unchanged after eccentric contractions of mouse muscle. Instead, the defect site is thought to be at the transverse-tubule–sarcoplasmic reticulum interface[21].

The appearance of low frequency fatigue after eccentric contractions also suggests that excitation-contraction coupling is impaired, as low frequency fatigue occurs as a result of reduced intracellular calcium concentration which, in turn, is probably a consequence of reduced calcium release. Low frequency stimulation with reduced calcium release will not induce sufficient change in myofibrillar calcium concentration to induce full contraction. The low frequency fatigue following eccentric contractions could also result from damage to contractile protein structures; this would increase compliance of the muscle at low frequencies of stimulation and reduce twitch amplitude at subtetanic frequencies[17]. However, while changes in resting muscle length or compliance may be a contributing factor to low frequency fatigue, the pattern of low frequency fatigue suggests that the main cause of exercise-induced low frequency fatigue is an impairment of excitation-contraction coupling[22].

Calcium ion overload

Initial structural injury to skeletal muscle from lengthening contractions, if severe enough, leads to a cascade of further damage. In humans, this is apparent from the delayed release of CK and other proteins, with serum CK activity reaching a maximum five or more days after an initial exercise bout[1,2,23]. Histological examination of damaged muscle indicates that more type II fibres than type I are damaged, and that type IIb fibres may be the most susceptible to damage[11].

Exercise-induced muscle damage is associated with a massive infiltration of the tissue by phagocytic cells and neutrophils, which may invade the muscle in response to release of substances from the damaged fibres. While the timecourse of infiltration of damaged muscle in rodents is relatively fast, with peak infiltration one to three days after induction of injury[5], it appears to be more delayed in humans, reaching a peak between four and seven days after eccentric exercise[8]. The extent of cellular infiltration in humans is variable between individuals, with some showing infiltration around the endomysium of affected fibres and others showing little evidence of infiltration[8].

Thus, inflammation appears to be delayed in onset and it is apparent that degenerative cellular processes are activated before inflammation within the muscle. The trigger for such autolytic damage may be an uncontrolled rise in intracellular calcium levels, either as a result of an influx of extracellular calcium via a mechanically damaged sarcolemma, or as a failure of calcium homeostasis within the cell resulting from damage to the sarcoplasmic reticulum. Indirect evidence for this is seen in the ultrastructural changes that occur within muscle after eccentric contractions, particularly the appearance of crystalline structures within the sarcoplasmic reticulum[23]. The increase in intracellular calcium is thought to:

- activate phospholipase A_2 to cause damage to the sarcolemma
- activate calpains (non-lysosomal calcium-activated proteases), which could digest myofibrillar proteins to produce cytoskeletal disruption[12].

Either or both mechanisms may be active, providing a link between the early mechanical damage induced during the bout and the later massive cellular infiltration of damaged muscle by inflammatory cells.

Role of free radicals in exercise-induced muscle damage

What are free radicals?

Free radicals are reactive molecules with an unpaired electron in their outer shell; they are implicated in a number of disease states. Oxygen-centred free radicals — called reactive oxygen species (ROS) — may be produced within the cell during oxidative phosphorylation. Although evolutionary adaptation to oxygen use has led to an effective set of antioxidant enzymes and antioxidant substances within cells to deal with such free radicals, ROS are still able to produce damaging effects within cells. The oxidative stress acts on membranes, where superoxide radical reactions with unsaturated fatty acids produce a cascade of events known as lipid peroxidation. Furthermore, free radicals can produce protein oxidation and can damage deoxyribonucleic acid within the cell, with subsequent deleterious effects on cell function.

Free radicals and muscle damage

There are many potential sources for free radicals within muscle. For example, mitochondrial oxidative phosphorylation is greatly increased during exercise, leading to a potential rise in free radical production although the mitochondrion has a well-developed antioxidant defence system. Xanthine oxidase metabolism within capillary endothelium in muscle tissue may also be a source of free radical production, in addition to the production of ROS by white blood cells attracted into muscle by muscle fibre damage. Moreover, free radicals may be produced as a result of calcium overload within the muscle fibre, since ROS generation within contracting muscle seems to be strongly influenced by the extracellular calcium concentration[24].

There is evidence, mostly indirect, that free radicals are produced within muscle during muscle damage subsequent to eccentric contractions. For example, Best *et al* recently reported a 25% increase in free radical production in rabbit tibialis anterior (measured using dichlorofluoroscin, which is oxidized by free radicals as a fluorescent probe) 24 hours after acute stretch injury[25]. An increase in antioxidant activity within the muscle was also noted, although there was no evidence of lipid peroxidation. In another study, vitamin E was shown to reduce efflux of CK from damaged rat muscle[26]. The difficulty of applying animal results to the human model is the potential role of neutrophils in producing ROS. Best *et al* reported significant polymorphonuclear cell infiltration of the damaged region 24 hours after injury. The differing timecourse of cellular infiltration in human muscle damage suggest that ROS produced by invading neutrophils may not be important 24 hours after eccentric contractions.

Studies of the role of ROS in human exercise have generally used indirect methods to examine blood or urinary markers of oxidative stress. For example, running a simulated half marathon produced a significant rise in serum malondialdehyde (a marker of lipid peroxidation immediately after exercise)[27] and downhill running produced a significant increase in thiobarbituric reactive substances (similar to but a less specific marker than malondialdehyde)[28]. However, as the source of oxidative stress during exercise could be tissues other than muscle, and the exercise regimens in these studies produced large elevations in metabolic rate during exercise, these indirect methods cannot provide conclusive evidence of ROS action in human muscle following eccentric contractions.

In contrast, the muscle biopsy technique can be used to directly measure markers of ROS activity in human muscle. There are a few disadvantages of muscle biopsy. For instance, as the procedure is of an invasive nature, repeated biopsies may not always be possible; also, muscle biopsy sites need to be distanced from each other since the biopsy itself can damage muscle tissue and affect the surrounding area. However, this technique is the only means of measuring the effects of ROS in human exercise.

A study was carried out to compare levels of markers of lipid peroxidation and protein oxidation in human muscle after eccentric and concentric muscle contractions[28]. Six volunteers, aged 21–30 years, performed one bout of eccentric muscle contraction and one bout of concentric contraction of the knee extensors of opposite legs, one week apart. Each bout consisted of 80 maximal voluntary contractions of the knee extensors performed on an isokinetic dynamometer. Muscle biopsies were performed five days before the first bout, and immediately and two days after each bout of muscle contractions. Malondialdehyde and protein carbonyl derivative levels were measured but an increase in lipid peroxidation or protein oxidation was not detected because of the action of ROS following eccentric muscle contractions (Figure 2)[29]. However, there was evidence of an increase in protein carbonyl derivatives immediately after

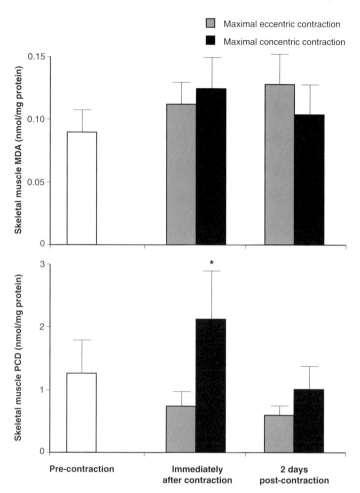

Figure 2

Results of malondialdehyde (MDA) and protein carbonyl derivatives (PCD) measurement immediately after and two days after 80 maximal eccentric and concentric muscle contractions of the knee extensors
Redrawn and reproduced with permission[29].

concentric muscle contractions, which suggested an increase in ROS generation during the concentric bout. Since concentric contractions are more metabolically demanding than eccentric contractions, these results indicate that ROS may be produced in muscle during metabolically demanding activities, but not during contractions leading to muscle damage. Thus, this human damage model did not demonstrate elevated ROS immediately after or two days after the bout.

ROS and secondary muscle damage

Initial primary damage to human muscle can be followed by more severe, secondary damage; the peak of secondary damage can occur four or more days after the initial

Table 1 *Biopsy results for muscle concentrations of markers of muscle damage and antioxidant status before and after a bout of stimulated eccentric muscle contractions*[8]

	Baseline	Day 4	Day 7
β glucuronidase (log pg phenolphthalein formed/h/g muscle wet weight)	4.94±0.04	5.17±0.06	5.42±0.11
Glucose-6-phosphate dehydrogenase (log pmol NADP+ reduced/min/g muscle wet weight)	4.72±0.15	5.07±0.06	5.36±0.19
Malondialdehyde (log pmol/g wet weight muscle)	5.07±0.15	4.72±0.06	5.36±0.19

bout, when the muscle becomes infiltrated by inflammatory cells. ROS could theoretically play a role in this process, either as a result of free radical production within the muscle fibre subsequent to calcium overload or as a result of respiratory burst release from activated neutrophils.

The possible role of ROS in secondary muscle damage was recently studied. It was hypothesized that the damage processes would result in increased lipid peroxidation and a compromised ability of the cellular antioxidant system to deal with ROS[8]. Eight untrained volunteers performed 70 maximal voluntary contractions of the knee extensors of a randomly selected leg; superimposed electrical stimulation was delivered during each contraction to maximize the force production. Biopsies were collected five days before and on the fourth and seventh days after the eccentric bout (Table 1). Substantial muscle damage was observed, including grossly elevated serum CK activity, loss of muscle contractile force and delayed muscle soreness. The extent of inflammatory action within the tissue was determined by the actions of β glucuronidase and glucose-6-phosphate dehydrogenase. Increased activities of both enzymes indicated cellular infiltration of the tissue on day seven after the eccentric contractions. However, there was no evidence of lipid peroxidation as both serum and muscle malondialdehyde levels remained unchanged. Furthermore, antioxidant capacity was enhanced seven days after the eccentric contractions, possibly reflecting the increase in inflammatory cells within the muscle tissue, since such cells have a strong antioxidant protection. The results did not provide evidence for the involvement of ROS in the human muscle damage process.

Enhanced antioxidant capacity and muscle damage

Another approach to determining the role of ROS in the muscle damage process is to enhance the antioxidant capacity of muscle by supplementation with dietary antioxidants. Studies in which vitamin E food supplements or injections were used to increase the antioxidant status of rat muscle have found no significant decrease in both initial or secondary damage determined by histological analysis and force measurement[26]. However, vitamin E may play a role in preserving membrane stability; one study revealed that vitamin E injection significantly lowered the increasing serum activity of muscle-derived enzymes[26].

ROS and fatigue

Antioxidants have been shown to influence force loss after eccentric contractions. In a study examining maximal force production in mouse muscle, treatment with a free radical scavenger (polyethylene glycol superoxide dismutase) reduced muscle force decline after eccentric contractions[30]. There is also evidence that treatment with vitamin C may reduce low frequency fatigue after eccentric contractions in humans[31]. ROS may promote low frequency fatigue by inhibiting excitation-contraction coupling at the transverse-tubule–sarcoplasmic tubule junction. This reduction in excitation-contraction coupling may be a result of ROS producing oxidation of key sulfydril groups on the excitation-contraction voltage sensors[32].

Conclusions

Although the exact mechanism by which muscle damage results from eccentric contractions is not fully understood, it is thought that initial sarcomere overstretch and subsequent calcium overload within the muscle play an important role. The relevance of ROS in generating muscle damage in humans after eccentric contractions still remains unclear. Studies on humans suggest no evidence for a major role of ROS in the damage process, although animal studies show that they are produced during the damage process. There is, as yet, no clear evidence that these free radicals are produced in sufficient quantities to overwhelm muscle antioxidant systems in human muscle.

Muscle damage is associated with a decline in the muscle ability to produce force; this may, in part, result from failure of excitation-contraction coupling. It is possible that ROS contributes to the failure of excitation-contraction coupling, and that this aspect of the muscle damage process may be influenced by dietary antioxidants. Further investigation is needed in this area.

Acknowledgements

Special thanks to Dr Steven Brown, Dr Robert Child, Mr Steven Day, Dr Helen Roper and Dr John Saxton for their immense contributions to this research.

References

1 Clarkson PM, Nosaka K, Braun B. Muscle function after exercise–induced muscle damage and rapid adaptation. *Med Sci Sports Exerc* 1992; **24**: 512–20.

2 Newham DJ, Jones DA, Clarkson PM. Repeated high force eccentric exercise: effects on muscle pain and damage. *J Appl Physiol* 1987; **63**: 1381–7.

3 MacIntyre D, Reid W, McKenzie D. Delayed muscular soreness: the inflammatory response to muscle injury and its clinical implications. *Sports Med* 1995; **20**: 24–40.

4 Brown SJ, Child RB, Donnelly AE *et al*. Changes in human skeletal muscle function following stimulated eccentric exercise. *Eur J Appl Physiol* 1996; **72**: 515–21.

5 McCully KK, Faulkner JA. Injury to skeletal muscle fibres of mice following lengthening contractions. *J Appl Physiol* 1985; **59**: 119–26.

6 Edwards RHT, Hill DK, Jones DA, Merton PA. Fatigue of long duration in human skeletal muscle after exercise. *J Physiol (Lond)* 1977; **272**: 769–78.

7 Child RB, Saxton JM, Donnelly AE. Comparison of eccentric knee extensor muscle actions at two muscle lengths on indices of damage and angle-specific force production in humans. *J Sports Sci* 1998; **16**: 301–8.

8 Child R, Brown S, Day S *et al*. Changes in indices of antioxidant status, lipid peroxidation and inflammation in human skeletal muscle after eccentric muscle actions. *Clin Sci* 1999; **96**: 105–15.

9 Apple FS, Rogers MA, Sherman WM, Ivy JL. Comparison of serum creatine kinase and creatine kinase MB activities post marathon race versus post myocardial infarction. *Clin Chim Acta* 1984; **138**: 111–8.

10 Apple FS, Rogers MA, Casal DC *et al*. Skeletal muscle creatine kniase MB alterations in women marathon runners. *Eur J Appl Physiol* 1987; **56**: 49–52.

11 Friden J, Lieber RL. Structural and mechanical basis of exercise-induced muscle injury. *Med Sci Sports Exerc* 1992; **24**: 521–30.

12 Lieber RL, Thornell L-E, Friden J. Muscle cytoskeletal disruption occurs within the first 15 minutes of cyclic eccentric contraction. *J Appl Physiol* 1996; **80**: 278–84.

13 Gleeson M, Blannin A, Zhu B *et al*. Cardiorespiratory, hormonal and haematological responses to sub maximal cycling performed 2 days after eccentric or concentric bouts. *J Sports Sci* 1995; **13**: 471–79.

14 Hikida RS, Staron RS, Hagerman FC *et al*. Muscle fibre necrosis associated with human marathon runners. *J Neurol Sci* 1983; **59**: 185–203.

15 Widrick JJ, Costill DL, McConnel GK *et al*. Time course of glycogen accumulation after eccentric exercise. *J Appl Physiol* 1992; **72**: 1999–2004.

16 Asp S, Daugaard JR, Richter EA. Eccentric exercise decreases glucose transporter GLUT 4 protein in human skeletal muscle. *J Physiol (Lond)* 1995; **482**: 705–12.

17 Jones DA, Newham DJ, Torgan C. Mechanical influences on long-lasting human muscle fatigue and delayed onset pain. *J Physiol (Lond)* 1989; **412**: 415–27.

18 Morgan DL. New insights into the behaviour of muscle during active lengthening. *Biophys J* 1990; **57**: 209–21.

19 Jones C, Allen T, Talbot J *et al*. Changes in the mechanical properties of human and amphibian muscle after eccentric exercise. *Eur J Appl Physiol* 1997; **76**: 21–31.

20 Saxton JM, Donnelly AE. Length-specific impairment of skeletal muscle contractile function after eccentric muscle actions in man. *Clin Sci* 1996; **90**: 119–25.

21 Ingalls CP, Warren GL, Williams JH *et al*. E-C coupling failure in mouse EDL muscle after in vivo eccentric contractions. *J Appl Physiol* 1998; **85**: 58–67.

22 Ratkevicius A, Skuvydas A, Lexell J. Submaximal exercise-induced impairment of human muscle to develop and maintain force at low frequencies of electrical stimulation. *Eur J Appl Physiol* 1995; **70**: 294–300.

23 Friden J, Lieber L. Ultrastructural evidence for loss of calcium homeostasis in exercised skeletal muscle. *Acta Physiol Scand* 1996; **158**: 381–2.

24 Supinski G, Nethery D, Stofan D, DiMarco A. Extracellular calcium modulates generation of reactive oxygen species by the contracting diaphragm. *J Appl Physiol* 1999; **87**: 2177–85.

25 Best TM, Fiebig R, Corr DT *et al*. Free radical activity, antioxidant enzyme and glutathione changes with muscle stretch injury in rabbits. *J Appl Physiol* 1999; **87**: 74–82.

26 Van der Meulen JH, McArdle A, Jackson MJ, Faulkner JA. Contraction induced injury to the extensor digitorum longus muscles of rats: the role of vitamin E. *J Appl Physiol* 1997; **83**: 817–23.

27 Child RB, Wilkinson DM, Fallowfield JL, Donnelly AE. Elevated serum antioxidant capacity and plasma malondialdehyde concentration in response to a simulated half-marathon run. *Med Sci Sports Exerc* 1998, **30**: 1603–7.

28 Maughan RJ, Donnelly AE, Gleeson M *et al.* Delayed-onset muscle damage and lipid peroxidation in man after a downhill run. *Muscle Nerve* 1989; **12**: 332–6.

29 Saxton JM, Donnelly AE, Roper HP. Indices of free radical mediated damage following maximum voluntary eccentric and concentric muscular work. *Eur J Appl Physiol* 1994; **68**: 189–93.

30 Zerba E, Komorowski TE, Faulkner JA. Free radical injury to skeletal muscles of young, adult and old mice. *Am J Physiol* 1990; **258**: C429–35.

31 Maxwell SRJ, Jakeman P, Thomason H *et al.* Changes in plasma antioxidant status during eccentric exercise and effects of vitamin supplementation. *Free Rad Res Comms* 1993; **19**: 191–202.

32 Posterino GS, Lamb GD. Effects of reducing agents and oxidants on excitation-contraction coupling in skeletal muscle fibres of rat and toad. *J Physiol (Lond)* 1996; **496**: 809–25.

Heat generation, accumulation and dissipation: effects on core temperature and fatigue

DR SUSAN SHIRREFFS

LECTURER IN PHYSIOLOGY, DEPARTMENT OF BIOMEDICAL SCIENCES, UNIVERSITY MEDICAL SCHOOL, FORESTERHILL, ABERDEEN, UK

Skin temperature can vary widely, depending mainly on environmental temperature. The temperature of deep tissues, however, must be maintained within a few degrees of the normal resting level (37 °C). Thus, the rate of heat gain by the body must be balanced by the rate of heat loss. When this does not happen, a change in body temperature occurs, where an increase to 41 °C or a decrease to 35 °C becomes a major cause of concern. These temperatures can be reached by marathon runners. This chapter will discuss heat generation and its effects during exercise on body temperature and fatigue.

Heat generation

Muscle mechanical work uses only about 25% of overall energy in stored or ingested fuel substrates — the remainder appears as heat. This apparent inefficiency is necessary to ensure the direction of the metabolic reactions. In homeothermic organisms, metabolic heat is important in maintaining body temperature at an appropriate level, although the resting rate of heat production is low.

There are several ways of expressing metabolic rate; in exercise studies it is usually referred to as oxygen uptake (VO_2), which may be expressed in absolute terms (l/min) or may be related to body mass (ml/kg/min). The typical human VO_2 at rest is about 4 ml/kg/min (250–300 ml/min). When considering thermal balance, however, it is more useful to express metabolic rate in terms of energy turnover, where resting metabolic rate is about 60 W.

During exercise, metabolic rate increases in proportion to the energy demand. In simple locomotor activities, such as walking, swimming, running or cycling, the energy demand is a function (linear at low speeds but exponential at higher speeds) of the rate of movement. Exercise intensity in most sporting or exercise situations is not constant but consists of intermittent activity of varying intensity and duration. In walking or running, where the body mass is moved against gravity at each step, body mass and speed determine the energy cost — air resistance becomes a factor at high speeds. The metabolic rate sustained during an event such as a marathon is determined primarily by the cardiovascular capacity and the availability of substrate. Elite athletes can sustain rates of heat production in the order of 1,200 W for about two hours, which is the average time taken to complete a marathon. To prevent a catastrophic rise in body temperature, the rate of heat loss from the body must be raised to match the increased rate of heat production. There is evidence to indicate that an individual's tolerance to a rise in body temperature as a result of exercise is not influenced by training[1], heat acclimatization[2] or exercise intensity[3].

If, for example, the heat capacity of human tissue was 3.47 kJ/°C/kg, and assuming a body mass of 65 kg, a 1,200 W rate of heat production would cause the body temperature to rise by 1 °C every three minutes; the runner would, therefore, exceed the upper limit of the tolerable core temperature within the first 10–5 minutes of the race. However, as core temperature very rarely rises above 40–1 °C, this does not happen[4]. Thus, running speed can be maintained only if the capacity for heat dissipation is high. Nielsen *et al* calculated that a marathon runner competing in a hot climate would be seriously disadvantaged. They suggested that a runner with a best time of two hours and 10 minutes (2:10:0) competing in warm conditions (35 °C, 60% relative humidity), typical of what was expected for the 1996 Olympic games in Atlanta, US, would not be able to complete the race faster than 3:20:0 due to the limited heat loss that would be possible[5]. The winner of the men's race at the 1996 Olympics finished in two hours, 12 minutes and 36 seconds (2:12:36) compared with his previous best time of 2:11:46. Thus, if there was an effect on performance it was likely to have been a very small one. This may have been due to environmental conditions not being as severe as those used by Nielsen in her equations (the actual temperature and relative humidity were 23 °C and 92% respectively), but it does indicate that the body is able to perform well even in adverse environmental conditions. Marathons held in temperatures of 20–5 °C are generally 6–10% slower than those completed in ambient temperatures of 10–2 °C[6,7].

Heat loss: conduction, convection, radiation and evaporation

Heat exchange with the environment occurs by conduction, convection and radiation. In addition, evaporation can cause heat loss from the body[8]. Conduction has little importance in marathon running when only the soles of the feet touch the ground. Convection and radiation are effective methods of heat loss when the skin temperature is high and the ambient temperature low; under these conditions, they will account for much of the heat loss even during intense exercise. Conversely, in high ambient temperature, radiant heat may be gained from the sun or road surface. However, as ambient temperature rises, the gradient from skin to environment falls and, above about 35 °C, is reversed so that heat is gained from the environment. Evaporation is the only means of heat loss in this situation. Ignoring the negligible exchange via conduction, the avenues of heat exchange can be described as follows:

$$\begin{array}{lll} \text{convective loss} & C = 8.3(T_{sk} - T_a)\sqrt{v} & W/°C/m^2 \\ \text{radiant loss} & R = 5.2(T_{sk} - T_{mrt}) & W/°C/m^2 \\ \text{evaporative loss} & E = 124(P_{sk} - P_a)\sqrt{v} & W/kPa/m^2 \end{array}$$

where:

T_{sk} = mean skin temperature (°C)

T_a = ambient temperature (°C)

T_{mrt} = mean radiant temperature (°C)

P_{sk} = mean skin water vapour pressure (kPa)

P_a = ambient water vapour pressure (kPa)

v = mean air velocity (m/s).

A high rate of evaporative heat loss is essential when the rate of metabolic heat production is high and there is little or no loss possible by other means. Although the potential for heat loss by evaporation from the skin is high, this will not be the case if the sweating rate is insufficient to wet the skin surface, or if the vapour pressure gradient between the skin and environment is low. The latter situation arises if the skin temperature is low or if the ambient water vapour pressure is high; clothing that restricts air flow will restrict water evaporation from the skin surface. A large body surface area and a high rate of air movement over the body surface also have a major impact on evaporative heat loss, but these factors will promote heat gain by convection when the ambient temperature is higher than skin temperature[8]. Smaller individuals have a high surface area relative to their body mass; they may, therefore, be at an advantage in hot conditions[9], although this depends on the relative rates of evaporative heat loss and heat gain by physical transfer.

The ability of athletes to complete events such as the marathon, even in adverse climatic conditions, with relatively little change in body temperature indicates that the thermoregulatory system is normally able to dissipate the associated heat load[10]. High rates of evaporation, therefore, require increased rates of sweat secretion onto the skin surface. This maintenance of temperature results in progressive loss of water and electrolytes in sweat.

Body temperature in the marathon: climatic influences

Hyperthermia is often thought to be the main thermoregulator concern associated with marathon running. This may be the case in marathons held in warm conditions. However, many large-scale marathons take place in cool conditions and it is evident that the core (rectal) temperature of runners can vary significantly. Maughan studied 59 runners of a marathon held in an ambient temperature of 12 °C and 75% relative humidity. Their finishing times ranged from two hours and 24 minutes (2:24) to 5:7 (the seconds were not recorded)[4], and body temperatures from 35.6 °C (in a runner who completed the race in 3:45) to 39.8 °C (in two runners who finished in 3:40 and

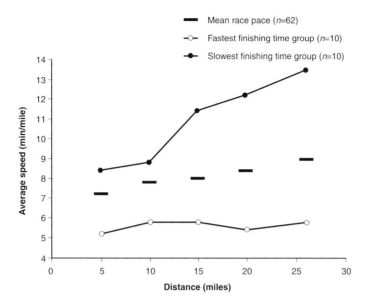

Figure 1

Relationship between running speed and distance of 62 male marathon runners

3:47). Although there was no significant relationship between the measured post-race rectal temperature and the time taken to complete the whole course, a correlation existed between the post-race rectal temperature and the time taken to cover the second half of the course — the lowest temperatures were recorded in individuals who ran most slowly over the latter part of the race. In addition, post-race rectal temperatures were <38 °C in 31% of the runners, clearly indicating that hyperthermia was not a cause for concern.

The relationship between running speed and post-race rectal temperature was investigated further in a group of 62 males competing in a marathon held at 9 °C[11]. The mean finishing time was 3:33, ranging from 2:17 to 5:11; their times to cover 5, 10, 15 and 20 miles were also recorded. The mean post-race rectal temperature was 38.7 °C, ranging from 35.6 °C to 40.3 °C. As in the previous study, there was no relationship between post-race rectal temperature and finishing time but the temperature was significantly correlated with the time taken to cover the last 6.2 miles of the race. There was a tendency for runners to reduce their running speed as the race progressed, but this did not apply to the faster runners (Figure 1). Furthermore, runners with the highest post-race rectal temperature showed slight progressive deceleration as the distance covered increased. In contrast, runners with the lowest post-race rectal temperature slowed down markedly in the closing stages of the race (Figure 2).

Hypothermia is clearly a potential situation at the end of a marathon. When runners slow down gradually throughout the race, their core temperature does not decline which can happen when runners have a rapid deceleration towards the end of the race.

113

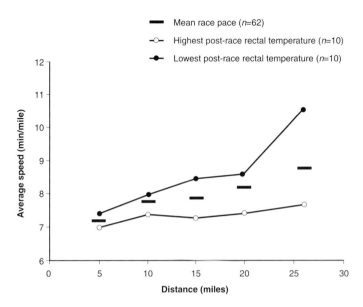

Figure 2

Relationship between post-rectal temperature and distance covered of 62 male marathon runners

Sweating: water and electrolyte losses

Evaporation of 1 l water from the skin removes about 2.4 MJ (580 kcal) heat from the body[12]. Variations in electrolyte content within the normal range of sweat composition have a small effect on the latent heat of vaporization, but this may become significant as the concentration of salt on the skin surface gradually increases as sweat evaporates. A runner with a body mass of 70 kg and who can complete the marathon in 2:30:0 would, thus, need sweat evaporated from the skin at a rate of 1.6 l/h in order to balance the rate of metabolic heat production by evaporative loss. At this high sweat rate, much of the sweat will drip from the skin without being evaporated — an approximate sweat secretion rate of 2 l/h would be needed to achieve this rate of evaporative heat loss. This is possible, but would result in the loss of 5 l body water, corresponding to a loss of >7% of body mass for a runner weighing 70 kg.

Even in cool conditions, sweat losses may be high when exercise intensity is increased or duration is long. This was determined in a marathon held on a cool (12 °C) day; the mean sweat losses of 59 male runners were estimated to be 3.5 l, with a large interindividual variability, even when the running speed was the same[4]. In warmer environments, sweat losses can be substantially greater, causing a reduction of as much as 8% in body mass during a marathon[13].

Some water will also be lost by evaporation from the respiratory tract; this contributes to heat dissipation. During hard exercise, respiratory water loss can be significant if the environment is of low humidity although it is not generally considered to be a major heat loss mechanism in man[14]. The 2–3 °C increase in body temperature that normally occurs during marathon running indicates that some of the heat produced is stored, but the effect on heat balance is minimal. For a 70 kg runner, a 3 °C rise in mean body temperature would reduce the total requirement for evaporation of sweat by <300 ml.

Sweat secreted onto the skin contains a variety of organic and inorganic solutes; significant losses of these will occur where large volumes of sweat are produced. The composition of sweat undoubtedly varies between individuals, but can also differ within the same individual depending on the rate of sweating, the level of fitness and the state of heat acclimatization[8]. In response to a standard heat stress, sweat rate increases and electrolyte content decreases with training and acclimatization. There is also a redistribution of sweating, with greater sweat rate on the limbs and relatively less on the trunk. These adaptations are thought to improve thermoregulation while conserving electrolytes, particularly sodium. An advantage of reducing sodium loss is a disproportionate loss of fluid from the intracellular space, thus helping to maintain plasma volume[15]. There are, however, some puzzling aspects; for example, where the sweat rate is sufficient to keep the skin wet, further rises in sweat rate will increase the amount of water that drips from the skin without evaporation but will not increase the rate of evaporative heat loss.

Despite the variations that occur, the main electrolytes in sweat, as in the extracellular fluid, are sodium and chloride, although their concentrations are lower than those in plasma (Table 1). As sweat is hypotonic with respect to body fluids, prolonged sweating will increase the plasma osmolality, which in turn may have a significant effect on the ability to maintain body temperature. A direct relationship between plasma osmolality and body temperature has been demonstrated during exercise[18,19]. Hyperosmolality of plasma, induced before exercise, has been shown to result in a decreased thermoregulatory effector response; the threshold for sweating is elevated and the cutaneous vasodilator response is reduced[20]. In short-term (30 minutes)

Table 1 *Concentrations (mmol/l) of the main electrolytes in sweat, plasma and intracellular water*[12,16,17]

Electrolyte	Sweat	Plasma	Intracellular water
Sodium	20–80	130–55	10
Potassium	4–8	3.2–5.5	150
Calcium	0–1	2.1–2.9	0
Magnesium	<0.2	0.7–1.5	15
Chloride	20–60	96–110	8
Bicarbonate	0–35	23–8	10
Phosphate	0.1–0.2	0.7–1.6	65
Sulphate	0.1–2.0	0.3–0.9	10

exercise, however, the cardiovascular and thermoregulatory response appears to be independent of changes in osmolality induced during the exercise period[21]. Changes in the concentration of individual electrolytes are more variable, but an increase in the plasma sodium and chloride concentrations is generally observed in response to both running and cycling exercise. Exceptions to this are rare and only occur when excessively large volumes of drinks low in electrolytes are consumed over long periods of time[22].

Differences in sweating function and in sweat composition between men and women have been reported[23], but the extent to which this apparent sex difference can be accounted for by changes in training and acclimatization status remains unclear.

Sweat loss and dehydration: effects on exercise performance

It is often reported that exercise performance is impaired when an individual is dehydrated by as little as 2% of body mass, and that >5% losses of body mass can decrease the capacity for work by about 30%[24]. Previous dehydration will impair the capacity to perform high-intensity exercise as well as endurance activities[25,26]. Nielsen *et al* showed that prolonged exercise, which resulted in a loss of fluid corresponding to 2.5% of body mass, reduced the ability to perform high-intensity exercise by 45%[25]. A fluid deficit of as little as 1.8% of body mass has recently been shown to impair exercise tolerance[27].

Fluid losses are distributed in varying proportions among the body fluid compartments, ie plasma and extracellular and intracellular water[28]. The decrease in plasma volume that accompanies dehydration may be particularly important in influencing an individual's work capacity; for example, blood flow to the muscles must be maintained at a high level to supply oxygen and substrates, but a high blood flow to the skin is also needed to convect heat to the body surface where it can be dissipated[29]. When the ambient temperature is high and blood volume has been decreased by sweat loss during prolonged exercise, it may be difficult to meet the requirement for a high blood flow to both these tissues. In this situation, skin blood flow is likely to be compromised, allowing central venous pressure and muscle blood flow to be maintained but reducing heat loss and causing body temperature to rise[30].

These factors have been investigated by Montain and Coyle and their results clearly demonstrate that increases in core temperature and heart rate during prolonged exercise are graded according to the level of hypohydration achieved[31]. They also showed that ingestion of fluid during exercise increases skin blood flow, and therefore thermoregulatory capacity, independent of raised circulating blood volume[32]. Expansion of plasma volume using dextran or saline infusion was less effective in preventing a rise in core temperature than was the ingestion of sufficient volumes of a carbohydrate electrolyte drink to maintain plasma volume at a similar level.

Other factors influencing marathon performance and fatigue

In addition to body temperature changes, either towards hyper- or hypothermia, and dehydration as a result of sweat losses, two other factors may be implicated in the fatigue of individuals during a marathon: muscle glycogen depletion and central fatigue.

Muscle glycogen depletion has been clearly established as a cause of fatigue in prolonged exercise when the exercise intensity is moderate to high. The evidence suggests that in warm environmental conditions there is increased reliance on carbohydrate as a substrate that causes enhanced carbohydrate oxidation and accelerates muscle glycogenolysis[33]. Fatigue in the heat, however, occurs before muscle glycogen levels become depleted to any great extent.

The central fatigue hypothesis proposes that fatigue is related to serotonergic activity in the brain, and that the uptake of the serotonin precursor, tryptophan, into the brain may be a key step. An increased level of serotonin in some parts of the brain can cause tiredness, and increased neuronal firing in these regions may raise sensitivity to fatigue. Measurement of blood prolactin levels has been used as an index of serotonin receptor activity and evidence is accumulating that higher levels of circulating prolactin are found when exercise is prolonged and results in an increased body heat content. It has been proposed that this is the cause of the increased feelings of tiredness and fatigue in these conditions[34], but the evidence currently available is by no means convincing.

Conclusions

The elite marathon runner can produce significant amounts of heat during the course of a marathon, but because the core temperature does not always rise to dangerously high levels, this heat must be capable of being dissipated. The effectiveness of the thermoregulatory system in these runners is demonstrated by the fact that during marathons in warm environments, exercise performance seems to be only marginally worse than performance in a cooler environment. Cool weather marathons generally pose no thermoregulatory stress on the elite runner.

The recreational marathon runner may, however, find him- or herself 'cold-stressed' in the final stages of a cool-weather marathon if fatigue causes him or her to slow rapidly in the latter stages of the race.

References

1 Sawka MN, Young AJ, Latzka WA *et al*. Human tolerance to heat strain during exercise: influence of hydration. *J Appl Physiol* 1992; **73**: 368–75.

2 Nielsen B, Hales JRS, Strange S *et al*. Human circulatory and thermoregulatory adaptation with heat acclimation in a hot dry environment. *J Physiol* 1993; **460**: 467–85.

3 Montain SJ, Sawka MN, Cadarette BS *et al*. Physiological tolerance to uncompensatable heat stress: effects of exercise intensity, protective clothing and climate. *J Appl Physiol* 1994; **77**: 216–22.

4 Maughan RJ. Thermoregulation and fluid balance in marathon competition at low ambient temperature. *Int J Sports Med* 1985; **6**: 15–9.

5 Nielsen B. Olympics in Atlanta: a fight against physics. *Med Sci Sports Exerc* 1996; **28**: 665–8.

6 Brown S. *A complete guide to running in the heat*. Hong Kong: Travel Publishing Asia, 1986: 23.

7 Frederick EC. Hot times. *Running* 1983; **9**: 51–3.

8 Leithead CS, Lind AR. *Heat stress and heat disorders*. London: Casell, 1964.

9 Dennis SC, Noakes TD. Advantages of a smaller body mass in humans when distance running in warm-humid conditions. *Eur J Appl Physiol* 1999; **79**: 280–4.

10 Sutton JR. Clinical implications of fluid imbalance. In: Gisolfi CV, Lamb DR, eds. *Perspectives in exercise science and sports medicine, vol 3. Fluid homeostasis during exercise*. Carmel, Inc: Cooper Publishing Group, 1990: 425–48.

11 Maughan RJ, Leiper JB, Thompson J. Rectal temperature after marathon running. *Br J Sports Med* 1985; **19**: 192–6.

12 Lentner C, ed. *Geigy scientific tables*. 8ᵗʰ ed. Basle: Ciba-Geigy Limited, 1981.

13 Costill DL. Sweating: its composition and effects on body fluids. *Ann N Y Acad Sci* 1977; **301**: 160–74.

14 Mitchell JW, Nadel ER, Stolwijk JAJ. Respiratory weight losses during exercise. *J Appl Physiol* 1972; **34**: 474–6.

15 Nadel ER, Mack GW, Nose H. Influence of fluid replacement beverages on body fluid homeostasis during exercise and recovery. In: Gisolfi CV, Lamb DR, eds. *Perspectives in exercise science and sports medicine. Volume 3: Fluid homeostasis during exercise*. Carmel: Benchmark, 1990: 181–205.

16 Pitts RF. *The physiological basis of diuretic therapy*. Springfield: CC Thomas, 1959.

17 Schmidt RF, Thews G, eds. *Human physiology*. 2nd edn. Berlin: Springer-Verlag, 1989.

18 Greenleaf JE, Castle BL, Card DH. Blood electrolytes and temperature regulation during exercise in man. *Acta Physiologica Polonica* 1974; **25**: 397 410.

19 Harrison MH, Edwards RJ, Fennessy PA. Intravascular volume and tonicity as factors in the regulation of body temperature. *J Appl Physiol* 1978; **44**: 69–75.

20 Fortney SM, Wenger CB, Bove JR, Nadel ER. Effect of hyperosmolality on control of blood flow and sweating. *J Appl Physiol* 1984; **57**: 1688–95.

21 Fortney SM, Vroman NB, Beckett WS *et al*. Effect of exercise hemoconcentration and hyperosmolality on exercise responses. *J Appl Physiol* 1988; **65**: 519–24.

22 Noakes TD, Goodwin N, Rayner BL *et al*. Water intoxication: a possible complication during endurance exercise. *Med Sci Sports Exerc*; **17**: 370–5.

23 Brouns F, Saris WHM, Schneider H. Rationale for upper limits of electrolyte replacement during exercise. *Int J Sports Nutr* 1992; **2**: 229–38.

24 Saltin B, Costill DL. Fluid and electrolyte balance during prolonged exercise. In: Horton ES, Terjung RL, eds. *Exercise, nutrition and metabolism*. New York: Macmillan, 1988: 150–8.

25 Nielsen B, Kubica R, Bonnesen A *et al*. Physical work capacity after dehydration and hyperthermia. *Scand J Sports Sci* 1981; **3**: 2–10.

26 Armstrong LE, Costill DL, Fink WJ. Influence of diuretic-induced dehydration on competitive running performance. *Med Sci Sports Exerc* 1985; **17**: 456–61.

27 Walsh RM, Noakes TD, Hawley JA, Dennis SC. Impaired high-intensity cycling performance time at low levels of dehydration. *Int J Sports Med* 1994; **15**: 392–8.

28 Costill DL, Cote R, Fink W. Muscle water and electrolytes following varied levels of dehydration in man. *J Appl Physiol* 1976; **40**: 6–11.

29 Nadel ER. Circulatory and thermal regulations during exercise. *Fed Proc* 1980; **39**: 1491–7.

30 Rowell LB. *Human circulation*. New York: Oxford University Press, 1986.

31 Montain SJ, Coyle EF. Influence of graded dehydration on hyperthermia and cardiovascular drift during exercise. *J Appl Physiol* 1992; **73**: 1340–50.

32 Montain SJ, Coyle EF. Fluid ingestion during exercise increases skin blood flow independent of increases in blood volume. *J Appl Physiol* 1992; **73**: 903–10.

33 Febbraio MA, Snow RJ, Hargreaves M *et al.* Muscle metabolism during exercise and heat stress in trained men: effect of acclimation. *J Appl Physiol* 1994; **76**: 589–97.

34 Pitsiladis YP, Galloway SDR, Strachan AT, Maughan RJ. Hyperprolactinaemia during prolonged exercise in the heat: evidence for a centrally mediated component of fatigue. *J Sports Sci* 1998; **16**: 479–80.

DISCUSSION

Dr Dan Tunstall Pedoe: The argument about whether or not the heart limits maximum performance intrigues me as a cardiologist. The heart tends to be blamed but pumps out what is returned to it. I have always been interested in resistance in major arteries as limiting arterial blood flow in maximum performance, through the development of turbulent blood flow[1,2] as the size varies considerably between active and inactive individuals, and active and inactive animals of the same size. Surely with training, each system adapts and is likely to be limiting at about the same point? How much of the actual limitation in maximum performance comes from the heart, and how much from other components of the cardiovascular system?

Professor Bengt Saltin: The cardiovascular system is very plastic and adaptation occurs rather quickly. You can have a doubling of the number of capillaries within four to six weeks, but then the number of capillaries will decrease when you are inactive. I do not think the resistance is in the capillary bed. I think the increase in capillaries produces a match of mean transit time within the active muscle. The resistance is in the small arteries, but I agree that even resistance in the larger vessels like the femoral artery may be limiting. When comparing the vessel size in tennis players, the dominant arm has a much larger artery. When we are looking at the diameter of the femoral artery in well trained and inactive men, there is a 95–6% correlation between the size of the femoral artery and the oxygen uptake of that leg. The femoral artery reduces from 8 to 12 mm diameter (11.8 was the highest value) so it is a 50% diameter difference between those with a high maximal oxygen uptake and those with a low. I think the resistance is a combination of smaller and possibly also the larger arteries.

Attendee: Does lactate cause muscle soreness, and how does training prevent muscle damage and delayed onset muscle soreness (DOMS)?

Dr Alan Donnelly: Muscle damage is most pronounced after eccentric contractions, which are not as metabolically demanding as concentric contractions, and is less likely to result in muscle lactate accumulation. Muscle damage is delayed, with peak damage occurring many days after exercise, long after lactate would have cleared from the muscle. There is no easy answer as to why training prevents muscle damage. There are a number of hypotheses. It might well be some form of motor control adaptation to eccentric contractions, but could also be structural alterations within muscle fibres.

Attendee: What sort of training is required in preventing DOMS?

Dr Alan Donnelly: I think the start of a training programme should be gradual in order to avoid muscle damage. Having severe muscle damage is not helpful. Eccentric exercise will only protect you against DOMS from eccentrics. It will only protect against further muscle damage; it would not necessarily improve function any other way. If you are trying to prevent muscle damage you would perform light eccentrics, not run down a hill at high velocity in order to induce as much damage as possible, and try to gradually increase the eccentric content.

Muscle damage protection is a very odd thing in that you could perform as few as 10 or 15 contractions and get perfect protection against a later bout of maybe 100 contractions. The adaptation occurs straightaway. It is unlike normal training. The explanation for it is still very unclear; although it might be some form of motor control adaptation, other explanations related to structural changes to the skeletal muscle fibres may exist.

Dr Dan Tunstall Pedoe: The most common muscle problem in a marathon is muscle cramp. Metabolic causes are unproven in runners and there is now a suggestion that it is associated with the muscle spindle gamma afferent loop and the spinal cord rather than the muscle itself[3]. Have the speakers any views on the causes of muscle cramps in runners?

Professor Eric Newsholme: There is no metabolic explanation.

Professor Bengt Saltin: It is difficult to find a metabolic or electrolyte cause, so a theory involving the muscle spindle loop is attractive. Of course you could say that micro changes in the environment of the muscle spindles could be a factor but we have not been able to study this in humans.

Dr Alan Donnelly: Antioxidant supplementation may work in two ways. First, it may prevent a free oxygen radical effect. Second, it may prevent the immune system from being able to cope with pathogens, tumours and other clinical conditions; thus, antioxidant supplementation could be bad in some ways. I think there has been a study of vitamin E supplementation in Finland, which found a negative effect of antioxidant supplementation — it increased death rates of cancer-prone individuals in the population. It would depend on the antioxidant that was being supplemented and the dosage, but very high supplementation could be counterproductive.

Mr Christopher Brasher: Should we stretch our muscles to try to prevent injuries? Should this be carried out before or after the warm up?

Dr Alan Donnelly: A recently published paper suggested that stretching is ineffective. Pre-exercise stretching in injury prevention is not really my field. Post-exercise stretching, I think, may alleviate muscle soreness to a certain extent, through a temporary analgesic effect.

Dr Dan Tunstall Pedoe: Stretching seems logical as an injury preventive before explosive events where muscles and joints are put through an extreme range of movement. It is of debatable value before relatively slow, steady pace running. After running, it is claimed to strengthen the muscle and prevent muscle shortening that classically occurs in distance runners as the muscle fibre length adapts to be most efficient for the usual range of movement at the joints, which is restricted in long-distance runners.

Professor Craig Sharp: Does eccentric contraction-induced muscle damage lead to muscle hypertrophy? Goldspink has suggested that it leads to splitting of myofibrils from z-line dislocation, forming daughter myofibrils[4]. He has provided evidence from electron microscopy.

Dr Alan Donnelly: Z-line streaming could lead towards splitting of myofibrils and production of daughter myofibrils. Whether or not the extreme muscle damage observed after eccentric exercise or marathon running would actually lead to an improvement in muscle mass and muscle cross-sectional area, is questionable.

Attendee: Some running magazines encourage people to take non-steroidal anti-inflammatory drugs to prevent muscle soreness during a marathon. Is there evidence that these are of benefit during the marathon?

Dr Dan Tunstall Pedoe: They are potentially dangerous whether or not they benefit soreness. There is an increased incidence of gastrointestinal haemorrhage in runners in endurance events, and to give something else that is well-known to cause this seems unwise.

References

1 Tunstall Pedoe DS. The velocity distribution of blood flow in major arteries of animals and man. *DPhil thesis, Oxford University* 1970.

2 Tunstall Pedoe DS. Arterial flow regimes in exercising athletes demonstrated by transcutaneous Doppler ultrasound blood velocity measurements. In: Lubich, ed. *Sports Cardiology*. Aulio Gaggi Bologna, 1978: 57–60.

3 Schwellnus MP, Derman EW, Noakes TD. Aetiology of skeletal muscle 'cramps' during exercise: a novel hypothesis. *J Sports Sci* 1997; **15**: 277–85.

4 Goldspink G. Ultrastructural changes in striated muscle fibres during contraction and growth with particular reference to the mechanism of myofibril splitting. *J Cell Sci* 1971; **9**: 123–38.

Role of haemoglobin, altitude training, and exposure to hypoxia for sea level performance in endurance events

PROFESSOR BENGT SALTIN

THE COPENHAGEN MUSCLE RESEARCH CENTRE,
RIGSHOSPITALET (UNIVERSITY HOSPITAL), COPENHAGEN, DENMARK

Since the work of Hill and Lupton and colleagues, maximal oxygen uptake (VO_{2max}) has been the preferred measure to characterize endurance athletes. Hill himself had a VO_{2max} of 4.06 l/min, much higher than what was and is observed even in regularly active people, but far from the 5–7 l/min (75–90 ml/kg/min) that international calliper endurance athletes achieve[1]. Such a high level appears to be a prerequisite for success when running a marathon. Other success criteria are running economy and the capacity to use a high percentage of the VO_{2max}. The question of what limits VO_{2max} has a history as long as its measurements. The factors discussed early last century are the same as those discussed today, ie the lungs, oxygen transport into the blood and cells of the human body, capacity of the heart as a pump, and the distribution of the cardiac output. In the early days, the oxygen-carrying capacity of blood was not clear although Hill and others observed that breathing oxygen-enriched gas mixtures also enhanced performance and in most studies caused an elevation in VO_{2max}. A direct focus on the haemoglobin (Hb) content and its saturation did not take place until the middle of the 20th century, when both total amount of Hb and Hb concentration ([Hb]) were well studied and related to exercise capacity and VO_{2max}[2] — this was followed a decade later by the first report on arterial desaturation during intense exercise. This chapter will highlight some of the important developments since this time regarding variation in red cell mass and VO_{2max}. Special emphasis will be placed on the means by which [Hb] can be varied including training or living at medium altitude or in a hypoxia house, and the mechanisms by which such preparation may cause an improved endurance performance at sea level.

[Hb] and VO_{2max}

The eye-opener for [Hb] playing a significant role for VO_{2max} was a study carried out in the 1950s in which anaemic patients were compared with healthy controls. The anaemic patients had an elevated cardiac output at light submaximal work, which compensated for the low oxygen content of the arterial blood, but peak performance and VO_{2max} were close functions of [Hb]. Later, in extensive studies of children and adults with varying [Hb], Hermansen questioned a decisive role of [Hb] for the VO_{2max}[3]. A limitation in this latter study was the large variation in other factors that are also important for an individual's exercise capacity. One example is the training status. Conclusive evidence for [Hb] affecting VO_{2max} is available from studies by Ekblom *et al* who reinfused, after four weeks, previously withdrawn red cells which elevated [Hb] from about 14.5 g to 16.0 g/100 ml. This resulted in a 5–10% increase in VO_{2max}, which has later been confirmed in similar studies and the conclusion is unambiguous[4].

[Hb] and endurance training

Several longitudinal endurance training studies were performed on healthy young subjects in the 1960s. VO_{2max} improved and the magnitude of change was largely related to the individual's pre-training VO_{2max}[5]. These or later studies do not show that training significantly altered [Hb] in healthy individuals with normal [Hb]. If a change or a trend does exist, it is towards lowering the [Hb]. This has also been

Table 1 *Summary of [Hb] and VO_{2max} data from studies of well-trained male endurance athletes of world-class performance (1960–90)*[7]

Scandinavian endurance trained athletes	[Hb] (g/100 ml)	VO_{2max} (ml kg/min)
1960–70 (*n*=23)		
Runners	14.8	78
Bicyclists	14.6	80
Cross-country skiers	14.5	83
Mean	14.7	80
Range	13.8–15.3	70–85
1970–80 (*n*=15)		
Runners	14.8	83
Cross-country skiers	14.6	80
Mean	14.7	81
Range	13.9–15.4	75–85
1980–92 (*n*=16)		
Runners	14.7	77
Cross-country skiers	14.8	84
Mean	14.8	80
Range	14.0–15.9	67–86

observed in training studies of middle-aged adults and in women, as well as in people who perform endurance training on a regular basis[6].

A further indication that training per se does not elevate [Hb] comes from cross-sectional studies of world and elite endurance athletes from the 1960s to 1980s (Table 1). A common mean value for these groups is <15 g/100 ml with an upper range of <16 g/100 ml — this pattern changed dramatically in the 1990s[7]. Videman et al recently summarized the situation within cross-country skiing[8]. Until an upper value of 18.5 g/100 ml was introduced for male skiers, individual values of as high as 20.0 g/100 ml were observed in connection with international competitions. After the upper [Hb] limit was set in 1997, the mean value has been 16.0–16.5 g/100 ml with no individual values >18.5 g/100 ml at the time of a competition. High values for [Hb] have also been reported in large cohorts of German male and female endurance athletes in the 1990s[7]. Specific reports on [Hb] in elite endurance runners are scarce. Kenyan runners covering distances from 1,500 m to the marathon have, at about 2,000 m above sea level (MASL), a group mean of 15.8 g/100 ml with only few runners having a [Hb] >16.0 g/100 ml. When competing in Europe at sea level they are in the range of 14.5–15.0 g/100 ml[7]. In running, as opposed to cycling and skiing, there is no upper allowed limit for [Hb] and, therefore, few tests.

It may be worth noting here that in well-controlled laboratory experiments, [Hb] has been elevated successfully with the use of erythropoietin (EPO). As in earlier studies where red blood cell mass and [Hb] have been increased, VO_{2max} is elevated as a function of the [Hb][9]. The elevation in VO_{2max} is of the same magnitude when the [Hb] is increased from 14.5 to 16.0 g/100 ml as it is from 17.0 to 18.5 g/100 ml. This is unexpected as the high red blood cell content could have been anticipated to hinder the flow through the capillaries due to a high viscosity as the haematocrit (Hct) is >50%. However, it appears that in exercise the beneficial effect of the high oxygen-carrying capacity compensates for possible adverse effects at the micro-circulatory level.

Living and training in hypoxic environments

Altitude

Aerobic power

The praxis of training at altitude was an important integrated part in the preparation for the 1968 Olympic games held in Mexico City, Mexico, at an approximate altitude of 2,100 MASL. Several athletes, although struggling in the games, felt they had an improved performance when they returned to sea level. One explanation for this could be that total Hb and [Hb] at altitude had increased, and with a lifetime of ≥100 days for red cells this adaptation would also remain for some time at sea level. Many investigations on this topic are being carried out, most of which demonstrate no trends for

Table 2   *Sea level VO$_{2max}$ (ml/kg/min) after living/training at moderate altitude*[10]

	Duration (weeks)	Altitude MASL	Pre-training	1–5	Post-training 6–13	20–30
Runners (n=14)	2	2,100	74	73	74	—
		Control: 0	68	69	69	—
Cross-country skiers (n=7)	4	(0)–2,700 no control group	76 —	76 —	77 —	79 —
Cross-country skiers (n=11)	2	1,600–1,800	80	81	—	—
		Control: 0	80	83	—	—
Runners (n=16)	4	1,800–2,000	73	74	—	—
		Control: 0	72	73	—	—

an alteration in VO$_{2max}$ after an altitude stay combined with training (Table 2)[10]. Although [Hb] is increased during the stay at altitude, a common finding is that it does not remain elevated on return to sea level[11]. Several explanations have been offered for [Hb] being unaltered post- versus pre-altitude. For example, an individual must be present at altitude for three to four weeks or longer for total Hb to be increased. It is true that [Hb] is also increased within a few days at medium altitude. This is, however, due to haemoconcentration as a result of an elevated diuresis and lowering of total and plasma water (Figure 1). At medium altitude, the rate of increase in total Hb is in the order of 20 g/week provided iron is in sufficient supply. Another and more important explanation for [Hb] being normal soon after (ie <1–3 days) return to sea level following an altitude sojourn is that the plasma volume quickly expands under normobaric conditions. Svedenhag *et al* demonstrated in cross-country skiers who had lived and trained at 2,100–2,700 MASL for four weeks that post-altitude plasma volume at sea level expanded by about 0.4–0.5 l within 48–72 hours, lowering the [Hb] and Hct levels to pre-altitude levels within a few days (Figure 2)[11]. The normalized [Hb] and Hct with expanded blood volume will improve filling conditions of the heart and lead to an enlarged stroke volume, cardiac output, and peak oxygen delivery during exhaustive exercise — this will improve performance.

An argument for altitude training being unsuccessful when performing at sea level is that training intensity and sometimes training duration are reduced in hypoxia. It has, therefore, been suggested that it is not the training at altitude that is important but the arterial hypoxia or desaturation per se that causes an elevation in red cell mass. Levine and Stray-Gundersen have carried out most research to test this hypothesis. The design consists of various combinations of living 'high' (2,500–3,000 MASL) and training 'low' (about 1,200 MASL), and vice versa. Their results have recently been summarized in a mini-review[12]. Average runners who performed standardized training

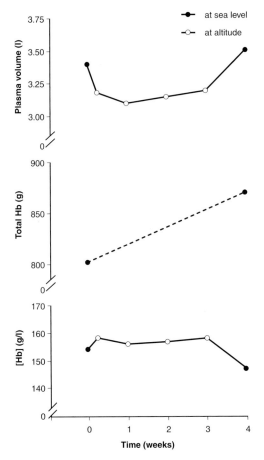

Figure 1

Plasma volume, total amount of Hb (CO-method) and [Hb] in Olympic level athletes at sea level and at altitude

Redrawn and reproduced with permission[10].

at sea level during a month are studied first and then again at sea level after they have trained for another month either at low (about 1,200 MASL) or high (about 2,700 MASL) altitude combined with living either low or high. These four alternatives produced no or a small gain in VO_{2max}, with those living high and training low obtaining an increase of 1.5 ml/kg/min, reaching a value in the upper 60s. Equally important is the fact that these runners could also perform at a higher steady state VO_{2max}. According to results by Gore *et al*, most well-trained athletes desaturate when active at 1,200 MASL[13]. Thus, the runners in the 'high-low' groups in Levine and Stray-Gundersen's studies experienced desaturation both when living at altitude and when training 'low'.

Early studies evaluating the 'high-low' concept did not include top-level athletes, although one later study did[14]. In this study, runners were brought to and lived at

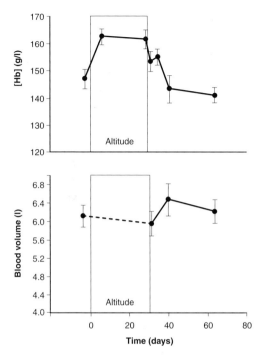

Figure 2

Blood volume (tagged albumin) and [Hb] in seven elite cross-country skiers before, during and after a stay at 2,100 MASL and with training at 2,700 MASL

Redrawn and reproduced with permission[11].

altitude, and trained with low intensity at 2,500–2,800 MASL and at high intensity at a lower altitude (about 1,200 MASL). These athletes improved their VO_{2max} by about 1–3% to 74.4 ml/kg/min and a 1.5% improvement in performance (3,000 m time trial) was recorded. This would have made some of these national calliper runners competitive on the international arena. These US-based studies appear to have no flaws. However, the results have not been confirmed by others. Gore *et al*, who in Australia have access to well-trained endurance athletes, have performed studies with a design similar to that used by Levine and Stray-Gundersen[15]. They did not observe an elevation in aerobic power of living high and training low as compared to other alternatives of combining living and training at sea level or at altitude. In the US studies there are non-responders, ie some do not improve although they live high and train low as reported by the US group. The proposed explanation is that there is an elevation in the red cell mass in responders but not in non-responders which, in turn, relates to less EPO increase in this group, although there is a difference between these groups in red cell mass. However, [Hb] is the same in responders and non-responders. This would indicate that elevations in blood volume and total amount of Hb, although small, significantly affect aerobic power. Svedenhag *et al* also observed a similar expansion of the blood volume of 0.4–0.5 l (and total Hb) post-altitude in top endurance athletes with a VO_{2max} >76 ml/kg/min; however, a significant elevation in VO_{2max} was not observed in their study. Four of the seven cross-country skiers had a post-altitude VO_{2max} higher than the error of method when measuring VO_{2max}. There was also a trend at the individual level for coupling between the magnitude of change in total blood volume and VO_{2max}. This leads to the question whether or not an increased plasma volume enlarges VO_{2max}. Kanstrup and Ekblom infused 700 ml dextran and observed an elevated stroke volume and cardiac output at peak exercise, but this was not large enough to counteract the lowering of the oxygen-carrying capacity[16]. This resulted in an unchanged systemic oxygen delivery and VO_{2max}. Later studies using only 300 ml infusion of a plasma expander have demonstrated an approximate 5% elevation in VO_{2max}[17]. A plasma volume expansion of up to 0.5 l on return to sea level after training/staying at medium altitude would be in the range of what may be beneficial for the oxygen delivery and VO_{2max}.

Another observation that deserves comment is that, in some studies, VO_{2max} remains or becomes elevated several weeks after an altitude-training period. In Svedenhag's study, VO_{2max} was 2.6 ml/kg/min in athletes who already had a mean value of 76 ml/kg/min. At this time, both [Hb] and blood volume are at pre-altitude levels. It is difficult to offer a physiological explanation for the causative mechanisms other than that more effective training can be performed on returning to sea level, especially in regard to its intensity.

Anaerobic power

Muscle glycogen storage is insensitive to hypoxia[10] and the V_{max} for enzymes such as muscle phosphorylase (a+b) and phosphofructokinase (PKF) is unaltered. Factors controlling the activity of these enzymes such as catecholamines (conversion of phosphorylase a-b), cytosolic adenosine diphosphate (ADP) and ADP/adenosine triphosphate (ATP) ratios (PFK activation) are most likely enhanced by exercise at altitude, increasing the rate by which anaerobic energy is released and lactate formed. Glucose uptake by muscle is also stimulated by hypoxia, but this has to be quite severe. The lactate dehydrogenase (LDH) activity in skeletal muscle behaves 'strangely' at altitude. As acute exposure to hypoxia accelerates glycogenolysis, it could be anticipated that the V_{max} for LDH would be elevated, primarily due to an increase in the activity of the LDH_{4-5} isoform. This does not happen. Instead LDH_{4-5} activity is significantly reduced and LDH_{1-2} is unchanged, resulting in a higher LDH_{1-2}/LDH_{4-5} ratio when staying at medium altitude. This adaptation is quite fast since it is observed after two weeks at 2,100 MASL and is not markedly higher when staying for four weeks. The change in LDH ratio does not appear to affect the peak blood lactate response at altitude. However, it cannot be excluded that lactate turnover is increased which could be of functional importance during submaximal exercise also on return to sea level[18]. It is the general belief that lactate production is minimal in prolonged exercise with a rather constant blood lactate concentration of 2.5 mmol/l and, thus, the subsequent turnover is quite small. This is not the case. Active leg muscles constantly produce and take up lactate. It is therefore a function of the muscles to consume blood lactate and maintain a stable and low lactate concentration[18]. The ability of the leg muscles in running to continuously produce and consume lactate at a speed using 85–90% VO_{2max} may be just as important for performance as high VO_{2max} and good running economy.

Muscle buffer capacity increases at altitude which could contribute to a larger anaerobic capacity[19,20]. The change is observed as early as after two weeks and appears to be maintained at sea level for up to two weeks. Data are not available for athletes after longer stays at altitude, but findings on mountaineers' arm and leg muscles indicate that muscle buffer capacity is increased after several months at altitude, but only to a slightly larger extent than at lower altitudes and of shorter duration. In the study by Svedenhag *et al*, control groups were included who trained similarly at sea level as those at altitude without any alteration in either LDH isoenzymes or muscle buffer capacity. This finding, as well as that for the climbers, could indicate that altitude (hypoxia) induces the changes. There also appears to be a coupling between the change in anaerobic exercise capacity and running performance. Mizuno and coworkers[19] carried out this test on cross-country skiers and found a relation between improved running time and change in muscle buffer capacity. An estimation of maximal oxygen deficit also revealed a coupling to performance. No changes were observed in muscle features in the US studies, and it was concluded that improved lactate metabolism or anaerobic exercise capacity are not at play to explain these runners' improved performances[12]. In contrast, Gore *et al*, being unable to confirm the US studies in regard to aerobic power, observed that the anaerobic exercise capacity was improved[20]. Together, several variables of significance for the anaerobic capacity appear to be increased as a result of exposure to hypoxia.

Other skeletal muscle adaptations

In addition to changes observed in some variables related to the anaerobic capacity, other features of muscle tissue that are important for peak as well as endurance

Table 3 *Mean muscle fibre sizes (μm^2 10^3) and mean capillary number per fibre ratio (vastus lateralis muscle) in groups of sea level residents before and after staying at various altitudes for different periods of time*[10]

Study	Altitude (MASL)	Physical duration (weeks)	Mean activity level at altitude	Fibre size Before	After	Capillary/fibre Before	After
A	c3,700	24	low	4.8	4.2*	1.3	1.2
B	c2,100–2700	2	very high	5.8	5.4*	2.6	2.7
C	c2,100	4	very high	5.9	5.5*	2.8	2.7
D	c2,100	2	very high	4.9	4.8	2.7	2.7

* significant

performance could be anticipated to occur[10]. Muscle fibre size and capillarization have been studied extensively, both in athletes and in climbers. There is a striking similarity in the findings. The number of capillaries per muscle fibre is unaltered by exposure to any altitude (Table 3). In contrast, muscle fibre size is reduced while at altitude. Hypotrophy is quite pronounced at extreme altitudes, but also present during a prolonged stay at a moderate altitude such as 2,000 MASL. With a reduction in muscle fibre size and an unaltered capillary per fibre ratio, there is an increase in number of capillaries/ mm^2 and the average diffusion area for a capillary is reduced using the Krogh model for estimation. The functional significance of these changes is in addition to the reduced diffusion distance that the mean transit time is lengthened at a given muscle blood flow, provided the capillary length is unaltered. These adaptations are important to optimize oxygen extraction at altitude when oxygen tension in the blood is low, but would enhance oxygen delivery to the muscle tissue also at sea level as long as muscle fibre sizes are subnormal. The return to normal muscle fibre size on return to sea level after a period at altitude has not been studied, but it is likely to be slow as muscle hypertrophy even with optimal strength training takes weeks to months.

Muscle mitochondrial capacity is fairly stable at altitude[10]. This is the result of studies using morphometric methods to estimate mitochondrial volume as well as using biochemical assays to determine V_{max} for mitochondrial enzymes in the respiratory chain, the β-oxidation or Krebs cycle. There is a consensus on this topic. In contrast, a small but significant elevation in mitochondrial enzyme activities has been reported in subjects training at simulated altitude or with insufficient blood supply. The study design includes training one leg while using the other as a control, or the inclusion of a control group, and training at equivalent exercise intensities at sea level. It was not possible until recently to explain the contrasting findings. Submaximal training loads were used in these latter studies. Based on srEMG amplitude measurements it was shown that muscle activation was more marked when oxygen availability was reduced. A greater number of fast twitch fibres were also recruited as demonstrated by the muscle glycogen depletion pattern. Thus, the enhancement of V_{max} for certain mitochondrial enzymes occurred in the fast twitch fibres. The data also confirm that training induced elevations can be obtained in mitochondrial capacity when training with a subnormoxic amount of oxygen made available to the active muscle. However, the data do not demonstrate that hypoxia is an additional stimulus to the ordinary training stimulus, although it appears to modulate motor unit recruitment.

Finally, what about skeletal muscle contractile characteristics or muscle fibre transformation when exposed to hypoxia? This topic is well explored and the myosin isoforms do not appear to be sensitive to hypoxia[10]. This is based on histochemical staining of myosin ATPase of samples obtained on athletes or climbers in connection with short or even long stays at various altitudes. Taken together, there are no indications that altitude exposure or training at medium altitude alters the oxidative capacity of the muscles.

Hypoxia house

The literature on altitude training does not provide a basis for a consensus statement — it is even harder to conclude when we consider the use of hypoxia houses in preparation for sea level performance. The literature is scarce, although hypoxia houses have been used for almost 10 years and quite extensively in some countries. Hahn, Gore and colleagues recently summarized their own studies and those of other researchers and compared the effect of living in hypoxia houses with that of a combination of genuine altitude stay, together with training low[21]. These studies primarily focus on whether or not living part (about 10 hours) of a full day at the equivalent of about 1,800–2,000 MASL is sufficient to elicit an EPO response followed by an elevation in reticulocytes and red cell mass. EPO is increased by 70–80%, whereas the latter two variables are not increased. Although the desaturation is small at this level of hypoxia, it is obviously of a magnitude large enough to enhance EPO production by and release from the kidneys. Why it does not result in a stimulation of red cell mass is not clear. It is important to note that the elevation in EPO is transient and not long-lasting as was first anticipated with intermittent hypoxia exposure. The present development in the use of hypoxia houses is to expose the athletes to the equivalent of 3,000 or even 4,000 MASL for brief periods of time during the day. As of yet, data are only available from acute exposure. They indicate a pronounced effect causing haemoconcentration and an EPO response[22]. Exercise performed during the hypoxia exposure does not augment this effect.

Conclusions

Endurance performance is enhanced in endurance athletes living at medium altitude, in a hypoxia house combined with training at medium or low-to-medium altitude, and especially when training is intense. The mechanisms by which this occurs are under debate. One possibility is that red blood cell mass is elevated due to an enlarged blood volume, as is VO_{2max} with no change in [Hb]. Another proposal is that anaerobic power is improved, primarily related to a larger muscle tissue buffer capacity. The improved prolonged exercise capacity could also be related to an enhanced muscle lactate consuming capacity as there is an altered LDH isoform pattern when exposed to hypoxia.

References

1 Saltin B. The physiological and biochemical basis of aerobic and anaerobic capacities in man; effect of training and range of adaptation. In: Maehlum S, Nilsson S, Renström P, eds. *An update on sports medicine*. Oslo: Astra-Syntex; 1987, 16-59.

2 Åstrand P-O. *Experimental studies of physical working capacity in relation to sex and age*. Copenhagen: Munksgaard, 1952.

3 Hermansen L. Oxygen transport during exercise in human subjects. *Acta Physiol Scand* 1973; (suppl 399): 1973.

4 Ekblom B, Goldbarg AN, Gullbring B. Response to exercise after blood loss and reinfusion. *J Appl Physiol* 1972; **33**: 175–80.

5 Saltin B, Blomqvist G, Mitchell JH *et al*. Response to exercise after bed rest and after training. A longitudinal study of adaptive changes in oxygen transport and body composition. American Heart Association. Monograph no 23. *Circulation* 1968; **37, 38**(suppl 5): VII1–78.

6 Saltin B. The ageing endurance athlete. In: Sutton JS, Brock RM, eds. *Sports medicine for the mature athlete*. Indianapolis: Benchmark Press, 1986: 59-80.

7 Doping I Danmark. En Hvidbog med bilag. The Danish Ministry of Culture, ISBN 87-90801-64–4, 1999 (to be found also at www.kum.dk).

8 Videman T, Lereim I, Hemmingsson P *et al*. Changes in hemoglobin values in elite cross-country skiers from 1987–1999. *Scand J Med Sci Sports* 2000; **10**: 98–102.

9 Berglund B, Ekblom B. Effect of recombinant human erythropoietin treatment on blood pressure and some haematological parameters in healthy men. *J Intern Med* 1991; **229**: 125–30.

10 Saltin B. Exercise and the environment: focus on altitude. *Res Quarterly Exerc Sport* 1996; **67**: 1–10.

11 Svedenhag J, Piehl-Aulin K, Skog C, Saltin B. Increased left ventricular muscle mass after long-term altitude training in athletes. *Acta Physiol Scand* 1997; **161**: 63–70.

12 Stray-Gundersen J, Levine B. 'Living high and training low' can improve sea level performance in endurance athletes. *Br J Sports Med* 1999; **33**: 150–1.

13 Gore CJ, Hahn AG, Scroop GC *et al*. Increased arterial desaturation in trained cyclists during maximal exercise at 580 m altitude. *J Appl Physiol* 1996; **80**: 2204–10.

14 Chapman RF, Stray-Gundersen J, Levine BJ. Individual variation in response to altitude training. *J Appl Physiol* 1998; **85**: 1448–56.

15 Hahn AG, Gore CJ. The effect of altitude on cycling performance: a challenge to traditional concepts. *Sports Med* 2000; in press.

16 Kanstrup IL, Ekblom B. Acute hypervolemia, cardiac performance and aerobic power during exercise. *J Appl Physiol* 1982; **52**: 1186–91.

17 Warren GL, Cureton KJ. Modelling the effect of alterations in hemoglobin concentration on Vo_2max. *Med Sci Sports Exerc* 1989; **21**: 526–31.

18 Hall Gv. Lactate as a fuel for mitochondrial respiration. *Acta Physiol Scand* 2000; **168**: 643–56.

19 Mizuno M, Juel C, Bro-Rasmussen T *et al*. Limb skeletal muscle adaptation in athletes after training at altitude. *J Appl Physiol* 1990; **68**: 496-502.

20 Gore CJ, Hahn AG, Aughey RJ *et al*. *Live high: train low changes muscle buffering capacity*. Int Council of Sport Science and Physical Education 2000 Pre-Olympic Congress, Book of Abstracts, 2000: 64.

21 Hahn AG, Gore CJ, Cartin DT *et al*. An evaluation of the concept of living at moderate altitude and training at sea level. *Comp Biochem Physiol* 2001; in press.

22 Rodríguez FA, Casas H, Casas M et al. Intermittent hypobaric hypoxia stimulates erythropoiesis and improves aerobic capacity. *Med Sci Sports Exerc* 1999; **31**: 264–8.

Diets to combat fatigue

PROFESSOR CLYDE WILLIAMS

PROFESSOR OF SPORTS SCIENCE, DEPARTMENT OF PHYSICAL EDUCATION, SPORTS SCIENCE & RECREATION MANAGEMENT, LOUGHBOROUGH UNIVERSITY, LEICESTERSHIRE, UK

One of the most frequently asked questions in sports nutrition is, 'What can I eat before the competition in order to improve my performance?'. The answer to this question has been the focus of an increasing amount of research over the past decade and has been reported at international consensus conferences[1–5]. From these studies it is clear that the endurance athlete in general and the marathon runner in particular are faced with the dual problems of eating sufficiently well to cover their daily energy expenditures but in doing so they have to avoid unnecessary weight gain. Low body fat is clearly an advantage to endurance runners, so it is not surprising that they are among the leanest of all athletes[6]. Low body fat in female runners, however, is associated with disturbances in their menstrual cycle[7]. Female endurance runners may regard an absence of regular menses as an advantage. However, long-term amenorrhoea carries with it the risk of decreased bone health that may eventually manifest itself in the occurrence of 'stress fractures'. The female endurance athlete must, therefore, try to maintain an adequate diet and a body mass that is optimum for both health and participation in sport.

Heavy and prolonged training and competition throughout the year is a real challenge to the immune system of endurance athletes, especially if their diet is insufficient to meet their needs for energy and essential nutrients (see Dr Pedersen's chapter)[8]. Thus, the need to achieve long-term energy balance should not be overlooked[9]. There are always 'new diets' that promise to decrease body mass and increase performance without detriment to long-term health that rely almost entirely on anecdotal evidence, rather than on evidence from controlled trials, for support. For example the Zone Diet recommends a daily energy intake of 40% carbohydrate, 30% protein and 30% fat. If the overall daily energy intake is maintained and protein intake is increased to meet the recommendations then the amount of carbohydrate consumed must decrease[10]. Thus, it would be interesting to know how athletes on this diet can train hard and recover quickly with a reduced carbohydrate intake. There is little published information in the scientific literature on the efficacy of this and other such diets[10]. The evidence-based dietary recommendation is that athletes should eat a high carbohydrate diet, composed of a wide range of foods that is of sufficient quantity to cover their daily energy expenditure[1]. Endurance athletes should pay particular attention to the carbohydrate content of their diets because of the link between carbohydrate depletion and the early onset of fatigue[11]. This chapter will summarize the reasons for this recommendation. It should be noted that most of the evidence underpinning the dietary advice for athletes is based on studies in which the subjects were men. There is evidence that female endurance athletes use less carbohydrate, spare more protein and oxidize more fat than men[12].

Energy demands of prolonged exercise

At present it is not possible to obtain routine comprehensive descriptions of the physiological responses of runners to the demands of endurance exercise during competitions. Laboratory studies on endurance exercise, therefore, continue to provide insight into the challenges faced by athletes in long-distance races[13]. In one such study, an experienced veteran marathon runner completed a simulated marathon race on a laboratory treadmill which was instrumented so that he controlled his speed using a lightweight hand-held switch. The chosen speed, distance and time elapse were shown on a computer screen in front of the treadmill. The athlete's aim was to match his best road running performance on the treadmill by selecting his own speed throughout the 42.2 km simulated race. He completed the marathon in two hours and 45 minutes, five minutes longer than his best time for the season. His overall energy expenditure was 8.9 MJ (2,120 kcal) which represented about two-thirds of his daily energy intake. Although he had free access to water, cold sponges and a towel, he drank only 92 ml water during the race and lost 1.9 kg that was equivalent to 3.5% of his pre-run 54.2 kg body mass. Surprising as it seems, it is not uncommon for runners to drink small amounts during long runs, even when water is freely available[14]. Running at an average exercise intensity of 79% maximal oxygen uptake (VO_{2max}), his total oxygen consumption was 436 l and ventilation was 12,000 l standard temperature pressure-dry (STPD). His running pace is similar to the exercise intensities of elite runners competing in long-distance races[15-7] and his physiological responses illustrate the severe demands of marathon racing.

Analysis of the results from indirect calorimetry clearly demonstrated that the contribution of fat to energy metabolism became greater than that of carbohydrate only during the latter part of the race, when he reduced his running speed (Figure 1). The relative contributions of fat and carbohydrate to energy metabolism were first described in studies using indirect calorimetry[18] and more recently using stable isotopes as metabolic tracers[19,20]. These techniques confirm that the fall in respiratory exchange ratio during prolonged submaximal exercise reflect the shift towards greater fat metabolism[21]. However, in this particular example of marathon running, it was only after the runner reduced his speed that the rate of fat oxidation exceeded that of carbohydrate. The reduction in running speed was most probably a consequence of a severe decrease in the runner's muscle glycogen stores[22]. In the absence of sufficient muscle glycogen, the rate of adenosine triphosphate (ATP) production in contracting muscle fibres cannot match the rate of ATP use, thus preventing these motor units from continuing to contribute to locomotion. When this occurs in a large number of motor units, the selected exercise intensity cannot be sustained and the runner slows down.

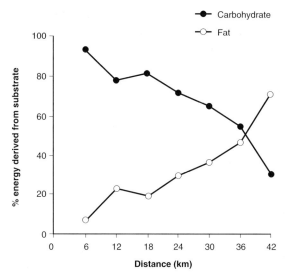

Figure 1

Relative contributions of fat and carbohydrate to energy production during the completion of a simulated marathon race on a laboratory treadmill (finishing time two hours and 40 minutes)

Carbohydrate nutrition and performance

Early studies on energy metabolism during prolonged cycling identified the severe reduction in muscle glycogen stores as the main cause of fatigue[23,24]. It is, therefore, not surprising that methods of increasing the glycogen stores before prolonged exercise have been pursued[25,26]. A rise in carbohydrate intake during the three to four days before prolonged heavy cycling exercise increases muscle and liver glycogen stores and improves endurance capacity[24,27]. Similarly, high carbohydrate diets lead to an increase in muscle glycogen following prolonged running[28–33].

Although the early studies on the benefits of carbohydrate loading used cycling rather than running, the methods were adopted by almost all endurance athletes in preparation for competition, irrespective of sport. The obvious question that follows is whether or not carbohydrate loading improves running performance. In order to try to answer this question it is helpful to consider the available evidence under two headings:

- the influence of carbohydrate loading on endurance running capacity — these studies assess performance as the time to exhaustion during constant pace running
- the studies in which performance is assessed as the time taken to complete a fixed distance.

Endurance running capacity

Using the original method of carbohydrate loading, Goforth *et al* reported a 9% improvement in endurance running capacity when their subjects ran on a treadmill at

80% VO_{2max} to exhaustion[29]. Both simple and complex carbohydrates are effective in increasing muscle glycogen stores in preparation for prolonged heavy exercise[34]. For example, Brewer et al showed that rice, pasta and confectionery products were equally effective in improving endurance running capacity when used for carbohydrate loading[30]. In this study, 15 men and 15 women completed a run to exhaustion on a level treadmill at 70% VO_{2max} after an overnight fast. The subjects were then divided into three groups and consumed their normal diets supplemented with either additional fat and protein, additional carbohydrate in the form of extra potatoes, rice and pasta, or additional carbohydrate in the form of confectionery products. These isocaloric diets were consumed over a 72-hour period after which the runners performed a second run to exhaustion. There was no improvement in running time for the group who ate the high protein diet but the runners on the two carbohydrate diets improved their endurance capacity by approximately 20%.

Madsen and colleagues also showed that glycogen supercompensation occurs in runners who adopted the strategy of reducing their training volume and increasing their carbohydrate intake during the week before treadmill running to exhaustion[33]. Although the three men and three women ran seven minutes longer after the high carbohydrate diet, the difference did not reach statistical significance. Furthermore, they ended their run with relatively well stocked glycogen stores, having used similar amounts of glycogen. There was no evidence to suggest that high rates of lactate accumulation contributed to the onset of fatigue even though the relative exercise intensity was between 75% and 80% VO_{2max}.

Using a similar diet and tapered training preparation as described by Sherman et al[26], Pizza and colleagues investigated the influence of carbohydrate loading on running performance at an intensity equivalent to VO_{2max}. In this study, the runners tapered their training during the week leading up to the endurance capacity test and increased their carbohydrate intake from 4.2 to 8.2 g carbohydrate/kg body weight/day for the last three days. On the morning of the test they arrived in the laboratory, after an overnight fast, and completed a 15-minute treadmill run at 75% VO_{2max}; this was followed by a run to exhaustion at an average speed of 15.5 km/h up a gradient of 3.3%. Run time was 303.9 s and 280.5 s for the carbohydrate group and mixed diet group respectively. The 23.4 s difference was reported to be statistically significant[35].

Endurance running performance

Carbohydrate loading, using the original diet and exercise method[25], improved performance of runners competing in a 30 km race by eight minutes compared with their performance after a mixed diet[28]. Post-race biopsy samples taken from the vastus lateralis muscles of the male runners, who ate a mixed diet before the race, had glycogen concentrations as low as those values reported after cycling to exhaustion[28]. Following carbohydrate loading, their pre-race muscle glycogen concentrations increased, demonstrating that a high carbohydrate diet following running to exhaustion leads to glycogen supercompensation. Furthermore, even though they completed the 30 km distance at a faster rate after the high carbohydrate diet, they had higher muscle glycogen concentrations at the end of the race than before the race when they were eating a mixed diet. Clearly, the high carbohydrate pre-race diet provided more than enough glycogen to cover the increased running speed.

In other studies that have not confirmed the benefit of increasing pre-exercise muscle glycogen concentrations, the distance over which the subjects ran may not have been long enough to fully challenge their carbohydrate stores. For example, Sherman and colleagues reported the results of three trials in which, after dietary preparation, six well trained male runners raced a distance of 20.9 km on an indoor 200 m track[26]. In two of the trials, subjects increased their pre-exercise muscle glycogen concentrations by tapering their training and increasing their carbohydrate intake for three days before the race, whereas the third trial was run without carbohydrate loading. There was no difference in the performance times (83 minutes) for the three races, even though more glycogen was available and used during the races following the carbohydrate loading.

Maughan *et al* studied the influence of carbohydrate loading on 10-km treadmill running performances[36]. Six runners prepared for two simulated treadmill races by eating a diet with a carbohydrate content equivalent to 40% of daily energy intake for the week before the first test. For the other occasion, two weeks later, the runners ate a diet containing 55% of daily energy from carbohydrate for four days and then increased their carbohydrate intake to 70% for the last three days before the simulated race. The high carbohydrate diet provided 482 g/day (6.8 g/kg body mass) for four days and 613 g/day (8.6 g/kg body mass) for the last three days before the treadmill 10 km race. On the low carbohydrate diet the runners consumed 350 g/day (4.9 g/kg body mass) for the seven days before the simulated race. The high and low carbohydrate diets were isocaloric with each other and with the runners' habitual diets. There was no difference between the performance times achieved after the high carbohydrate(48.8 minutes) and low carbohydrate (48.6 minutes) diets. The diet described as low carbohydrate provided almost 5 g/kg body mass and so was not low in carbohydrate. The authors point out that the availability of carbohydrate was probably not a limiting factor during the race because there was no difference in running times even though less carbohydrate was oxidized on the low carbohydrate diet[36].

Diet and training

Eating a high-carbohydrate diet throughout training improves endurance capacity to a greater extent than training on a high-fat diet. Helge and colleagues studied the responses to training of 20 untrained men who were allocated equally to either a high-carbohydrate or high-fat diet for seven weeks. Before training began, the subjects' VO_{2max} and endurance cycling capacities were assessed. They were required to cycle to volitional fatigue at approximately 81% VO_{2max}, and then trained three to four times a week for the subsequent seven weeks. Training loads were increased appropriately as endurance fitness of the subjects improved. The high-carbohydrate and high-fat diets contained 65% and 62% daily energy from carbohydrate and fat foods respectively. At the end of the seven-week training, the endurance cycling capacities of the subjects were assessed at the same absolute exercise intensity as that used at the beginning of training[37].

After seven weeks of training, VO_{2max} values of both groups increased by approximately 11%. The endurance cycling capacity increased from 35 to 102 minutes in the carbohydrate diet group and from 35 to 65 minutes in the high-fat group. At the end of the seventh week of training the subjects on the fat diet switched to the high-carbohydrate diet for one week to assess whether or not the greater endurance capacity of the latter diet group was simply the result of the recent intake of carbohydrate. At the end of the eighth week of training both groups again completed an endurance test to exhaustion. The high-fat diet group increased its endurance time, after a week on the high-carbohydrate diet, from 65 to 77 minutes whereas the high-carbohydrate diet group had no further improvement in its performance.

At the end of the seven weeks of training, the muscle glycogen concentration of the high-carbohydrate and high-fat diet groups was 611 and 511 mmol/kg dw respectively. However, after a further week on a high-carbohydrate diet, the carbohydrate group had no further increase in muscle glycogen concentration (561 mmol/kg dw). In contrast the muscle glycogen concentration of the high-fat diet group increased by 44% (from 511 to 738 mmol/kg dw). However, the cycling time to exhaustion was 25 minutes longer for the carbohydrate group than the high-fat diet group. Furthermore, there was a similar amount of glycogen used during the prolonged cycling test. Thus, neither inadequate glycogen stores nor low blood glucose was responsible for the earlier onset of fatigue in subjects on the high-fat diet. The authors suggest that changes in calcium availability in the active muscle sarcoplasm of the fat-diet group may have contributed to the earlier onset of fatigue — the high-fat diet may have caused changes in the phospholipid composition of the muscle membranes, referred to as the 'leaky membrane hypothesis[38]. If this phenomenon also occurs within the sarcoplasmic reticulum then it could have had a profound influence on calcium release and sequestration. This, in turn, would influence muscle fibre recruitment and contribute to the onset of fatigue.

Helge and colleagues repeated their training and diet study and recorded the responses of two groups of untrained subject to four weeks of endurance training[38]. Endurance capacity and VO_{2max} of the high-fat and high-carbohydrate diet groups were determined at the end of two and four weeks of training. There was no difference in pre-training endurance cycling time to exhaustion at 80% VO_{2max} between the two groups (about 30 minutes). At the end of the first two weeks of training, the high-carbohydrate diet group increased its endurance capacity by 87% whereas the high-fat diet group showed an increase of 62% which did not reach the prescribed level of statistical significance. At the end of four weeks of training, the high-carbohydrate and high-fat diet groups had raised their endurance cycling capacities by 150% and 166% respectively. However, there was no difference in the times to exhaustion for the two groups. The four weeks on the high-carbohydrate diet increased muscle glycogen concentration by 33% (from 487 to 651 mmol/kg dw) whereas the high-fat diet showed an increase of only 4% (from 442 to 460 mmol/kg dw). It is interesting to note that both groups recorded similar exercise times to exhaustion (79 vs 78 minutes), even though the muscle glycogen concentration of the high-carbohydrate diet group was significantly higher than that of the high-fat diet group. In contrast, muscle triacylglycerol concentration of the high-fat diet group increased from 42 to 78.3 mmol/kg dw (86%), whereas the values for the high-carbohydrate diet group did not change (51 vs 43 mmol/kg dw).

The authors conclude from their studies on diet and training that the duration of the dietary period is all-important. After four weeks on a high-fat diet, there appears to be no detriment to performance when compared with a high-carbohydrate diet; however, poorer performances begin to appear after four weeks on a high-fat diet. Previous observations on high-fat diets and performance have been carried for only a few weeks[39] or have excluded carbohydrate completely from the experimental diet[40].

Diet before exercise

Dietary preparation during the week before competition or heavy training is designed to increase muscle and liver glycogen stores. This involves tapering training and increasing the amount of carbohydrate in the diet during the three to four days before heavy exercise[26]. The recommended pre-exercise meal is one that is high in easy to digest carbohydrate-containing foods and low in fat. The nature of carbohydrate in this meal may influence subsequent endurance performance. Some studies report that pre-exercise ingestion of low glycaemic index carbohydrates improves cycling endurance capacity[41,42], while others report no improvements in exercise performance during cycling[43] or running[44]. In all but the running study reported by Wee and colleagues, high and low glycaemic index carbohydrates were ingested within the hour before exercise. Furthermore, these studies used single carbohydrates such as lentils, glucose, potatoes and sweetened rolled oats. However, Wee and colleagues provided their subjects with isocaloric meals containing carbohydrate, fat and protein that only differed in the glycaemic index of the carbohydrate. Furthermore, the meals were consumed three hours before exercise in order to simulate the custom and practice of sportsmen and women preparing for competition. Therefore, the available evidence does not suggest that eating pre-exercise meals that contain mainly low glycaemic index carbohydrates improve subsequent exercise performance.

Carbohydrate intake during the hour before exercise has been discouraged on the grounds that it decreases fat metabolism and accelerates the depletion of the muscle's limited glycogen stores[45]. This common recommendation is based on results from a study that examined the influence of high plasma fatty acid concentrations on muscle glycogen use during 30 minutes of submaximal treadmill running[46]. The study found that drinking a 25% glucose solution 45 minutes before exercise resulted in a rise and then sharp fall in blood glucose concentrations early in the run. Furthermore, it appeared that a greater degradation of muscle glycogen occurred than when the runners drank only water. Drinking a concentrated glucose solution during the hour before exercise does cause an increase and then sharp reduction in blood glucose concentrations during the first 10–20 minutes of exercise. In some individuals, blood glucose concentrations will fall to hypoglycaemic values but they rarely experience the hypoglycaemic symptoms that often appear when the same glucose concentrations occur at the end of exercise. Although an early study reported that ingesting a 25% glucose solution 30 minutes before cycling to exhaustion, at approximately 84% VO_{2max}, reduced endurance capacity by 19%[47], subsequent studies failed to confirm this result[48].

Increasing fat metabolism reduces the rate of carbohydrate use during prolonged exercise and thus helps delay the onset of fatigue. To this end, several studies have examined the benefits of ingesting medium chain triglycerides (triacylglycerols) before and during exercise. The fat in our diet is mainly present as long-chain fatty acids, ie 18–25 carbon atoms that are combined with glycerol as triglycerides. Medium-chain fatty acids contain about six to eight carbon atoms and are semi-synthetic oil mixtures produced from coconut oil. The medium-chain fatty acids are then re-esterified with glycerol to form medium chain triglycerides (MCT). These MCT enter the systemic circulation more quickly than long chain triglycerides because they are transported across the small intestine, whereas long chain triglycerides enter the systemic circulation via the lymphatic system. The medium-chain fatty acids released from MCT have a further advantage over long-chain fatty acids in that they enter mitochondria without the help of the carnitine shuttle and are, thus, oxidized more quickly than an equivalent amount of long-chain fatty acids. The value of MCT as a means of increasing fat metabolism during exercise has been explored in a number of recent studies. In one study, supplementation with MCT during prolonged cycling improved performance[49] but these benefits have not been confirmed by more recent studies[50,51]. Furthermore, ingestion of >30g MCT causes gastrointestinal distress and it is unlikely that small amounts have any influence on fat metabolism. For example, a recent study has shown that ingesting a tolerable amount (about 25 g) of MCT does not reduce the rate of glycogen degradation during 30 minutes of cycling at 84% VO_{2max}[52].

Carbohydrate intake during exercise

Prolonged exercise is a challenge to human temperature regulation, especially in a hot and humid environment. Drinking on the run clearly helps to delay the onset of severe dehydration and prevent premature fatigue (see Professor Maughan's chapter).

Dehydration will cause fatigue in the presence of adequate glycogen stores[53]. Drinking well-formulated carbohydrate-electrolyte solutions provides athletes with both fluid and fuel, and improves endurance capacity during prolonged submaximal exercise[54]. For example, treadmill marathon performance times were improved as a result of ingesting a well-formulated sports drink[17]. In a 30 km road race, experienced runners also improved their performance times when they consumed a sports drink[55]. Although cycling studies clearly show that drinking a carbohydrate solution improves endurance capacity, there is little evidence to suggest that glycogen sparing is responsible for the improved performance[56]. However, ingesting a sports drink during prolonged submaximal running improves endurance capacity, and this is clearly associated with glycogen sparing in type 1 fibres[57].

Recovery diets

Early studies on post-exercise glycogen resynthesis recommended that the optimum amount of carbohydrate is about 1 g/kg body weight, consumed immediately after exercise and at two-hour intervals until the next meal[58]. Carbohydrates that stimulate a large insulin response, as a consequence of increased blood glucose concentration (high glycaemic index carbohydrates), are preferable to those that evoke only a low glycaemic response[59]. When the recovery period lasts two to three days rather than a day or less, the nature of the carbohydrate is not as important as the amount of carbohydrate[30]. When the recovery period is only 22–4 hours, the amount of carbohydrate consumed must be about 9–10 g/kg body mass in order to replace glycogen stores. Carbohydrate can be provided in liquid or solid form during the first five hours of recovery with equal benefit[60].

Although there is good evidence to support the recommendation that a high carbohydrate diet during the 24 hours following prolonged heavy exercise will restore muscle glycogen to normal values, there is relatively less information on whether or not exercise capacity is restored when these dietary recommendations are implemented. Nevertheless, there are at least two running studies which show that eating a high carbohydrate diet (9–10 g/kg body weight) following prolonged heavy exercise restores exercise capacity during continuous submaximal running[61] and following prolonged intermittent high-intensity running[62]. Eating the high carbohydrate recovery diet not only restored endurance capacity during the intermittent high-intensity exercise but also improved on the previous day's performance[62].

During prolonged exercise, intramuscular triglycerides appear to contribute to fat metabolism and may even make up for a shortfall in the delivery of fatty acids from adipose tissue to muscle[20,63]. However, not all authors agree that intramuscular triglycerides play an active role as substrate for energy production during prolonged exercise[64,65]. For example, Kiens and Richter reported that, whereas intramuscular triglycerides were not used during prolonged exercise, they were used during recovery, contributing to energy production while muscle glycogen resynthesis progressed to completion.

Costill *et al* measured the intramuscular triglyceride concentrations before and after 120 minutes submaximal cycling (65% VO_{2max}) and found no change in this substrate. Thereafter, their seven endurance-trained men consumed either a high carbohydrate diet (83% energy intake) or a high fat diet (68% energy intake) for the succeeding 12 hours. After a 12-hour overnight fast, the subjects returned to the laboratory where they undertook a cycling test that required them to complete 1,600 kJ as fast as possible[66]. Intramuscular triglyceride concentrations were significantly (36%) higher after the 24-hour recovery on the high fat diet and fast (44.7±2.4 mmol/kg dry wt) than on the high carbohydrate diet and overnight fast (27.5±2.1 mmol/kg dry wt). The high carbohydrate diet restored 93% of the muscle glycogen used during the 120 minutes of cycling, while the value for the high fat diet was only 13%. Total time to complete the 1,600 kJ self-paced cycling test was significantly longer after the high fat diet (139±7.1 minutes) than after the high carbohydrate diet (117±3.2 minutes). This study, therefore, endorses the performance benefits of high pre-exercise muscle glycogen, rather than high intramuscular triglycerides.

When recovery is only a few hours, then complete glycogen resynthesis is unachievable. Even so carbohydrate intake still has a beneficial effect on subsequent performance. For example, implementing the recommendation to consume 1 g/kg body weight of carbohydrate immediately after exercise, and again two hours later before running to exhaustion, improved running time by 20 minutes. On one occasion, runners consumed the recommended amount of carbohydrate in the form of a sports drink and on another occasion they drank an artificially sweetened placebo solution[67]. The slightly more practical recommendation of simply drinking the equivalent of 50 g carbohydrate immediately after exercise and water for the rest of the four-hour recovery period is also more beneficial than drinking water alone[68]. Paradoxically, consuming a greater amount of carbohydrate during a four-hour recovery does not improve subsequent exercise capacity beyond what can be achieved with a single intake of 50 g[69] or 1 g/kg body weight[70]. In order to rehydrate during a short recovery period, approximately 150% of the body fluid lost should be ingested[71], which is more than recommended from earlier studies. There is some suggestion that ingesting a mixture of carbohydrate and protein, in the ratio of 3:1, increases the rate and amount of muscle glycogen resynthesis[72]. However, this has yet to be confirmed.

After prolonged exercise, especially after endurance races, there is clear evidence of muscle damage as reflected by increases in the appearance of muscle enzymes, such as creatine kinase, in blood[17]. This delayed onset of muscle soreness appears to involve not only mechanical damage to muscle fibres but also secondary metabolic effects involving free radical activity and an inflammatory response[73]. Muscle damage impairs the resynthesis of muscle glycogen and thus slows the recovery process (see Dr Donnelly's chapter)[74,75]. This subclinical damage to muscle fibres, which is experienced as soreness during the days following exercise, may cause a decrease in the availability of glucose transporter proteins, principally GLUT-4[76,77]. There are, as yet, no clear nutritional recommendations to help accelerate the repair of skeletal muscle during recovery. However, there is some evidence that carbohydrate intake decreases the amount of nitrogen lost during recovery from heavy resistance training[78]. Furthermore, ingestion of amino acids following resistance exercise appears to change the balance between protein synthesis and degradation in favour of greater synthesis[79,80]. This is an aspect of recovery that clearly deserves more attention.

Conclusions

The available evidence suggests that endurance athletes should continue to pay attention to the composition of their diets such that they obtain about 60% of their daily energy intake from carbohydrates (approximately 4–5 g/kg body mass). They should also obtain about 12–5% from protein (1.2–1.5 g/kg body mass); fat intake should be <30% of daily energy intake, although it is the intake of saturated fats that must be reduced.

References

1 Devlin J, Williams C. Foods, nutrition and sports performance; a final consensus statement. *J Sports Sci* 1991; **9**: 3.

2 Maughan R, Goodburn R, Griffin J *et al*. Fluid replacement in sport and exercise: a consensus statement. *Br J Sports Med* 1993; **27**: 34–5.

3 Ekblom B, Williams C. Foods, nutrition and soccer performance: final consensus statement. *J Sports Sci* 1994; **12**(special issue): S3.

4 Maughan R, Horton E. Current issues in nutrition in athletics: final consensus statement. *J Sports Sci* 1995; **13**(special issue): S1.

5 Joint position statement: nutrition and athletic performance. American College of Sports Medicine, American Dietetic Association and Dieticians of Canada. *Med Sci Sport Exerc* 2000; **32**: 2130–45.

6 Dennis SC, Noakes T. Advantages of a smaller bodymass in humans when distance-running in warm humid conditions. *Eur J Applied Physiol* 1999; **79**: 280–4.

7 Rosetta L, Williams C, Brooke-Wavell C, Norgan NG. Diet and body composition of female distance runners of differing menstrual status. *J Sports Sci* 1998; **16**: 629–37.

8 Gleeson M, Bishop N. Modification of immune responses to exercise by carbohydrate, glutamine and antioxidant supplements. *Immunol Cell Biol* 2000; **78**: 554–61.

9 Melby C, Commerford R, Hill J. Exercise, macronutrient balance and weight control. In: Lamb D, Murray R, eds. *Exercise, nutrition and weight control*. Indianapolis: Cooper Publishing Group, 1998: 1–55.

10 Cheuvront S. The zone diet and athletic performance. *Sports Med* 1999; **27**: 213–28.

11 Williams C. Dietary macro- and micronutrient requirements of endurance athletes. *Proc Nutr Soc* 1998; **57**: 1–8.

12 Tarnopolsky M. Nutritional implications of gender differences in energy metabolism. In: Driskell J, Wolinsky I, eds. *Energy-yielding macronutrients and energy metabolism in sports nutrition*. London: CRC Press, 2000: 245–62.

13 Costill DL. Physiology of marathon running. *J Am Med Assoc* 1972; **221**: 1024–9.

14 Bebb J, Brewer J, Patton A, Williams C. Endurance running and the influence of diet on fluid intake. *J Sports Sci* 1984; **3**: 198–9.

15 Costill D, Winrow E. Maximum oxygen intake among marathon runners. *Arch Phys Med Rehab* 1970; **51**: 317–20.

16 Williams C, Brewer J, Patton A. The metabolic challenge of the marathon. *Br J Sports Med* 1984; **18**: 245–52.

17 Tsintzas O, Williams C, Singh R *et al*. Influence of carbohydrate-electrolyte drinks on marathon running performance. *Eur J Appl Physiol* 1995; **70**: 154–68.

18 Christensen EH, Hansen Arbeitsfahigkeit und ehrnahrung. *Skand Arch Physiol* 1939; **81**: 160–75.

19 Romijn J, Coyle E, Hibbert J, Wolfe R. Comparison of indirect calorimetry and a new breath 13C/12C ratio method during strenuous exercise. *Am J Physiol* 1992; **263**: E64–71.

20 Romijn J, Coyle E, Sidossis L *et al*. Regulation of endogenous fat and carbohydrate metabolism in relation to exercise intensity and duration. *Am J Physiol* 1993; **265**: E380–91.

21 Jansson E. On the significance of the respiratory exchange ratio after different diets during exercise in man. *Acta Physiol Scand* 1982; **114**: 103–10.

22 Tsintzas O, Williams C, Boobis L, Greenhaff P. Carbohydrate ingestion and single muscle fiber glycogen metabolism during prolonged running in men. *J Appl Physiol* 1996; **81**: 801–9.

23 Bergstrom J, Hultman E. A study of the glycogen metabolism during exercise in man. *Scand J Clin Lab Invest* 1967; **19**: 218–28.

24 Ahlborg B, Bergstrom J, Brohult J *et al*. Human muscle glycogen content and capacity for prolonged exercise after different diets. *Forsvarsmedicin* 1967; **3**: 85–99.

25 Astrand P-O. Diet and athletic performance. *Fed Proc* 1967; **26**: 1772–7.

26 Sherman W, Costill D, Fink W, Miller J. Effect of exercise-diet manipulation on muscle glycogen and its subsequent utilization during performance. *Int J Sports Med* 1981; **2**: 114–8.

27 Bergstrom J, Hultman E. A study of glycogen metabolism during exercise in man. *J Clin Lab Invest* 1967; **19**: 218–28.

28 Karlsson J, Saltin B. Diet, muscle glycogen and endurance performance. *J Appl Physiol* 1971; **31**: 203–6.

29 Goforth HW, Hodgdon JA, Hilderbrand RL. A double blind study of the effects of carbohydrate loading upon endurance performance. *Med Sci Sport Exerc* 1980; **12**: 108A.

30 Brewer J, Williams C, Patton A. The influence of high carbohydrate diets on endurance running performance. *Eur J Appl Physiol* 1988; **57**: 698–706.

31 Williams C, Brewer J, Walker M. The effect of a high carbohydrate diet on running performance during a 30 km treadmill time trial. *Eur J Appl Physiol* 1992; **65**: 18–24.

32 Sherman W, Costill D, Fink W, Miller J. Effect of exercise-diet manipulation on muscle glycogen and its subsequent utilization during performance. *Int J Sports Med* 1981; **2**: 114–8.

33 Madsen K, Pedersen P, Rose P, Richter E. Carbohydrate supercompensation and muscle glycogen utilization during exhaustive running in highly trained athletes. *Eur J Appl Physiol* 1990; **61**: 467–72.

34 Roberts K, Noble E, Hayden D, Taylor A. Simple and complex carbohydrate-rich diets and muscle glycogen content of marathon runners. *Eur J Appl Physiol* 1988; **57**: 70–4.

35 Pizza F, Flynn M, Duscha B *et al*. A carbohydrate loading regimen improves high intensity, short duration exercise performance. *Int J Sport Nutr* 1995; **5**: 110–6.

36 Pitsiladis Y, Duignan C, Maughan R. Effect of alterations in dietary carbohydrate intake on running performance during a 10 km treadmill time trial. *Br J Sports Med* 1996; **30**: 226–31.

37 Helge J, Richter E, Kiens B. Interaction of training and diet on metabolism and endurance during exercise in man. *J Physiol* 1996; **492**: 293–306.

38 Helge J, Wulff B, Kiens B. Impact of a fat-rich diet on endurance in man: role of dietary period. *Med Sci Sports Exerc* 1998; **30**: 456–61.

39 Lambert E, Speechly D, Dennis S, Noakes T. Enhanced endurance in trained cyclists during moderate intensity exercise following 2 weeks adaptation to a high fat diet. *Eur J Appl Physiol* 1994; **69**: 287–93.

144

40 Phinney S, Bistrian B, Evans W *et al*. The human metabolic response to chronic ketosis without caloric restriction: preservation of submaximal exercise capability with reduced carbohydrate oxidation. *Metabolism* 1983; **32**: 769–76.

41 Thomas D, Brotherhood J, Brand J. Carbohydrate feeding before exercise: effect of glycemic index. *Int J Sports Med* 1991; **12**: 180–6.

42 Kirwan J, O'Gorman D, Evans W. A moderate glycemic meal before endurance exercise can enhance performance. *J Appl Physiol* 1998; **84**: 53–9.

43 Febbraio M, Stewart K. CHO feeding before prolonged exercise: effect of glycemic index on muscle glycogenolysis and exercise performance. *J Appl Physiol* 1996; **82**: 1115–20.

44 Wee S-L, Williams C, Gray S, Horabin J. Influence of high and low glycemic index meals on endurance running capacity. *Med Sci Sport Exerc* 1999; **31**: 393–9.

45 Wootton S. *Nutrition for sport*. London: Simon & Shuster Ltd, 1989.

46 Costill D, Coyle E, Dalsky G *et al*. Effects of elevated plasma FFA and insulin on muscle glycogen usage during exercise. *J Appl Physiol* 1977; **43**: 695–9.

47 Foster C, Costill D, Fink W. Effects of pre-exercise feedings on endurance performance. *Med Sci Sports Exerc* 1979; **11**: 1–5.

48 Chryssanthopoulos C, Hennessy L, Williams C. The Influence of pre-exercise glucose ingestion on endurance running capacity. *Br J Sports Med* 1994; **28**: 105–9.

49 Van Zeal C, Lambert E, Hawley J *et al*. Effects of medium chain triglyceride ingestion on carbohydrate metabolism and cycling performance. *J Appl Physiol* 1996; **80**: 2217–25.

50 Goedecke J, Elmer-English R, Dennis S *et al*. Effects of medium-chain triacylgycerol ingested with carbohydrate on metabolism and exercise performance. *Int J Sport Nutr* 1999; **9**: 35–47.

51 Jeukendrup A, Theilen J, Wagenmakers A *et al*. Effect of MCT and carbohydrate ingestion on substrate utilization and cycling performance. *Am J Clin Nutr* 1998; **67**: 397–404.

52 Horowitz J, Mora-Rodriguez R, Beyerley L, Coyle E. Preexercise medium-chain triglyceride ingestion do not alter muscle glycogen use during exercise. *J Appl Physiol* 2000; **88**: 219–25.

53 Gonzalez-Alonso J, Calbet J, Nielsen B. Metabolic and thermodynamic responses to dehydration-induced reduction in muscle blood flow in exercising humans. *J Physiol* 1999; **520**: 577–89.

54 Maughan R. Physiological responses to fluid intake during exercise. In: Maughan R, Murray R, eds. *Sports drinks: basic science and practical aspects*. London: CRC Press, 2000: 129–51.

55 Tsintzas K, Liu R, Williams C *et al*. The effect of carbohydrate ingestion on performance during a 30-km race. *Int J Sport Nutr* 1993; **3**: 127–39.

56 Coyle E, Hodgkinson B. Influence of dietary fat and carbohydrate on exercise metabolism and performance. In: Lamb D, Murray R, eds. *The metabolic basis of performance in exercise and sport*. Indianapolis: Cooper Publishing Group, 1999: 165–98.

57 Tsintzas K, Williams C. Human muscle glycogen metabolism during exercise: effect of carbohydrate supplementation. *Sports Med* 1998; **25**: 7–23.

58 Ivy JL. Muscle glycogen synthesis before and after exercise. *Sports Med* 1991; **11**: 6–19.

59 Burke L, Collier G, Hargreaves M. Glycemic index — a new tool in sports nutrition. *Int J Sport Nutr* 1999; **8**: 401–15.

60 Keizer H, Kuipers H, van Kranenburg G. Influence of liquid and solid meals on muscle glycogen resynthesis, plasma fuel hormone response, and maximal physical working capacity. *Int J Sports Med* 1987; **8**: 99–104.

61 Fallowfield J, Williams C. Carbohydrate intake and recovery from prolonged exercise. *Int J Sport Nutr* 1993; **3**: 150–64.

62 Nicholas C, Green P, Hawkins R, Williams C. Carbohydrate intake and recovery of intermittent running capacity. *Int J Sport Nutr* 1997; **7**: 251–60.

63 Horowitz J, Klein S. Lipid metabolism during endurance exercise. *Am J Clin Nutr* 2000; **72**(suppl): 558S–63S.

64 Turrcotte L, Richter E, Keins B. Lipid metabolism during exercise. In: Hargreaves M, ed. *Exercise metabolism*. Leeds: Human Kinetics, 1995: 99–130.

65 Kiens B, Richter E. Utilization of skeletal muscle triacylglycerol during postexercise recovery in humans. *Am J Physiol* 1998; **275**: E332–7.

66 Starling R, Trappe T, Parcell A *et al*. Effect of diet on muscle triglyceride and endurance performance. *J Appl Physiol* 1997; **82**: 1185–9.

67 Fallowfield J, Williams C, Singh R. The influence of ingesting a carbohydrate-electrolyte solution during 4 hours recovery from prolonged running on endurance capacity. *Int J Sport Nutr* 1995; **5**: 285–99.

68 Wong S, Williams C, Adams N. Effects of ingesting a large volume of carbohydrate-electrolyte solution on rehydration during recovery and subsequent exercise capacity. *Int J Sport Nutr Exerc Metab* 2000; **10**: 375–93.

69 Wong S, Williams C. Influence of different amounts of carbohydrate on endurance running capacity following short term recovery. *Int J Sports Med* 2000; **21**: 444–52.

70 Fallowfield J, Williams C. The influence of a high carbohydrate intake during recovery form prolonged constant pace running. *Int J Sport Nutr* 1997; **7**: 10–25.

71 Shirreffs S, Maughan R. Rehydration and recovery of fluid balance after exercise. *Exerc Sport Sci Rev* 2000; **28**: 27–32.

72 Zawadski KM, Yespelkis BB, Ivy JL. Carbohydrate-protein complex increases the rate of muscle glycogen storage after excercise. *J Appl Physiol* 1992; **72**: 1854–9.

73 Clarkson P, Sayers S. Etiology of exercise-induced muscle damage. *Can J Appl Physiol* 1999; **24**: 234–48.

74 Costill DL, Pascoe DD, Fink WJ *et al*. Impaired muscle glycogen resynthesis after eccentric exercise. *J Appl Physiol* 1990; **69**: 46–50.

75 O'Reilly K, Warhol M, Fielding R *et al*. Eccentric exercise-induced muscle damage impairs muscle glycogen repletion. *J Appl Physiol* 1987; **63**: 252–6.

76 Ivy JL, Kuo C-H. Regulation of GLUT 4 protein and glycogen synthase during muscle glycogen synthesis after exercise. *Acta Physiol Scand* 1998; **162**: 293–304.

77 Asp S, Daugaard J, Richter E. Eccentric exercise decreases glucose transporter GLUT4 protein in human skeletal muscle. *J Physiol* 1996; **482**: 705–12.

78 Roy B, Tarnopolsky M, Macdougall J *et al*. Effect of glucose supplement timing on protein-metabolism after resistance training. *J Appl Physiol* 1997; **82**: 1882–8.

79 Biolo G, Tipton K, Klein S, Wolfe R. An abundant supply of amino acids enhances the metabolic effect of exercise on muscle protein. *Am J Physiol* 1997; **273**: E122–9.

80 Tipton K, Ferrando A, Phillips S *et al*. Postexercise net protein synthesis in human muscle from orally administered amino acids. *Am J Physiol* 1999; **276**: E628–34.

Sports drinks before, during and after running

PROFESSOR RON MAUGHAN

PROFESSOR OF HUMAN PHYSIOLOGY, DEPARTMENT OF BIOMEDICAL SCIENCES,
UNIVERSITY MEDICAL SCHOOL, FORESTERHILL, ABERDEEN, UK

Water is the largest component of the human body, accounting for about 60% of body mass in the average adult and more than this in very lean individuals. It also has a very high turnover rate — an athlete training or competing in a hot environment may exchange 25% of total body water per day[1]. Fluid losses, mainly due to sweating, may be >2 l/h. Total water loss during a marathon held in cool conditions is typically 1–6% of body mass[2], and may reach 8% of body mass in races run in warm environments[3]. A reduction of even 2% body water will impair exercise performance — this has important implications for the marathon runner. Serious incapacity occurs when the body water deficit reaches about 10%. If not corrected, this level of hypohydration can lead to heat illness, coma and even death, indicating the need for tight regulation of body fluid balance. As electrolyte balance is associated with water balance and distribution among the body water compartments, intake and excretion of the major electrolytes must also be regulated.

Several factors influence the body's fluid and electrolyte balance. For the healthy individual, the stress of physical exercise, especially when undertaken in a hot environment, poses a great challenge to homeostasis. Heat illness, which may be fatal, is not uncommon when physically demanding events take place in warm weather[4], and the risk is greatly magnified if dehydration develops. The rise in body temperature that accompanies exercise in the heat can be attenuated by sweating, but large sweat losses result in hypohydration and loss of electrolytes which may also have serious consequences. This chapter will focus on the effects of fluid and electrolyte replacement before, during and after exercise.

Thermoregulation and sweat loss

The rate of metabolic heat production during running is determined mainly by body mass and running speed. Heat production results in a rise in core temperature unless the rate of heat loss is also increased. In cool conditions, heat loss is achieved by the physical transfer of heat to the environment, but when the ambient temperature exceeds skin temperature heat is gained by this route[5]. Sweating becomes the only avenue of heat loss in such circumstances and can limit the rise in core temperature, but only at the expense of water and electrolyte loss from the body. The progressive dehydration that follows will impair both exercise performance and thermoregulatory capacity[6]. Many electrolytes are lost in sweat and must be replaced either during or after exercise. Some negative effects associated with large sweat losses can be alleviated by ensuring that the individual is well hydrated at the start of exercise and by ingesting fluid during exercise[7]. Restoration of fluid and electrolyte balance following exercise is an important part of the recovery process, especially in training. Published literature shows that pre-existing hypohydration has a strong negative effect on exercise performance[8], and it is important to appreciate the factors that normally act to regulate body water balance. The thermoregulatory response to exercise and the control of body fluid balance are discussed in more detail in Dr Shirreffs' chapter.

Fluid intake and thirst regulation

Except during periods of restricted intake, daily fluid intake in the form of food and drink is greater than obligatory water loss; renal excretion of excess fluid is the main mechanism for regulating body water content[9]. However, the ability of the kidneys to conserve water or electrolytes only reduces the rate of loss — it cannot compensate for inadequate intake. The sensation of thirst initiates the desire to drink and is, therefore, important in controlling fluid intake and balance. Although thirst appears to be an insensitive index of acute changes in hydration status in humans[10], the long-term stability of total body water volume indicates that the desire to drink is an effective regulatory factor.

The need to drink is perceived as thirst, but drinking itself may not always be driven by a physiological requirement for water intake. Drinking behaviour can be initiated by habit or ritual, by a desire for sensory experience or intake of nutrients or stimulants (eg caffeine), or by a perceived need for a warming or cooling effect. Many thirst-associated sensations are learned in early life, with signs such as dryness of the mouth or throat inducing drinking, while distention of the stomach can stop ingestion before a fluid deficit has been restored. However, thirst is controlled separately by the osmotic pressure and volume of the body fluids, and is regulated by the same mechanisms that affect water and solute reabsorption in the kidneys and control central blood pressure.

The physiological responses to fluid intake and the physiological and behavioural consequences of drinking are described in detail elsewhere[11]. The regulation of body fluid content and distribution involves regulation of plasma osmolality sodium concentration and of blood volume and arterial blood pressure. The end result of any excursion from normal is a stimulation of fluid intake via an increased thirst, or an increased loss of fluid and/or solute in the urine. The regulatory processes that mediate these effects have been the subject of a recent comprehensive review[12]. It is important to recognize, however, that all of the physiological mechanisms involved are subject to behavioural factors and conscious control, which may cause inappropriate drinking behaviour.

Fluid and electrolyte replacement: best composition of sports drinks

Importance of carbohydrate

To maintain a high rate of work output, an adequate supply of carbohydrate substrate should be available to the working muscles and, in addition to replacing water and electrolytes lost in sweat, drinks consumed during exercise should provide a source of carbohydrate fuel to supplement the body's limited stores. The composition of drinks that meet these objectives most effectively has been the subject of much debate. Although it is a common belief among athletes that plain water is the best drink during exercise, scientific evidence does not support this view. This belief is justified to some extent by a Position Statement on the prevention of thermal injuries in distance runners published by the American College of Sports Medicine in 1984[13]. This statement recommended that cool water was the optimum fluid for distance runners. The evidence is now overwhelming that the addition of carbohydrate[14], electrolytes[15] and flavouring[16] can all confer benefits over plain water. There is, however, no single formulation that will best meet the needs of each individual in all situations[17].

Increasing the carbohydrate content of drinks raises the rate at which oxidizable substrates can be delivered to the working muscles, but will reduce the rate at which water can be made available[18]. Where provision of water is first priority, the carbohydrate content of drinks will be low. Thus, the composition of drinks to be taken is influenced by the importance of the need to supply fuel and water. Carbohydrate depletion will result in fatigue and a decrease in the exercise intensity that could normally be sustained, but is not usually a life-threatening condition. Disturbances in fluid balance and temperature regulation have potentially more serious consequences, suggesting that endurance runners should give priority to maintaining fluid and electrolyte balance.

Although the American College of Sports Medicine stated in 1984 that cool water is the best fluid to drink during endurance exercise[13], more recently it has been shown that plain water is not the best rehydration drink for most runners, and that ingestion of drinks containing added substrate and electrolytes may be more beneficial[19]. For example, addition of carbohydrate to drink improves performance in prolonged exercise; glucose, sucrose and oligosaccharides have all been shown to enhance endurance capacity[7]. Some studies suggest that long-chain glucose polymer solutions are used more readily by muscles during exercise than are glucose or fructose solutions[20], but others have found no difference in the oxidation rates of ingested glucose or glucose polymer[21,22]. Massicote *et al* demonstrated that ingested fructose was less readily oxidized than glucose or glucose polymers[21]. Fructose is poorly absorbed in the small intestine, so drinks with high fructose concentrations should be avoided because of

149

the risk of gastrointestinal upset, although inclusion of small amounts with other sugars does not seem to have adverse effects[14]. The argument in favour of fructose ingestion during exercise — that it provides a readily available energy source but does not stimulate insulin release and consequent inhibition of fatty acid mobilization — is not well founded as insulin secretion is suppressed during exercise[23].

The optimum concentration of sugar to be added to drinks will depend on individual circumstances. Factors influencing the maximum level include: ambient temperature and humidity; individual sweating characteristics; and biochemical, nutritional and physiological factors that influence substrate use in exercise. High carbohydrate concentrations will delay gastric emptying and will, therefore, reduce the amount of fluid available for absorption; very high concentrations will cause secretion of water into the intestine which will increase the risk of dehydration[24]. High sugar concentrations (>10%) may also result in gastrointestinal disturbances but will increase the delivery of carbohydrate to the site of absorption in the small intestine.

Importance of sodium

The only electrolyte that should be added to drinks consumed during exercise is sodium (Na^+), which is usually added in the form of sodium chloride but also often as sodium citrate to regulate drink pH. Na^+ stimulates sugar and water uptake in the small intestine and helps maintain extracellular fluid volume[25]. Most soft drinks of the cola or lemonade variety contain virtually no Na^+ (1–2 mmol/l), sports drinks commonly contain 10–25 mmol/l, and oral rehydration solutions used for treating diarrhoea-induced dehydration have 30–90 mmol/l. A high Na^+ content, although it may stimulate jejunal absorption of glucose and water, tends to make drinks unpalatable, and it is important that drinks intended for ingestion during or after exercise have a pleasant taste to stimulate consumption. Thus, effective formulations for specialist sports drinks must balance the aims of efficacy and palatability.

In extreme endurance events lasting more than three to four hours, adding Na^+ to drinks may avoid the danger of hyponatraemia which has been reported when large volumes of low-Na^+ drinks have been ingested. The fluid intakes of runners in endurance events are generally low, and a progressive fluid deficit is normally observed. It is recognized that failure to ingest an adequate fluid volume may lead to dehydration and heat illness in prolonged exercise in high ambient temperatures. Runners are, therefore, advised to drink more than the level dictated by thirst. The low Na^+ content of sports drinks is sufficient in most situations, but may not be when sweat losses and fluid intakes are particularly high.

Hyperthermia associated with dehydration and hypernatraemia is common in endurance events held in the heat and often affects slower participants. However, it is now clear that some runners in prolonged events may suffer from hyponatraemia, which may be associated with either hyperhydration[26–8] or dehydration[29]; only a small number of cases have been reported and these are mostly associated with ultramarathon or prolonged triathlon events. Noakes *et al* reported four cases of exercise-induced hyponatraemia in which the race times were between seven and 10 hours and post-race serum Na$^+$ concentrations were between 115 and 125 mmol/l[26]. Estimated fluid intakes were between six and 12 litres, and consisted of water or drinks containing low levels of electrolytes; estimated total sodium chloride intake during the race was 20–40 mmol. Frizell *et al* reported even more astonishing fluid intakes of 20–4 l fluids (almost 2.5 l/h sustained for many hours, which is in excess of the maximum gastric emptying rate reported) with a mean Na$^+$ content of only 5–10 mmol/l in two runners who collapsed after an ultramarathon run and were found to be hyponatraemic (serum Na$^+$ concentration 118–23 mmol/l)[28].

The dangers of ingesting excessive volumes of fluid without adding Na$^+$ have long been recognized in various industrial settings, including foundry workers and ships' stokers. Hyponatraemia as a consequence of ingesting large volumes of fluids with a low Na$^+$ content has also been recognized in resting individuals. Flear *et al* reported the case of a man who drank nine litres of beer with a Na$^+$ content of only 1.5 mmol/l in 20 minutes; his plasma Na$^+$ level fell from 143 mmol/l to 127 mmol/l, although he appeared unaffected[30]. Noakes has suggested that, in these situations, a significant amount of Na$^+$ moves into the unabsorbed fluid in the intestinal lumen, thereby causing hyponatraemia[31,32]. Hyponatraemic competitors in the Hawaii Ironman triathlon have also been reported to be dehydrated[29]. Fellmann *et al* reported a small but statistically significant decrease (from 141 to 137 mmol/l) in serum Na$^+$ concentration in runners who completed a 24-hour run, but food and fluid intakes were neither controlled nor measured[33]. Supplementation with sodium chloride in amounts greater than those normally found in sports drinks may be needed in prolonged events where large sweat losses can be expected and where it is possible to consume large volumes of fluid. It remains true, however, that electrolyte replacement during exercise is not a priority for most runners in most sporting events. Most collapsed runners in marathons will have hypernatraemia, but particularly in longer events, and in runners who have a high venous pressure and no postural blood pressure drop this may not be true. Giving large volumes of low-sodium intravenous fluids without measuring plasma sodium may cause or even exacerbate pre-existing hyponatraemia.

Amino acid theories

There are often suggestions that addition of other ingredients may enhance the efficacy of sports drinks, and a variety of different amino acids have been proposed. Among these are glycine, glutamine and the branched-chain amino acids (BCAA).

Glycine and other actively transported amino acids offer the prospect of enhancing the rate of intestinal water uptake by adding solute that will use an alternative transport pathway and thus increase both solute drag and osmotic flux. The limited data that are available, however, do not support this proposition[34]. Glutamine can act as an energy substrate for cells of the immune system; the plasma glutamine level may fall after hard exercise, leading to the proposal that glutamine supplementation may enhance immune function in athletes during periods of hard training. Although this is an attractive hypothesis, the available evidence does not support it and well-controlled studies of glutamine supplementation have failed to show a beneficial effect[35]. The lack of stability of glutamine in acid solution would also seem to be an insuperable difficulty to its addition to sports drinks.

The addition of BCAA to sports drinks is based on the central fatigue hypothesis which has been championed by Newsholme and colleagues[36]. This theory proposes that an increased uptake of tryptophan (Trp), the amino acid precursor or the neurotransmitter 5-hydroxytryptamine (5-HT or serotonin) into central serotonergic neurones is associated with an increased susceptibility to fatigue signals arising in the periphery. The BCAA compete with Trp for uptake into the brain, and it is argued that increasing BCAA availablity will decrease brain Trp uptake and thus reduce the subjective sensation of fatigue. Well-controlled laboratory trials of BCAA supplementation, however, do not support an ergogenic effect[37].

Chilled drinks

Early experimental evidence suggests that drinking chilled (4 °C) fluids is advantageous as it accelerates gastric emptying and thus improves the availability of ingested fluids[38]. More recent evidence reveals that the gastric emptying rate of hot and cold beverages is not markedly different[25]. Despite this, there may be advantages in taking chilled drinks as the palatability of most carbohydrate-electrolyte drinks is improved at low temperatures — this has the effect of stimulating consumption and helps the exercising athlete to feel better. Such effects on the athlete's sense of well being cannot be ignored. The impact of significant volumes of cool fluids on body heat content is another factor that cannot be overlooked. Although this effect is relatively small, it helps delay the point at which a critical core temperature will be reached.

Fluid and electrolyte replacement: cardiovascular, metabolic and performance benefits

Many of the published studies investigating the effects of fluid ingestion on exercise performance have used carbohydrate-electrolyte beverages, thereby making it difficult to separate the effects of water replacement and substrate provision. One study that did separate these drink components demonstrated improved exercise performance when plain water was ingested than when no fluids were consumed, although further performance improvements were observed when carbohydrate and electrolytes were also present[39]. Similar results have been revealed in other studies with different exercise models, including continuous and intermittent running and cycling, laboratory time trials, and simulated or real race performances. Many extensive reviews have addressed this issue[40–2].

Some studies have reported either no effect or a beneficial effect of fluid ingestion on exercise performance[43-5]. Hyperthermia and cardiovascular drift have been shown to be reduced during prolonged moderate-intensity exercise, which is attributed to fluid replacement during exercise[46]. Improved maintenance of blood glucose, which can be used by exercising muscles and consequently reduce the need for mobilization of the limited liver glycogen reserves, appears to be the main benefit of carbohydrate consumption during exercise[47]. There may also be benefits for thermoregulatory function from ensuring that the blood glucose level is maintained; these may derive from a lower circulating catecholamine level when carbohydrate is ingested[48]. The studies that have reported adverse effects of fluid ingestion on exercise performance have generally been those in which the fluid ingestion has resulted in gastrointestinal disturbances.

A well-controlled study was recently carried out to distinguish between the effects of carbohydrate provision and the water replacement properties of a drink. Eight men undertook the same cycle ergometer exercise on four separate occasions[49]. After 50 minutes of exercise at 80% of maximal oxygen uptake (VO_{2max}), a performance test at a higher exercise intensity (ie completion of set amount of work as quickly as possible) was completed; the test lasted about 10 minutes. On each of the four trials, a different beverage consumption protocol was followed during the 50-minute exercise; nothing was consumed during the performance tests. The beverages were electrolyte-containing water in a large (1,330 ml) and small (200 ml) volume, and carbohydrate-electrolyte solutions (79 g) in the same large and small volumes; the electrolyte content of each beverage was the same and amounted to 619 mg (27 mmol) and 141 mg (3.6 mmol) of Na^+ and potassium ions (K^+) respectively. The results indicated that performance was 6.5% better after consuming the large volume of fluid compared to the smaller volume, and 6.3% better following carbohydrate-containing rather than carbohydrate-free beverage consumption; the fluid and carbohydrate independently enhanced performance and the two improvements were additive. The mechanism for the improvements in performance with the large fluid replacement versus the small fluid replacement was attributed to a lower heart rate and oesophageal temperature when the large volume was consumed. The mechanism by which carbohydrate ingestion improved performance has yet to be determined.

Pre-exercise hydration

A small degree of temporary hyperhydration occurs when drinks with high (100 mmol/l) Na^+ concentrations are ingested, but this does not seem beneficial for performance carried out in heat because of the high osmolality that follows[50]. An alternative strategy, which has recently been the subject of much interest, attempts to induce an expansion of the blood volume before exercise by adding glycerol to ingested fluids. In high concentrations, glycerol has little metabolic effect but exerts an osmotic action. Although its distribution in the body water compartments is variable, glycerol will expand the extracellular space, and some of the water ingested with the glycerol will be retained rather than being lost in the urine[51]. The elevated osmolality of the extracellular space will result in intracellular dehydration and the implications of this are currently unknown[52]. It might be expected, however, that the raised plasma osmolality would have negative consequences for thermoregulatory capacity[50,53], although current evidence indicates that this is not the case[54,55]. Studies investigating the effects of glycerol feeding on exercise performance before or during exercise have shown mixed results. It has recently been suggested that performance improves following glycerol and water administration before prolonged exercise[55], but earlier research has clearly indicated that the capacity to perform prolonged exercise is not improved[53,56].

Post-exercise rehydration

Post-exercise replacement of water and electrolyte losses is particularly important if repeated bouts of exercise are to be performed. This does not apply to the marathon runner in competition, but is important when training twice or even three times a day. Carbohydrate ingestion immediately after training is also necessary when the exercise has resulted in a significant reduction in the body's liver and muscle glycogen stores. The need for such replacement depends on the extent of losses incurred during exercise, but will also be influenced by the time and nature of subsequent exercise bouts. Rapid rehydration is important in events where competition is by weight category. Competitors in sports such as wrestling, boxing and weightlifting are segregated by body mass and they frequently undergo acute thermal- and exercise-induced dehydration to allow them to compete in a lighter weight category. This practice should be discouraged as it reduces exercise performance even when some restoration of the deficit is achieved[57] and increases the risk of heat illness[4]. However, competitors in these sports are convinced that the benefits of weight reduction outweigh the disadvantages, and the practice will persist. Rapid rehydration is essential in athletes training in hot, humid conditions where recovery time between training is limited.

In an early study where a moderately severe dehydration (4% of body mass) was induced by heat exposure, fluid consumption over three hours in a volume equal to the sweat lost did not restore plasma volume or serum osmolality within four hours[58]. Ingestion of a glucose-electrolyte solution, however, resulted in greater restoration of plasma volume than did plain water; this was accompanied by a greater urine production in the water trial. Where the electrolyte content of drinks is the same, addition of carbohydrate (100 g/l) or carbonation does not seem to affect plasma volume restoration over a four-hour period after sweat loss corresponding to approximately 4% of body weight[59]. Gonzalez-Alonso et al have shown that a dilute carbohydrate-electrolyte solution (60 g/l carbohydrate, 20 mmol/l Na^+, 3 mmol K^+) is more effective in promoting post-exercise rehydration than either plain water or a low-electrolyte diet cola[60]. As the two drinks produced different volumes of urine, it was suggested that the caffeine content of the diet cola might have exerted a negative effect because of its diuretic properties.

Ingestion of plain water in the post-exercise period results in a rapid fall in plasma Na^+ concentration and plasma osmolality[61]. These changes reduce thirst and stimulate urine output, both of which delay the rehydration process. Nose *et al* studied subjects exercising at low intensity in the heat for 90–110 min who, after inducing a mean dehydration of 2.3% of body mass, rested for one hour before drinkng[61]. Plasma volume was not restored until after 60 minutes when plain water was ingested together with sucrose capsules. When sodium chloride capsules were ingested with water to give a saline solution with an effective concentration of 0.45% (77 mmol/l), plasma volume was restored within 20 minutes. Voluntary fluid intake was higher and the urine output less in the sodium chloride trial; 71% of the water loss was retained within three hours compared with 51% in the plain water trial. Delayed rehydration in the water trial appeared to be a result of Na^+ loss, accompanied by water, in the urine caused by reduction in plasma renin activity and aldosterone levels[62].

An evaluation of the effects of replacing a fixed volume of fluid with different Na^+ concentrations demonstrated that urine output over the few hours following ingestion was inversely related to the Na^+ content of the ingested fluid[63]. In this study, subjects were dehydrated by intermittent exercise in the heat until 2% of body mass was lost, and then consumed a volume of fluid equivalent to 1.5 times the sweat loss — the drinks contained 0, 25, 50 or 100 mmol/l Na^+. These studies confirm that rehydration after exercise can only be achieved if both Na^+ and water are consumed. It might be suggested that rehydration drinks should have a Na^+ concentration similar to that of sweat, but no single formulation can meet this requirement for all individuals in all situations since the Na^+ content of sweat varies widely. The upper end of the normal range for Na^+ concentration (80 mmol/l), however, is similar to that of the oral rehydration solutions recommended by the World Health Organization in cases of severe diarrhoea (90 mmol/l).

The need for Na^+ replacement stems from its role as the major ion in the extracellular fluid. Inclusion of K^+, the main cation in the intracellular space, should enhance the replacement of intracellular water after exercise and thus promote rehydration[64]. K^+ has been shown to be as effective as Na^+ in retaining water ingested after exercise-induced dehydration, despite the low levels of K^+ lost in sweat. Addition of either ion was shown to significantly increase the fraction of the ingested fluid retained over the post-exercise period[65]. There was no additive effect of including both ions, which would be expected if they acted independently on different body fluid compartments, but this may be the result of the small volume of fluid ingested and the difficulty in further reducing the urine output. To achieve effective rehydration, the composition of the fluid should be considered and the volume ingested must be greater than the sweat volume lost[66]. The ingested electrolytes are not necessarily derived from the beverage itself — effective rehydration can ensue if solid food is consumed with an adequate fluid volume (eg with water or a soft drink)[67].

References

1 Saris WHM, van Erp-Baart MA, Brouns F *et al*. Study on food intake and energy expenditure during extreme sustained exercise. *Int J Sports Med* 1989; **10**(suppl 1): S26–31.

2 Maughan RJ. Thermoregulation and fluid balance in marathon competition at low ambient temperature. *Int J Sports Med* 1985; **6**: 15–19.

3 Costill DL. Sweating: its composition and effects on body fluids. *Ann N Y Acad Sci* 1977; **301**: 160–74.

4 Sutton JR. Clinical implications of fluid imbalance. In: Gisolfi CV, Lamb DR, eds. *Perspectives in exercise science and sports medicine. Vol 3. Fluid homeostasis during exercise*. Carmel: Benchmark Press, 1990: 425–48.

5 Leithead CS, Lind AR. Heat stress and heat disorders. Casell: London, 1964.

6 Montain SJ, Coyle EF. Influence of graded dehydration on hyperthermia and cardiovascular drift during exercise. *J Appl Physiol* 1992; **73**: 1340–50.

7 Maughan RJ. Effects of CHO-electrolyte solution on prolonged exercise. In: Lamb DR, Williams MH, eds. *Perspectives in exercise science and sports medicine. Volume 4. Ergogenics — enhancement of performance in exercise and sport*. Carmel: Benchmark Press, 1991: 35–85.

8 Armstrong LE, Costill DL, Fink WJ. Influence of diuretic-induced dehydration on competitive running performance. *Med Sci Sports Exerc* 1985; **17**: 456–61.

9 Zambraski EJ. Renal regulation of fluid homeostasis during exercise. In: Gisolfi CV, Lamb DR, eds. *Perspectives in exercise science and sports medicine. Volume 3. Fluid homeostasis during exercise*. Carmel: Benchmark Press, 1990, 247–80.

10 Adolph ED & associates. Physiology of man in the desert. New York: Interscience, 1947.

11 Maughan RJ, JB Leiper, SM Shirreffs. Fluids and electrolytes during exercise. In: Garrett WE, ed. *Textbook of sports medicine*. Baltimore: Williams and Wilkins, 2000: 413–24.

12 Stricker EM, Sved AF. Thirst. *Nutrition* 2000; **16**: 821–6.

13 American College of Sports Medicine. Position stand on prevention of thermal injuries during distance running. *Med Sci Sports Exerc* 1984; **16**: 9–14.

14 Aragon-Vargas LF. Metabolic and performance responses to carbohydrate intake. In: Maughan RJ, Murray R, eds. *Sports drinks: basic science and practical aspects*. Boca Raton: CRC Press; 2000: 153–82.

15 Maughan RJ. Physiological responses to fluid intake during exercise. In: Maughan RJ, Murray R, eds. *Sports drinks: basic science and practical aspects*. Boca Raton: CRC Press; 2000: 129–52.

16 Passe D. Physiological and psychological determinants of fluid intake. In: Maughan RJ, Murray R, eds. *Sports drinks: basic science and practical aspects*. Boca Raton: CRC Press; 2000: 45–88.

17 Hubbard RW, Szlyk PC, Armstrong LE. Influence of thirst and fluid palatability on fluid ingestion. In: Gisolfi CV, Lamb DR, eds. *Perspectives in exercise science and sports medicine. Vol 3. Fluid homeostasis during exercise*. Carmel: Benchmark Press, 1990: 39–95.

18 Vist GE, Maughan RJ. The effect of osmolality and carbohydrate content on the rate of gastric emptying of liquids in man. *J Physiol* 1995; **486**: 523–31.

19 American College of Sports Medicine. Position stand on exercise and fluid replacement. *Med Sci Sports Exerc* 1996; **28**: 1–7.

20 Noakes TD. The dehydration myth and carbohydrate replacement during prolonged exercise. *Cycling Sci* 1990; **2**: 23–9.

21 Massicote D, Peronnet F, Brisson G *et al*. Oxidation of a glucose polymer during exercise: comparison with glucose and fructose. *J Appl Physiol* 1989; **66**: 179–83.

22 Rehrer NJ. Limits to fluid availability during exercise. Harlem: De Vrieseborsch, 1990.

23 Newsholme EA, Leech AR. *Biochemistry for the medical sciences*. Chichester: Wiley, 1983.

24 Leiper JB, Maughan RJ. Absorption of water and electrolytes from hypotonic, isotonic and hypertonic solutions. *J Physiol* 1986; **373**: 90P.

25 Maughan RJ. Physiology and nutrition for middle distance and long distance running. In: Lamb DR, Knuttgen HG, Murray R, eds. *Perspectives in exercise science and sports medicine. Vol 7. Physiology and nutrition for competitive sport*. Carmel, Cooper Publishing, 1994: 329–72.

26 Noakes TD, Goodwin N, Rayner BL *et al*. Water intoxication: a possible complication during endurance exercise. *Med Sci Sports Exerc* 1985; **17**: 370–5.

27 Noakes TD, Norman RJ, Buck RH *et al*. The incidence of hyponatremia during prolonged ultraendurance exercise. *Med Sci Sports Exerc* 1990; **22**: 165–70 .

28 Frizell RT, Lang GH, Lowance DC, Lathan SR. Hyponatraemia and ultramarathon running. *JAMA* 1986; **255**: 772–4.

29 Hiller WDB. Dehydration and hyponatraemia during triathlons. *Med Sci Sports Exerc* 1989; **21**: S219–21.

30 Flear CTG, Gill CV, Burn J. Beer drinking and hyponatraemia. *Lancet* 1981; **2**: 477.

31 Noakes TD. The hyponatremia of exercise. *Int J Sports Nutr* 1992; **2**: 205–28.

32 Noakes TD. Hyponatraemia during distance running: a physiological and clinical interpretation. *Med Sci Sports Exerc* 1993; **24**: 403–5.

33 Fellmann N, Sagnol M, Bedu M *et al*. Enzymatic and hormonal responses following a 24 h endurance run and a 10 h triathlon race. *Eur J Appl Physiol* 1988; **57**: 545–53.

34 Shi X, Summers R, Schedl HP *et al*. Effects of carbohydrate type and concentration and soultion osmolality on water absorption. *Med Sci Sports Exerc* 1995; **27**: 1607–15.

35 Rohde T, MacLean DA, Pedersen BK. Effect of glutamine supplementation on changes in the immune system induced by repeated exercise. *Med Sci Sports Exerc* 1998; **30**: 856–62.

36 Newsholme EA, Acworth IA, Blomstrand E. Amino acids, brain neurotransmitters and a functional link between muscle and brain that is important in sustained exercise. In: Benzi G, ed. *Advances in biochemistry*. London: John Libbey Eurotext, 1987: 127–47.

37 van Hall G, Raaymakers JS, Saris WH, Wagenmakers AJ. Ingestion of branched-chain amino acids and tryptophan during sustained exercise in man: failure to affect performance. *J Physiol* 1995; **486**: 789–94.

38 Costill DL, Saltin B. Factors limiting gastric emptying during rest and exercise. *J Appl Physiol* 1974; **37**: 679–83.

39 Maughan RJ, Bethell LR, Leiper JB. Effects of ingested fluids on exercise capacity and on cardiovascular and metabolic responses to prolonged exercise in man. *Exp Physiol* 1996; **81**: 847–59.

40 Coyle EF, Coggan AR. Effectiveness of carbohydrate feeding in delaying fatigue during prolonged exercise. *Sports Med* 1984; **1**: 446–58.

41 Lamb DR, Brodowicz GR. Optimal use of fluids of varying formulations to minimize exercise-induced disturbances in homeostasis. *Sports Med* 1986; **3**: 247–74.

42 Murray R. The effects of consuming carbohydrate-electrolyte beverages on gastric emptying and fluid absorption during and following exercise. *Sports Med* 1987; **4**: 322–51.

43 Bosch AN, Dennis SC, Noakes TD. Influence of carbohydrate ingestion on fuel substrate turnover and oxidation during prolonged exercise. *J Appl Physiol* 1994; **76**: 2364–72.

44 McConell G, Fabris S, Proietto J, Hargreaves M. Effect of carbohydrate ingestion on glucose kinetics during exercise. *J Appl Physiol* 1994; **77**: 1537–41.

45 Maughan RJ, Fenn CE, Leiper JB. Effects of fluid, electrolyte and substrate ingestion on endurance capacity. *Eur J Appl Physiol* 1989; **58**: 481–6.

46 Gonzalez-Alonso J, Calbet JA, Nielsen B. Muscle blood flow is reduced with dehydration during prolonged exercise in humans. *J Physiol* 1998; **513**: 895–905.

47 Hamilton MT, Gonzalez-Alonso J, Montain SJ, Coyle EF. Fluid replacement and glucose during exercise prevent cardiovascular drift. *J Appl Physiol* 1991; **71**: 871–7.

48 Mora-Rodriguez R, Gonzalez-Alonso J, Below PR, Coyle EF. Plasma catecholamines and hyperglycaemia influence thermoregulation in man during prolonged exercise in the heat. *J Physiol* 1996; **491**: 529–40.

49 Below RP, Mora-Rodriguez R, Gonzalez-Alonso J, Coyle EF. Fluid and carbohydrate ingestion independently improve performance during 1 h of intense exercise. *Med Sci Sports Exerc* 1995; **27**: 200–10.

50 Fortney SM, Wenger CB, Bove JR, Nadel ER. Effect of hyperosmolality on control of blood flow and sweating. *J Appl Physiol* 1984; **57**: 1688–95.

51 Riedesel ML, Allen DL, Peake GT, Al-Qattan K. Hyperhydration with glycerol solutions. *J Appl Physiol* 1987; **63**: 2262–8.

52 Gleeson M, Maughan RJ, Greenhaff PL. Comparison of the effects of pre-exercise feeding of glucose, glycerol and placebo on endurance and fuel homeostasis in man. *Eur J Appl Physiol* 1986; **55**: 645–53.

53 Thecomata A, Nagashima K, Nose H, Morimoto T. Osmoregulatory inhibition of thermally induced cutaneous vasodilation in passively heated humans. *Am J Physiol* 1997; **273**: R197–204.

54 Montner P, Stark DM, Riedesel ML *et al.* Pre-exercise glycerol hydration improves cycling endurance time. *Int J Sports Med* 1996; **17**: 27–33.

55 Latzka WA, Sawka MN, Matott RP *et al. Hyperhydration: physiologic and thermoregulatory effects during compensable and uncompensable exercise-heat stress.* Natich, Massachusetts, US Army Technical Report, 1996: 1–107.

56 Miller JM, Coyle EF, Sherman WM *et al.* Effect of glycerol feeding on endurance and metabolism during prolonged exercise in man. *Med Sci Sports Exerc* 1983; **15**: 237–42.

57 Burge CM, Carey MF, Payne WR. Rowing performance, fluid balance, and metabolic function following dehydration and rehydration. *Med Sci Sports Exerc* 1993; **25**: 1358–64.

58 Costill DL, Sparks KE. Rapid fluid replacement following thermal dehydration. *J Appl Physiol* 1973; **34**: 299–303.

59 Lambert CP, Costill DL, McConnell GK *et al.* Fluid replacement after dehydration: influence of beverage carbonation and carbohydrate content. *Int J Sports Med* 1992; **13**: 285–92.

60 Gonzalez-Alonso J, Heaps CL, Coyle EF. Rehydration after exercise with common beverages and water. *Int J Sports Med* 1992; **13**: 399–406.

61 Nose H, Mack GW, Shi X, Nadel ER. Role of osmolality and plasma volume during rehydration in humans. *J Appl Physiol* 1988; **65**: 325–31.

62 Nose H, Mack GW, Shi X, Nadel ER. Involvement of sodium retention hormones during rehydration in humans. *J Appl Physiol* 1988; **65**: 332–36.

63 Maughan RJ, Leiper JB. Effects of sodium content of ingested fluids on post-exercise rehydration in man. *Eur J Appl Physiol* 1995; **71**: 311–9.

64 Nadel ER, Mack GW, Nose H. Influence of fluid replacement beverages on body fluid homeostasis during exercise and recovery. In: Gisolfi CV, Lamb DR, eds. *Perspectives in exercise science and sports medicine. Volume 3. Fluid homeostasis during exercise.* Carmel: Benchmark, 1990: 181–205.

65 Maughan RJ, Owen JH, Shirreffs SM, Leiper JB. Post-exercise rehydration in man: effects of electrolyte addition to ingested fluids. *Eur J Appl Physiol* 1994; **69**: 209–15.

66 Shirreffs SM, Taylor AJ, Leiper JB, Maughan RJ. Post-exercise rehydration in man: effects of volume consumed and drink sodium content. *Med Sci Sports Exerc* 1996; **28**: 1260–71.

67 Maughan RJ, Leiper JB, Shirreffs SM. Restoration of fluid balance after exercise-induced dehydration: effects of food and fluid intake. *Eur J Appl Physiol* 1996; **73**: 317–25.

Running shoe design: protection and performance

DR MARTYN SHORTEN

MANAGING PARTNER, BIOMECHANICA, LLC, OREGON, USA

During the course of a marathon race, a runner experiences approximately 25,000 impacts with the ground. The repeated impact loading of the body during running is a factor in the development of overuse injuries, and has been directly implicated in the aetiology of lower extremity stress fractures, tibial stress syndrome (shin splints) and lower back pain. However, many common running injuries are associated with secondary effects, eg rapid joint motions, soft tissue stresses and muscle forces induced by impact between the foot and the surface. Injuries of the latter type include common knee pain syndromes, Achilles tendinitis and plantar fasciitis.

The evolution of athletic shoes has shadowed that of the surfaces on which athletes perform. In ancient Greece, Olympians competed barefoot on clay surfaces dusted with sand. We can surmise that Pheidippides, the first marathon runner of legend, ran across natural surfaces either barefoot or wearing the leather sandals in common use at the time. Running shoes with protective features are a relatively recent invention, paralleling development of distance running on hard roads as a popular activity. Although Abebe Bikila ran barefoot to victory in the 1960 Olympic marathon, most modern runners prefer, like Bikila in his 1964 win, to wear shoes.

The shoe is the primary interface between the runner and the road and, therefore, has a potentially important role to play in the management of repetitive impact loads. Over the past 20 years, running shoe designs have changed significantly. This chapter aims to explore how our changing understanding of running injury mechanisms and lower extremity biomechanics has been reflected in altering running shoe designs.

Surveys of running injuries and running shoes in the 1970s and 1980s

Before 1978, little was known about the frequency or cause of overuse injuries among runners. Surveys conducted by *Runner's World Magazine* in the 1970s, and summarized by Cavanagh[1], revealed what is now a familiar list of complaints: >20% of the runners surveyed complained of knee pain, 18% of Achilles tendinitis, 10% of shin splints and 7% of injury to the arch of the foot. An early clinical survey found similar results, with knee pain reported by >25% patients and Achilles tendinitis, shin splints and plantar fasciitis among the most frequently reported injuries[2].

Although a characteristic profile of running injuries had been identified by 1980, mechanisms underlying the injuries were still unclear. It was believed that repeated impact loading was an important factor. The notion that excessive pronation of the subtalar joint was involved in running injuries became popular, but no definitive clinical or biomechanical results were obtained.

Running shoes of the late 1970s reflected some of this uncertainty. Shoes given top ratings by *Runner's World Magazine* in 1980 were very similar in design. Typical running shoes featured a cushioned midsole of ethylene vinyl acetate (EVA) foam, woven nylon uppers with suede reinforcements and moulded rubber outsoles. The editors' selection criteria included price, weight, shock absorption, flexibility and durability — stability and motion control had yet to emerge as important issues. Some shoes, notably those from the Brooks Shoe Company, incorporated a 4° varus wedge in the midsole. At the time, the concept was controversial and was criticized as a form of unprescribed treatment. In retrospect, it is now recognized as an early and effective pronation control device.

Injury surveys post-1980

The pattern of running injuries, established by early, ad hoc surveys, was confirmed by comprehensive surveys carried out in the 1980s[3]. Running accounted for 37% of the >10,000 injuries treated at one sports medicine clinic, more than any other recreational activity[4]. The distribution of 1,819 running injuries was documented over a two-year period and risk factors associated with the different types were identified[3]. Shoes and surfaces were each implicated as risk factors in about 5% of injuries. 'Training errors' (behaviours resulting in a sudden increase in the loads imposed on the body) were implicated in 75% of Achilles tendon injuries[3] and 60–75% of tibial stress fractures[5]. Examples of training errors include a sudden increase in duration or intensity of training runs, persistent high-intensity training, a severe training bout or race, and the sudden return to training after a period of inactivity.

Other reports also confirmed the significance of subtalar joint pronation as a risk factor in running injuries. Of the runners diagnosed with the four most common overuse injuries (patello-femoral pain, tibial stress syndrome, Achilles tendinitis and plantar fasciitis)[3], 66% were rated with moderate or severe varus alignment of the lower extremity; stress fractures have also been linked to varus alignment of the forefoot, rearfoot or tibia[6].

It is now generally acknowledged that varus alignment of the lower extremity and training errors are the most prevalent risk factors associated with overuse injuries among runners. Varus alignment and other anatomical factors predispose an athlete to injury by amplifying the impact-induced internal stresses on bone and soft tissue. Training errors produce increases in the load on the body, to which tissues are unable to adapt, thereby triggering injuries.

Functional over-pronation and common overuse injuries

During normal running, the foot contacts the ground beneath the centre of mass of the body to facilitate balance. Consequently, the foot naturally makes initial ground contact in a slightly supinated position (Figure 1a). Supination at contact typically ranges from 0–10° relative to the lower leg. Pronation occurs as the foot rotates to make flat contact with the ground, reaching a maximum angle of pronation about midway through the ground contact period (Figure 1b). Although pronation combines eversion and abduction of the foot by rotation about the talo-calcaneal (subtalar) joint and dorsiflexion of the ankle, its dominant component is calcaneal eversion that can be measured using two-dimensional kinematic methods. The total range of eversion from first contact to mid-stance is usually 10–20°, although this may exceed 25° in some individuals. In runners with an inherent varus alignment of the lower extremity, the foot contacts the ground in a more supinated position and undergoes a greater range of motion (functional over-pronation) in order to achieve flat contact with the ground.

Significantly, the talo-calcaneal joint is oriented in a manner that links pronation with internal tibial rotation. This mechanism in the ankle joint has been classically described as an oblique hinge[7]. Although recent studies show the mechanism to be slightly more complex, the link between pronation and tibial rotation is believed to play a role in running injury mechanisms.

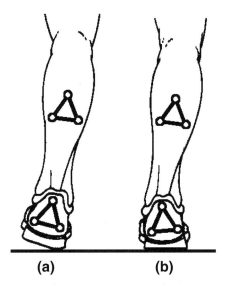

(a)　　　　　(b)

Figure 1

Rear view of the orientation of the right foot and lower leg during ground contact in running showing (a) supination of the talo-calcaneal joint at initial heel contact and (b) pronated talo-calcaneal joint at mid-stance

The four most common overuse injuries incurred by runners are associated with varus alignment of the lower extremity. In each case, the purported biomechanical link between impact and injury involves functional over-pronation.

In patello-femoral pain syndrome (or 'runner's knee'), for instance, excessive pronation and the associated internal tibial rotation is thought to cause the patella to move slightly from its normal alignment relative to the femoral condyles. The resulting increase in contact pressure in the patello-femoral joint leads to painful symptoms. In extreme cases, the high pressures cause degradation of the cartilage and underlying bone (chondromalacia patella).

Excessive pronation has also been implicated in some types of tibial stress syndrome, eg shin splints[8]. Functional over-pronation is thought to increase the tension in the Achilles tendon, overloading the insertion of the soleus where breakdown of the tibial surface may occur. Similarly, purported mechanisms of Achilles tendinitis include excessive pronation as a risk component. Violent motion of the tendon during impact may lead to micro-tears and tissue degeneration. It has also been suggested that functional over-pronation and internal tibial rotation produce torsional stresses in the tendon, with vascular impairment as a possible consequence[9]. Torsional stresses due to excessive pronation are also implicated in the aetiology of plantar fasciitis[10,11].

Pronation control in running shoes

Since the early 1980s, most running shoe manufacturers have included anti-pronation or motion control features in some or all of their products. Such features include stiffer cushioning, stiff heel counters, insole boards, medially posted midsoles, varus wedges and proprietary cushioning geometries. Some of these work by stiffening the shoe upper and midsole to physically restrain movement of the subtalar joint; others modify the geometry of the cushioning to reduce the lever arm of the ground reaction force about the subtalar joint — this reduces the torque that tends to promote pronation. Firmer, wider midsoles offer a greater lever arm to the ground reaction force, increasing angular displacement and pronation velocity. Softer midsoles increase shock attenuation and reduce angular velocity at the expense of greater rearfoot motion[12].

Shoes with a soft lateral border combined with a firmer medial post have been found to be effective at controlling pronation[13]. The soft lateral border is compressed on contact and attenuates shock and reduces the lever arm of the ground reaction force, while the firmer medial border resists excessive pronation. Upper constructions that encourage a close fit between the heel and the shoe also contribute to motion control[14].

The excessive pronation hypothesis is commonly used in shoe design and medical diagnoses. Treatments for running injuries, using orthotics, or specifically designed shoes to reduce pronation are often effective in relieving symptoms. Conventionally, athletes with pes planus are considered more likely to have hypermobile feet which hyperpronate and require 'stable shoes'. Conversely, those with pes cavus are more likely to have hypomobile feet that pronate less and require more cushioned shoes.

Detailed mechanisms of injury and treatment through pronation control, however, are still not well understood. For instance, the movement coupling between eversion of the calcaneus and tibial rotation is not absolute. An in vitro study revealed that only 14–66% of calcaneal eversion was transferred to tibial rotation[15]. The situation is further complicated by the observation that movement coupling is less for athletes with pes planus and greater for those with pes cavus[16]. Recent studies suggest that variability in coupling may be more important than the degree of coupling per se[17]. It is also known that the talo-calcaneal joint has variable anatomy, with both two- and three-faceted joints commonly found[18,19]. An individual may have a different number of facets on left and right sides.

These findings add to the difficulty in making individual footwear prescriptions and confound the running shoe manufacturers' problem of having to meet the needs of a large population of customers with relatively few shoe models. Historically, the manufacturers' strategy was to make shoes with varying degrees of pronation control, offer some guidance on shoe selection and allow consumers to choose. Products increasingly have cushioning systems with integrated anti-pronation mechanisms that make the stability properties of a shoe more independent of the cushioning properties. These sophisticated shoe designs respond to increasing medial loads by stiffening, intending to provide greater resistance to pronation 'on demand'. Such designs aim to meet the needs of a wider range of runners with different foot types and pronation mechanics.

Shoe inserts

Shoe inserts are commonly used to correct lower extremity alignment problems and pronation. They reduce rearfoot motion by 1–2° (slightly less than the effect of a stability-oriented running shoe), particularly when combined with a stability shoe[20], but recent research into their effectiveness is equivocal. Nigg et al[21] compared the effects of six different orthotic inserts on rearfoot motion during running; none were significantly different from the non-insert condition. Stacoff et al[22] measured three-dimensional calcaneal and tibial rotations using markers placed on intra-cortical pins. Orthotics were found to have only small effects on tibio-calcaneal motions which were inconsistent among subjects, indicating that any effects are highly individual. It has been suggested that the proper role of shoe inserts is to reduce muscular work instead of aligning the skeleton or limiting motion[23].

Cushioning in running shoes

The impact between the foot and the ground during a running step has a peak force magnitude in excess of two times the athlete's bodyweight, and generates a shock wave that is transmitted through the musculoskeletal system. The impact shock wave has a typical magnitude of five to 15 times the acceleration due to gravity (5–15 g) at the level of the tibia, but is attenuated to between 1 and 3 g at the level of the head. Impact forces and shock magnitudes are influenced by body mass, running speed, touchdown kinematics, shoe properties, surface properties and gradient. Muscle actions in the lower extremity can act to reduce peak impact loads and peak loading rates[24].

Loading is thought to be a risk factor for many running injuries, including stress fractures, shin splints, cartilage disease and osteoarthritis. Although direct impact injuries (eg metatarsal and tibial stress fractures) are reported by <5% injured runners[3], there are no published injury surveys from the pre-cushioning era, nor studies directly comparing injury rates in shod and barefoot running.

The first 'technical' running shoes of the 1970s incorporated a foam rubber midsole between the outsole and the upper to cushion the impact between the shoe and ground. Cushioning systems increased comfort, reduced the occurrence of painful feet, and allowed many people who would not otherwise have participated to enjoy the 'jogging boom'. They also attenuate skeletal shock transients and reduce peak plantar pressures. Shock-absorbing inserts in non-athletic shoes have been shown to relieve heel pain and Achilles tendinitis[25], and to reduce the incidence of stress fractures in military recruits[26].

Many different materials have been incorporated into modern running shoes. These include foamed polymers, viscoelastic materials, air, gases, gels and moulded springs. Materials are generally selected on the basis of their shock attenuation, energy

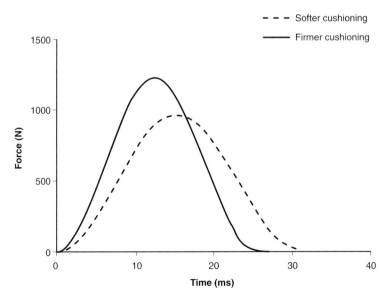

Figure 2

Effect of cushioning on force–time during impact

absorption, weight and durability. The addition of a layer of compliant material between the foot and the ground distributes impact forces, both temporally (reducing peak forces) and spatially (reducing peak pressures).

Figure 2 compares the results of in vitro impact testing of arbitrarily soft and firm cushioning systems. The force–time curve of the two impacts illustrates the basic mechanics of cushioning. The more compliant shoe undergoes greater deformation when impacted, increasing the duration of the impact. The decelerating impulse is thus applied over a longer period of time. This temporal redistribution of the impact force results in lower peak forces and the peak rate of force increase is also lower.

A cushioning system results in spatially distributed load. Figure 3 compares peak pressures on the plantar surface recorded during running at 5 m/s under different cushioning conditions. Data were collected using an array of pressure sensors in the insole of the shoe. Typically during running, peak pressures are focused under the heel, metatarsal heads and hallux. With increasing cushioning, however, loads are distributed over a greater area of the plantar surface, reducing the magnitude of local peak pressures.

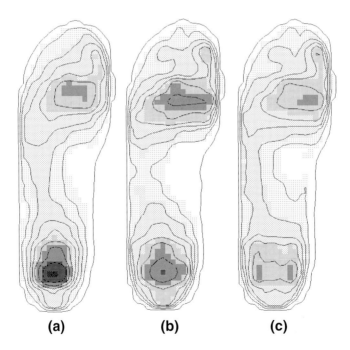

(a) (b) (c)

Figure 3

Peak plantar pressure distribution during running at 5 m/s under different cushioning conditions: (a) minimally cushioned shoe (b) moderately cushioned shoe (c) well-cushioned shoe. Each map is the grand mean of 60 running steps (five steps from each of 12 subjects) and the pressure contour interval is 50 kPa

Running shoes and running performance

Distance running performance is primarily determined by physiological factors. For example, maximal oxygen uptake (VO_{2max}), fractional use of VO_{2max}, lactate threshold and muscle fibre type have all been shown to correlate with successful distance running performance[27,28]. The main functional role of running shoes is to provide protection from contact with the running surface. There is little evidence to suggest that choice of footwear, within normal bounds, has an effect on performance great enough to outweigh primary physiological factors. That noted, footwear has been shown to influence the sub-maximal aerobic demand at a given running speed ('running economy'). Increasing the weight of a shoe, for example, increases oxygen consumption at moderate running speeds by approximately 1% per 100 g added weight[29]. Cushioning properties also have an effect, with soft-soled shoes reportedly reducing oxygen cost by 1–2% compared with hard-soled shoes[30]. Reducing the flexibility of the forefoot of a shoe lowers energy dissipation at the metatarsalphalangeal joints[31], but this effect has not been linked to improvements in distance running performance.

Although there has been some popular interest in the concept of 'energy return' in feet and footwear[32], the elastic energy stored and recovered in conventional cushioning systems is thought to be too small to have a direct influence on running economy[33]. The mechanism by which cushioning influences running economy is believed to be a kinematic adaptation to the compliance of the shoe sole[34]. Runners are thought to adapt to harder cushioning systems by changing their running style to one that compensates for the reduced shock attenuation, eg by increasing knee flexion velocity[35]. These adaptations require muscle action and incur an energy penalty; the 'cost of cushioning'. Conversely, greater shock attenuation in the sole reduces the metabolic cost of cushioning with consequent small reductions in the oxygen consumption.

Shoe selection

The great anatomical, physiological and kinematic variation among runners renders it difficult to make general prescriptions for the selection of appropriate running shoes. Athletes should select shoes that fit well, are comfortable and have cushioning that feels neither too hard nor too soft. Subjective assessments of fit, comfort and shock attenuation are generally reliable guides to the actual mechanical properties of the shoes. However, stability properties of shoes cannot be perceived reliably. Runners requiring pronation control must, therefore, rely on identifying features, such as firm cushioning, medial posting and heel fit, which are known to influence pronation.

It is common practice to select different shoes for competition and for training. In the case of marathon events, this may be inadvisable for several reasons.

- Although racing shoes are lighter than training shoes (by as much as 100 g/shoe), they are less protective. The added weight in a training shoe is mainly due to additional cushioning and support features.
- During training, the runner's body acclimatizes to the mechanical load levels experienced. Suddenly changing the load regimen by switching to a lighter, less cushioned shoe could constitute a 'training error', increasing the likelihood of injury if other risk factors are present.
- Weight savings may reduce oxygen cost of running by 1%; however, the saving is partly or wholly compensated for by the increased cost of cushioning and the net performance benefit may be minimal. It is up to the individual runner to balance the value of this small potential advantage with the increased risk of injury. That balance, in turn, will depend on whether the subject is an elite athlete with a possibility of winning the race or a recreational runner hoping to complete his or her first marathon.

Conclusions

Since the first London marathon, our knowledge of running injury mechanisms has greatly enhanced. From an initial focus on impact as a primary cause of overuse injuries, attention has shifted to the role of secondary effects and internal stresses caused by instability and excessive motion of the joints of the lower extremity. We also know that injury risk is increased by hyperpronation, muscular insufficiency, injury history and training habits. Current research suggests that injury mechanisms are variable and highly individual.

The sports shoe business is driven by the need to produce new products that are competitive, profitable and fashionable. Despite these demands, major athletic shoe manufacturers have generally responded to new knowledge about running injuries and injury mechanisms by introducing new designs and components intended to make their products more functional. The first cushioning systems were developed in response to concerns about the effect of repeated impacts between the foot and the ground. As the pronation hypothesis linking peripatellar knee pain and other injuries to excessive rearfoot motion became more popular, shoe designs intended to reduce pronation were developed. Currently, as our awareness of the individuality and specificity of injury mechanisms increases, shoe manufacturers are responding by developing models that allow more customization to meet individual needs.

Despite these advances, it is not known to what extent running shoes reduce the risk of running injury, mainly because definitive experiments would require, unacceptably, increasing the injury risk of some subjects. Indirect evidence can be found in the laboratory, where shoes have been shown to affect the hypothetical causes of injury (eg by reducing impact shock, plantar pressure and rearfoot motion). Such evidence is only as good as the purported injury aetiology however, and more research is necessary in this area.

References

1   Cavanagh PR. *The running shoe book*. Mountain View (CA): Anderson World, 1980.

2   James SL, Bates BT, Osternig LR. Injuries to runners. *Am J Sports Med* 1978; **6**: 40–9.

3   Clement DB, Taunton JE, Smart GW, McNicol KL. A survey of overuse running injuries. *Phys Sportsmed* 1981; **9**: 47–58.

4   Garrick JG. Characterization of the patient population in a sports medicine facility. *Phys Sportsmed* 1985; **13**: 73–6.

5   McBryde AM. Stress fractures in runners. *Clin Sports Med* 1985; **4**: 737–52.

6   Taunton JE, Clement DB, Webber D. Lower extremity stress fractures in athletes. *Phys Sportsmed* 1981; **9**: 77–86.

7   Inman VT. *The joints of the ankle*. Baltimore: Williams and Wilkins, 1976.

8   Viitasalo JT, Kvist M. Some biomechanical aspects of the foot and ankle in athletes with and without shin splints. *Am J Sports Med* 1983; **11**: 125–30.

9   Clement DB, Taunton, JE, Smart GW. Achilles tendinitis and peritendinitis: etiology and treatment. *Am J Sports Med* 1984; **12**: 179–84.

10 Taunton JE, Clement DB, McNicol K. Plantar fasciitis in runners. *Can J Appl Sport Sci* 1982; **7**: 41–4.

11 Warren BL. Plantar fasciitis in runners: treatment and prevention. *Sports Med* 1990; **10**: 338–45.

12 Stacoff A, Denoth J, Kaelin X, Stuessi E. Running injuries and shoe construction: some possible relationships. *Int J Sports Biomech* 1988; **4**: 342–57.

13 Nigg BM, Bahlsen HA. Influence of heel flare and midsole construction on pronation, supination and impact forces in heel–toe running. *Int J Sports Biomech* 1988; **4**: 205–19.

14 Van Gheluwe B, Kerwin D, Roosen P, Tielemans R. The influence of heel fit on rearfoot motion in running shoes. *J Appl Biomech* 1999; **15**: 361–72.

15 Hinterman B, Nigg BM, Sommer C *et al*. Transfer of movement between calcaneus and tibia in vitro. *Clin Biomech* 1994; **2**: 60–6.

16 Nigg BM, Cole GK, Nachbauer W. Effects of arch height of the foot on angular motion of the lower extremities in running. *J Biomech* 1999; **26**: 909–16.

17 Hamill J, van Emmerik REA, Heiderscheit BC *et al*. A dynamical systems approach to lower extremity injuries. *Clin Biomech* 1999; **14**: 297–308.

18 Bruckner J. Variations in the human subtalar joint. *J Orthop Sports Phys Ther* 1987; **8**: 481–94.

19 Forriol Campos F, Gomez Pellico L. Talar articular facets (facies articulares talares) in human calcanei. *Acta Anat (Basel)* 1989; **134**: 124–7.

20 Cairns MA. Effects of orthotics in altering rearfoot motion. In: Gregor RJ, Zernicke RF, Whiting WC, eds. *Proc XII International Congress of Biomechanics, Los Angeles (CA)*. Dept Kinesiology, University of California Los Angeles, 1989.

21 Stacoff A, Reinschmidt C, Nigg BM *et al*. Effects of foot orthoses on skeletal motion during running. *Clin Biomech* 2000; **15**: 54–64.

22 Nigg BM, Khan A, Fisher V, Stefanyshyn D. Effect of shoe insert construction on foot and leg movement. *Med Sci Sports Exerc* 1998; **30**: 550–5.

23 Nigg BM, Nurse MA, Stefanyshyn DJ. Shoe inserts and orthotics for sport and physical activities. *Med Sci Sports Exerc* 1999; **31**: S421–28.

24 Gerritsen KGM, van den Bogart AJ, Nigg BM. Direct dynamics simulation of the impact phase in heel–toe running. *J Biomech* 1995; **28**: 661–8.

25 Maclellan GE, Vyvyan B. Management of pain beneath the heel and Achilles tendonitis with visco-elasic heel inserts. *Br J Sports Med* 1981; **15**: 117–21.

26 Milgrom C, Giladi M, Kashtan H *et al*. A prospective study of the effect of a shock absorbing orthotic device on the incidence of stress fractures in military recruits. *Foot Ankle* 1985; **6**: 101–4.

27 Costill DL. Physiology of marathon running. *JAMA* 1971; **221**: 1024–9.

28 Basset DR, Howley ET. Limiting factors for maximum oxygen uptake and determinants of endurance performance. *Med Sci Sports Exerc* 2000; **32**: 70–84.

29 Morgan DW, Martin PE, Krahenbuhl GS. Factors affecting running economy. *Sports Med* 1989; **7**: 310–30.

30 Frederick EC, Howley ET, Powers SK. Lower oxygen demands of running in soft soled shoe. *Res Quart Ex Sport* 1983; **57**: 174–7.

31 Stefanyshyn DJ, Nigg BM. Influence of midsole bending stiffness on joint energy and jump height performance. *Med Sci Sports Exerc* 2000; **32**: 471–6.

32 Ker RF, Bennett MB, Bibby SR *et al*. The spring in the arch of the human foot. *Nature* 1987; **325**: 147–9.

33 Shorten MR. The energetics of running and running shoes. *J Biomech* 1993; **26**(suppl 1): 41–51.

34 Frederick EC. Kinematically mediated effects of sports shoe design. *J Sports Sci* 1986; **4**: 169–84.

35 McMahon TA, Valiant GA, Frederick EC. Groucho running. *J Appl Physiol* 1987; **62**: 2326–37.

DISCUSSION

Attendee: Do modern shoes prevent hyperpronation and consequently prevent problems such as shin splints and anterior knee pain?

Dr Martyn Shorten: We do not want to stop pronation as it is one of the body's natural cushioning mechanisms. The aim is to reduce the probability of excessive pronation, which is implicated in injuries. Shoes with stabilizing features reduce the measured pronation by a few degrees and, more importantly, reduce the rate at which the foot pronates. Experiments on injury prevention are difficult to carry out because it is ethically difficult to put athletes or experimental subjects into an environment where they are risking injury. In about 50–60% of cases of anterior knee pain or Achilles tendonitis, the use of a medial posting orthotic or of an appropriately designed shoe will relieve the symptoms.

Attendee: Different substances are used for cushioning in shoes, and different parts of shoes are cushioned with varying materials. Increasing cushioning does not necessarily mean that you are going to reduce the peak impact force — it can actually increase the speed of impact so that the peak forces are higher if cushioning is too much with certain materials. How much research do other manufacturers carry out and how much consideration is taken when looking at cushioning in different parts of the shoe?

Dr Martyn Shorten: You are correct. Soft material can only compress to a certain extent before it starts to bottom out. With a typical foam material, the densification occurs when the cell walls within the foam start to contact one another and the material starts to behave more like a solid material. The stiffness increases and the peak shocks on the impact test and in in vivo measurements will also increase. That has been known for a long time and properly designed shoes have stiffness in the cushioning adjusted so that does not happen. As we move into more regional cushioning systems, the first thing you do is to use pressure distribution information to calculate what stiffness of material you need in the different regions of the foot in order to stay within the limit of densification, so that that phenomenon that you are talking about does not occur.

Heat stress and related thermal disorders

DR WILLIAM O ROBERTS

MINNHEALTH FAMILY PHYSICIANS, WHITE BEAR LAKE, MINNESOTA, USA

'Emergencies' associated with runners who collapse during or immediately after road racing can vary from being fatal to easily reversible[1]. Cardiac arrest due to arrhythmia from coronary or congenital heart disease, hyponatraemia, exertional hyperthermia, hypothermia, exertional heat stroke (EHS) and exercise-associated collapse (EAC) are the usual causes of syncope or near syncope in the finish area and on the course.

Preventing 'emergencies' during the event is the responsibility of the race medical operation and the race administration. Primary interventions are the most effective means of decreasing casualties in road races, and require the race administration to define hazardous environmental conditions that pose a threat to the athlete's safety beyond the inherent risk of the running. Two common examples are high ambient temperature combined with high humidity and lightning. The race administration should develop contingencies for high-risk settings that include parameters for

Table 1 *Wet bulb globe temperature (WBGT)* cascades*

Temperature (°C/°F)	Flag	ACSM road race[2]	Military guide
<10/50	White	Increased hypothermia risk	
10/50 to 18/65	Green	Low risk of hyperthermia and hypothermia	
18/65 to 23/73	Yellow	Caution (hyperthermia risk moderate)	
23/73 to 26/78	Red	Extreme caution (hyperthermia risk high)	Caution for heat stroke
>28/82	Black	Extreme high hyperthermia risk; cancel or postpone	Discretion unseasoned — no heavy exercise
>30/85			Suspend exercise <3 weeks training
>31/88			Curtail <12 weeks hot weather training
>32/90			Suspend all training and exercises

* WBGT = 0.7 wet bulb (WB) + 0.2 black bulb (BB) + 0.1 dry bulb (DB)
ACSM = American College of Sports Medicine

cancelling, postponing or modifying the race (Table 1)[2]. This chapter will focus on heat stress, and the disorders related to heat stress and activity.

Body core and shell temperature measurement in the race medical facility

Definitions

For the purpose of describing heat transfer and distribution, the body can be divided into the core volume and the shell. The core is the central volume of the body encompassing the vital organs necessary for survival. At a minimum, it contains the brain, heart, kidneys, liver and central large vessels, and its average temperature is that of the blood in the central vessels. The core volume can expand to nearly the entire body as the central temperature rises and heat is conducted towards the surface of the shell. The skin is the outer level of the shell, which interfaces with the environment for heat exchange. The shell can include the skin, subcutaneous tissues, muscle mass and other noncritical tissues. It expands or contracts during centrally and peripherally controlled temperature regulation to either increase or decrease the insulation value of the shell, and preserves or expedites the transfer of body heat. The boundary between the core and the shell has no definite tissue demarcation and varies with the core and environmental temperatures. During and after exercise, the temperature difference between the core and the shell can be 5 °C (8 °F) in EHS and hyperthermia with the shell temperature in the normal range, while in cold conditions it may differ by as much as 20 °C (36 °F)[3].

Measurement methods

Core temperature during and immediately after exercise normally ranges between 36.5–40 °C (97–104 °F). The most reliable field core temperature measurement site is the rectum, which correlates with oesophageal temperature; both the diagnostic and treatment criteria for heat and cold injury are based on rectal temperature[3]. Other readily accessible field temperature measurement sites include the oral cavity, axilla and aural canal, all of which are attractive for modesty reasons. However, these measurement sites are biased by shell temperature and are, therefore, not very reliable[4].

The aural canal infrared temperature measurement devices (also referred to as tympanic membrane (TM) thermometers) have been popularized by advertizing campaigns based on the inaccurate assumption that TM temperature correlates well with hypothalamic temperature. The infrared temperature scanner device is generally a precise measurement tool, but it is not accurate in determining core temperature in sweating athletes because it detects aural canal temperature that is in the shell. The field use of the aural canal infrared thermometer in both hyperthermia and hypothermia often underestimates the core temperature by several degrees centigrade and can result in using the incorrect treatment protocol for a collapsed athlete[3,5]. The confusion surrounding aural canal and TM temperatures can be traced back to the original publications of Benzinger describing the method of measuring TM temperature. In 1959,

171

Benzinger first described the method of TM temperature measurement and stated that it 'may' reflect hypothalamic temperature[6]. He later said, in 1961, that 'TM is near the hypothalamus and shares a common blood supply with it from the internal carotid artery'[7] and, in 1969, the TM is 'located midway between the surface of the head and the sagittal midplane, close to the stem of the internal carotid artery (the mainline of blood supply to the brain including the thermoregulatory centers)...'[8].

The temperature gradient of the aural canal varies, with the highest temperature at the innermost locations of the canal, and may be adequate for estimating the tympanic temperature[9]. The external carotid artery, except for a small, minor terminal branch of the caroticotympanic artery of internal carotid artery origin, supplies blood to the TM; the TM is separated from the hypothalamus by several centimetres of bone and middle ear air. The TM is metabolically inert and heated by its blood supply, while the hypothalamus is a metabolic centre and is cooled by its blood supply. McCaffery demonstrated that TM temperature is influenced by facial temperature, and hypothalamic temperature follows the oesophageal temperature by simultaneously warming one side of the face while cooling the other side. He showed a concurrent increase and decrease of the respective ipsilateral TM temperatures with no effect on the oesophageal temperature[10]. The most convincing evidence came from Shiraki *et al* who showed that brain temperature followed the oesophageal and left ventricle core temperatures, while simultaneous tympanic temperature measurement followed the facial shell temperature by measuring concurrent brain, oesophageal and tympanic temperatures with body heating and face cooling[11]. Deschamps revealed that TM temperature is rapidly changed by skin temperature and may underestimate the extent of hyperthermia in athletes[5]. Rectal temperature is probably the highest temperature in the body after prolonged exercise. Use of this during athletic events will reduce the risk of accidentally missing EHS, although the true core temperature may be slightly lower[12]. Aural canal temperature measured by infrared temperature scanners will be less than core if sweat evaporation or a cold environment cools the face. The disparity between aural canal temperature and rectal temperature in EHS may reflect a functioning heat loss system that is overwhelmed by the intrinsic heat produced by muscle work during running. The athlete with a normal aural canal temperature may be inadequately treated if a rectal temperature is not measured[12].

Heat balance and heat stress

The mechanisms of heat exchange (ie conduction, convection, radiation and evaporation) transfer excess heat from the exercising athlete to the environment, and are discussed in detail in Dr Shirreff's chapter. Body heat is produced at rest and during exercise. The muscle energy efficiency during exercise is poor, with only 25% contributing to work, leaving the remaining 'waste' heat to be removed from the body. At rest, basal heat production is 70 kcal/h, which will increase body temperature by 0.8 °C/h if the excess heat is not dissipated. During moderate work, muscles produce heat at a rate of 200–350 kcal/h that will raise body temperature by 5 °C/h without normal dissipation of the heat energy; this would be similar to the heat load of running in a plastic suit. With intense work, the body can generate 1,000 kcal/h to cause a 15–25 °C/h increase in body temperature. Body temperature increases to higher levels in the same environment with faster race pace due to the increased muscle work and the resulting increased 'waste' heat[13,14].

Heat loss during activity is augmented by vasodilatation of surface vessels for heat exchange, by increased cardiac output for heat transfer from core to shell, and by increased sweat production and release for evaporative heat loss. When conductive, convective and radiant heat loss mechanisms become ineffective in temperatures >35 °C, heat transfer becomes dependent on evaporation. However, when evaporation is suppressed by high humidity, and exercise is continued, heat begins to accumulate in cells and tissues elevating the core body temperature.

Temperature regulation is under central control from temperature sensitive receptors in the preoptic hypothalamus, and peripheral control from temperature sensitive receptors in the skin[15]. Heat dissipation begins as heat storage in tissues induces the heat transfer system. Nonthermal components in temperature regulation include circadian factors relating to the time of day, and individual factors of absolute blood volume (hydration status), aerobic physical condition and heat acclimatization status that affect the athlete's ability to withstand heat stress. Temperature regulation and muscle work are in conflict during conditions that require heat removal from the body. Although cutaneous vasodilatation increases the demand for cardiac output and decreases effective blood volume available for exercise, working muscle and vascular volume take precedent for cardiac output resulting in a decrease in the effective volume available for heat transfer, causing body temperature to rise and allowing continued performance.

Pathophysiology of heat stroke

The energy depletion model of heat stroke can explain much of the pathophysiology encountered in an overheated athlete[16]. Excess heat accumulation in individual cells disrupts carbohydrate metabolism and energy pathways. The loss of energy in the cell induces malfunction of normal cellular operations and allows accumulation of intracellular heat. This in turn increases the transmembrane sodium leak, which leads to overuse of the energy dependent sodium-potassium pump and drains the cell of its remaining energy store. This produces loss of normal organ function, including the central nervous and cardiovascular systems, and results in rising core temperatures, loss of central thermoregulatory control, and pathophysiology of heat stroke. The central nervous changes due to cerebral cell hyperthermia produce the central nervous system (CNS) depression of heat stroke and can lead to coma. The most severe manifestation of EHS is hypothalamic failure that will result in anhidrosis and the central manifestations of 'classic' heat stroke. Cardiovascular collapse is due to decreased cardiac output from direct myocardial injury, volume depletion and peripheral vasodilatation. Rhabdomyolysis occurs when overheated muscle cells leak cell content into the circulation and cause damage to the kidney and other organs. Overheated intestinal cells may leak bacterial endotoxin into the circulation and produce the shock signs and symptoms common to heat stroke victims.

Running performance

Individual heat tolerance varies during exercise, and several marathon runners have had measured rectal temperatures of 42 °C without collapse[17]. There appears to be a general upper limit of rectal temperature to heat strain in fit, hydrated, acclimatized subjects, with nearly 100% discontinuing exercise at 40 °C rectal temperature and rare dropouts at <38 °C rectal temperature[17]. When the same subjects were hypohydrated to an 8% volume deficit, they stopped exercise at a lower core temperature with a reduced heart rate at exhaustion, and the exercise times were of shorter duration[17]. This indicates that hydration status influences performance in the heat, and it has been shown that a large fluid intake versus no fluid intake increases heat tolerance and decreases rectal temperature by 1 °C[18]. Dehydration is linearly associated with increased rectal temperature, decreased cardiac output and increased heart rate which are all physiological indicators of heat stress[18]. Sweat rates in athletes usually range from 1–2 l/h, and dehydration can occur rapidly during strenuous activity. Fluid replacement during activity is essential to optimize performance and thermoregulation. Some athletes have sweat rates in the 2–4 l/h range, which produces the 'heavy sweating' paradox where the maximum gastric emptying of 1–2 l/h limits fluid absorption and results in a large deficit in fluid replacement compared to sweat losses.

Running performance in the heat is slower with increased wet bulb globe temperature (WBGT)[14]. Whole body cooling before running improves performance in hot, humid conditions[19]. The optimum environment temperature for peak performance and lowest medical risk is in the 8–10 °C (45–50 °F) range, and the odds of requiring medical assistance increase above 12 °C (55 °F) in the marathon[20].

Adaptation to environmental heat stress

Athletes employ behavioural and physiological adaptation to heat stress. For instance, they will stop activity when training in hot conditions and will move to air conditioned areas when heat stress becomes uncomfortable. Normal behavioural responses are 'removed' or suppressed in athletic competition, so the safety of the competitive arena is the responsibility of the event administration. It is the duty of the event administration to modify or cancel events when confronted with hot, humid conditions that put the athlete at excessive risk for heat stroke.

Physiological adaptation to heat stress is called acclimatization and results in decreased heart rate, skin blood flow, sodium ion losses, core body temperature and perceived exertion, and increased plasma volume, sweating, earlier sweating and exercise tolerance time[21]. Acclimatization to heat occurs within 10–4 days of initial exposure and is at its maximum in eight to 12 weeks[21]. Induction of heat adaptation occurs more rapidly with increased training intensity, higher initial training level and greater maximal oxygen uptake[21]. Maintaining acclimatization requires daily heat exposure of half an hour and, if this is not possible, can be lost in a few days to weeks[21]. Replacing fluid losses to maintain normal expansion of plasma volume enhances acclimatization[21]. During heavy exercise loads, a salt intake of <3 g/day for the first three to five days of heat exposure reduces the acclimatization response and increases the risk of heat illness and, possibly, exercise-induced muscle cramps[21].

For optimum performance and safety in the heat, athletes should exercise in cool environments, choose the coolest part of the day to perform intense workouts, monitor hydration during activity, emphasize rehydration after activity, add extra salt in the first few days of heat exposure, and maintain daily heat exposure[21]. It appears, in the athletic setting, that cardiovascular stability is achieved in the first five days of heat exposure. Acclimatization is improved by training at >50% maximal oxygen uptake and can be induced with heavy clothing in cool environments[21].

Hyperthermia

Hyperthermia in athletes is defined by a core temperature >40 °C (104 °F) and can result in increased cell metabolism and destruction. The greatest risk for hyperthermia occurs when increased heat production in fast-paced races is combined with impaired heat dissipation in hot and humid environments[13,14]. The race administration should measure the environmental heat stress using an ambient temperature-relative humidity chart or the WBGT, and cancel the race if heat stress is in the dangerous range[2,22]. The WBGT is a combination of wet bulb (WB), dry bulb (DB) and black globe (BG) temperatures calculated using the equation: WBGT = 0.7WB + 0.2BG + 0.1DB. The relative risk based on WBGT is outlined in Table 1[2,23]. Hyperthermia risk is also increased in athletes who are hypohydrated, not acclimatized, salt depleted or older. In addition, those taking medications, supplements or recreational drugs that affect fluid and electrolyte balance, vascular tone, sweating, cardiac output or CNS function are at greater risk[24–6]. Skin disorders that cause sweat gland dysfunction, like sunburn, also affect heat dissipation[24]. Runners with exertional hyperthermia are often relatively 'asymptomatic' and specifically have no CNS signs of heat stroke. These athletes are treated like exercise exhaustion casualties with the addition of monitoring temperature and simple cooling measures[27].

Exertional heat stroke

EHS is a true medical emergency which occurs when endogenous heat production plus exogenous heat gain is greater than heat dissipation to the environment. Heat damage to cells and organs produces a multisystem disorder; complications include: seizure, rhabdomyolysis, renal failure, hepatic necrosis, lactic acidosis, disseminated intravascular coagulation, adult respiratory distress syndrome, cerebellar syndrome, cardiac damage (eg myocardial depression and myocardial infarction), immune system suppression and death[24,28]. Future heat intolerance risk is probably not increased in 80–90% of athletes who experience EHS[29], but the risk is increased with a family or personal history of malignant hyperthermia[30,31]. The mortality in road racing is very low, with isolated case reports in the lay press and medical literature. The 7.1 mile Falmouth Road Race in Falmouth, MA, US, is scheduled and run in moderate to high-risk heat conditions with a medical team trained for EHS care; no deaths have been reported in >200 EHS casualties (personal communication).

Diagnosis

The diagnostic criteria for EHS are a rectal temperature >40 °C (104 °F) associated with CNS dysfunction[29]. The clinical presentation is varied, and symptoms may include fatigue, impaired judgment, weakness, flushing, chills, hyperventilation and dizziness. Signs of CNS depression are the most important marker of this condition and include bizarre behaviour, loss of memory from the time of body temperature elevation, loss of lower limb function with unsteady gait, collapse, delirium, stupor, seizure and coma. If a seizure occurs in a race setting, cardiac arrest must immediately be excluded as a cause, and if the core temperature is normal, especially with a prolonged seizure, hyponatraemia should be excluded. The skin is usually sweaty in EHS, and its colour is ashen due to circulatory collapse. Use of dry skin as a screening marker for EHS will fail to recognize most EHS cases in athletes. Simple laboratory markers for field recognition are not available, but blood glucose, oxygen saturation, haematocrit and serum sodium may help with the onsite management and the decision to transfer care of the runner to an offsite emergency facility.

Treatment

The most effective and fastest field treatment for EHS is immediate body cooling by immersion in a cold 0–18 °C (32–65 °F) water tub — the cooling procedure should be integrated into the EAC protocol (discussed later)[27,29,32]. Immersion methods include trunk and limbs or trunk only placed into an ice water tub producing field body core cooling rates averaging 8 °C/h (17 °F/h)[27]. The hydrostatic pressure of immersion also improves blood pressure and functional cardiac output. If a tub is not available, alternative, but less effective and slower, cooling methods can reduce core temperature. These techniques include placing ice packs or ice water-soaked towels in the major body heat loss areas (eg neck, axilla and groin), sponging with wet, cold towels, or spraying atomized mist with fanning[27,33]. The rectal temperature should be monitored every five to 10 minutes during and after cooling therapy to check treatment effectiveness and to prevent overcooling. The endpoint for cooling therapy is 39 °C (102 °F) to minimize excessive cooling.

The athlete will require supportive care during the field treatment of EHS. One matter of particular concern is hydration during and after cooling. Dehydration is less likely in shorter races, and the hydrostatic pressure of tub immersion will usually augment blood pressure until the athlete can ingest oral fluids. In longer races, such as the marathon, intravenous (iv) fluids may be required. During the cooling process it may be prudent to limit the iv fluids to one litre in the first hour in the absence of severe dehydration signs[34–6]. The recommended fluid types are dextrose 5% and normal saline ($D_{5\%}$-NS), NS, dextrose 5% and one-half NS ($D_{5\%}$-½NS), or ½NS, although many medical teams stock only $D_{5\%}$-NS and NS out of concern for hyponatraemia. It is probably best not to use fluids containing potassium unless serum potassium is measured before administration of iv fluid[29]. Diazepam 1–5 mg iv push and/or magnesium sulphate 2–5 g iv push can be used to relieve muscle cramp and shivering, or to treat seizure[29,37]. Dantrolene sodium may also be effective for reversing muscle rigidity and decreasing heat production[38,39].

The prognosis for EHS is good if the athlete is treated with rapid cooling in the 'golden hour' (within one hour of onset), and athletes are often able to walk away from field treatment site without evaluation in another medical facility[40]. Prognosis is less assured if there is delayed recognition or deferred body cooling treatment prolonging the cell and tissue exposure to elevated temperatures.

Exercise-related exhaustion

Exercise-related exhaustion, commonly known as heat exhaustion, is defined as the inability to continue exercise and is the most common form of athlete collapse in the heat. It may be more related to exercise volume and intensity than exposure to heat as it occurs in cool environments and without an increase in core temperature. The frequency of exercise exhaustion seems to increase in hot conditions, probably due to the energy expenditure required for body cooling to maintain a normal core body temperature.

Classification

There are two classic descriptions of heat exhaustion: water depletion and salt depletion. Water depletion heat exhaustion is characterized by hypohydration symptoms including intense thirst, fatigue, impaired judgment, weakness, flushing, chills, hyperventilation and dizziness. Physical signs of water depletion exhaustion include rectal temperatures in the normal to 39 °C range, irritability, lethargy, muscular incoordination and oliguria. The presumed pathophysiology includes dehydration, peripheral blood pooling, decreased venous return and reduced blood flow to vital organs[34,41–5]. Ingesting oral fluids during activity prevents water depletion exhaustion. Salt depletion heat exhaustion is characterized by large volumes of sweat replaced by water alone and occurs most frequently in the first five to 10 days of activity in the heat[45]. Symptoms include weakness, frontal headache, anorexia, nausea, vomiting, diarrhoea and muscle cramps. These athletes do not report thirst, have no weight loss, and the clinical presentation resembles exercise-associated hyponatraemia. Body temperature is usually normal or lower than normal. Salt depletion exhaustion is prevented by consumption of salted fluids.

Treatment

The field treatment of exercise exhaustion includes water and salt replacement with oral or iv fluids as outlined in the EAC protocol. Muscle spasm can be controlled with neuromuscular inhibition techniques, salt replacement or the medications used in the heat stroke protocol for muscle contractions. Runners can usually return to full activity after rehydration and resolution of fatigue.

Exercise-associated collapse

EAC is a clinical classification and treatment system based on a three by three matrix for body temperature and symptom/sign severity at the time of collapse[41]. The presenting signs allow placement on the matrix based on normal or abnormal body temperature, CNS and mental status changes (eg unconscious, altered mental status and ambulation status), heart rate, leg muscle spasms, and extra fluid losses (eg vomiting and diarrhoea). The matrix allows rapid classification and expedites the treatment cascade during high-volume race medical triage situations. Temperature measurement is important, as symptoms do not always reflect body temperature. Most casualties have rapid recovery and discharge from the medical area.

Definitions and aetiology

EAC is defined as requiring assistance during or after endurance activity for full or near collapse. The matrix includes common causes of collapse such as EHS, exercise exhaustion, exercise-associated muscle (heat) cramps, heat syncope and hypothermia. EAC specifically excludes cardiac arrest, chest pain, insulin shock, asthma, anaphylaxis, seizure disorder, trauma, musculoskeletal problems and skin problems. The aetiology of EAC, other than the readily identifiable heat and cold related causes, is undetermined but is probably multifactorial. Several proposed mechanisms include a vasovagal response to discontinuing exercise, loss of the leg muscle pump augmenting blood return to the heart, dehydration, depletion of energy store with muscle fatigue, internal fluid shifts, temporary malfunction of temperature regulation, neural fatigue and CNS 'failure'[41–3].

The location of collapse can provide the first clue in the evaluation of the runner. For instance, collapse before the finish line increases the likelihood of cardiac arrest, EHS, severe hyponatraemia, insulin shock and anaphylaxis[42]. Collapse after the finish line will probably be due to EAC, although the other causes can precipitate collapse after the race has been completed[42]. The presenting symptoms are nonspecific and include: exhaustion, fatigue, feeling hot or cold, nausea, stomach cramps, lightheadedness,

Table 2 *EAC classification matrix*

	Severity of EAC		
	Mild	Moderate	Severe
Hyperthermic	T ⩾ 39.5 °C (103 °F)	T ⩾ 40.5 °C (105 °F)	T ⩾ 41 °C (106 °F)
Normothermic	97 °F < T < 103 °F	97 °F < T < 103 °F	97 °F < T < 103 °F
Hypothermic	T ⩽ 36 °C (97 °F)	T ⩽ 35 °C (95 °F)	T ⩽ 32 °C (90 °F)
Shared signs and symptoms	Any symptom or sign	No oral intake	CNS changes
	Walk with or without assistance	Extra fluid loss	Heart rate >100 bpm
	Heart rate <100 bpm	Unable to walk	
		Muscle spasm	
		Heart rate >100 bpm	

headache, leg cramps or palpitations. Downed or ill runners are placed in the classification scheme outlined in Table 2, where rectal temperature is measured at presentation and severity rating is based on body temperature, pulse rate and signs or symptoms common to all of the temperature classes.

Management

The management protocol for EAC is simple to follow and decreases the recovery time of collapsed runners, saving the most aggressive interventions for the more severe casualties. The initial step is diagnosis and documentation. Medical staff should initiate a medical record, similar to that shown in Figure 1. A standard medical form for a road race will allow medical staff to easily record presenting symptoms (ie vital signs including a rectal temperature, blood pressure, pulse and respirations), mental status and orientation, walking status, other physical examination findings, and treatment measures with a time log[3]. There are three main steps to treating EAC.

Fluid redistribution and replacement

A runner placed in the supine position with the legs and buttocks elevated will often recover without any other intervention. Oral fluid replacement is the safest means of restoring race losses and should be administered in all mild and moderate cases. Intravenous fluids may be needed in severe collapse cases, and in a few moderate collapse cases who do not respond to oral fluids or are unable to tolerate oral fluids. The recommended oral fluids are simple sugar-electrolyte drinks or water. The initial iv fluids contain $D_{5\%}$-½NS or $D_{5\%}$-NS, with the latter being the fluid of choice for races longer than four hours[37]. If glucose levels are high (>150 mg/100 ml (8.3 mmol/l)) after administration of the first litre of fluid, normal saline should be used for additional iv fluid replacement.

Intrinsic energy stores may be depleted after a long race and replacing the fuel supply appears to speed recovery of many collapsed runners. Oral glucose solutions should be offered to runners who are able to ingest fluids. The first litre of iv fluid should

Race Medical Form
Side one
TWIN CITIES MARATHON MEDICAL RECORD - CONFIDENTIAL   **1999**

Race # _____ Location: Finish / Aid Station Mile _____ **Arrival time** _____
Name _____ Age _____ Gender M / F **Discharge time** _____
Finish Time _____ Best previous time _____ Finished _____ Weekly Mileage _____
Previous marathons: Entered _____ Finished _____
Pre-race injury/illness: Yes / No Describe _____
Medical History

Symptoms:	Exhaustion	Fatigue	Lightheaded	Hot	Cold
Mobility:	Independent	Assistance	Wheelchair		
Mental Status:	Alert	Confused	Unresponsive		
Neuro symptoms:	Headache	Syncope	Weak		
Orientation:	Person	Place	Time		
Cardiac symptoms:	Chest pain	Tachycardia	Palpitations		
Resp symptoms:	SOB	Wheeze	Cough		
GI status:	Nausea Vomiting	Diarrhea	Stomach cramps		
Muscle cramps: Y / N	Location:	Calf	Thigh	Abdomen	Back
Skin:	Hot	Cold		Sweaty	Dry

Lab: O$_2$ Sat (ra) #1 _____ % #2 _____ % Na$^+$ #1 _____ #2 _____

Time	Temp (rectal)	BP	Pulse (R/Irr)	Glucose check	Meds/Rx

PO Fluids:
IV Fluids: **IV #1** 1L D$_5$NS   **IV #2** 1L D$_5$NS or NS   **IV #3** 1L D$_5$NS or NS
D$_{50}$W: #1 _____ #2 _____
Discharge status: Home   ER transfer   (ER Follow-up: Admit   Home)
Notes:

Diagnosis
EAC: Hyperthermic:Normothermic:Hypothermic - mild / mod / severe
Exercise Assoc Cramps   **Other:** _____
Signature: _____   **MD**   ©Wm Roberts MD

Side 2
Race # _____ Arrival Time _____ Discharge time _____
Skin, Bones, &Joints
Complaint: Pain Blister Abrasion Bleeding Swelling
Other
Tissue: Skin Muscle Tendon Ligament Bone
Other

Location:	Toe	R / L	Knee	R / L
	Foot	R / L	Thigh	R / L
	Ankle	R / L	Hip	R / L
	Calf	R / L	Back	R / L
	Other			

Diagnosis:	Blister	Abrasion
	Sprain	Tendinitis
	Strain	Stress Fx (suspected)
	Other	

Notes:

Treatment:	**Musculoskeletal**	**Skin**	**General**
	Ice pack	Prep	Fluids
	Compression	Lance	D/C instruction sheet
	Elevation	Bacitracin	
	Stretching	Dressing	
	Massage		
	Phys Rx		
	Other		

Treatment Refused

Signature: _____   **MD/DPM/RN/EMT**   ©Wm Roberts MD

Figure 1

Race medical form

contain 5% dextrose solution, and subsequent litres can continue to infuse dextrose if the blood glucose is not high. Blood glucose can be measured with a home glucose metre using blood from the toe or ear lobe, and dextrose 50% in water can be infused if the glucose is low, the response to iv hydration is slow, muscle cramps persist or if temperature correction is slow.

Temperature correction and maintenance

This intervention becomes the first priority when runners experience elevated rectal temperature combined with CNS changes. Most runners who seek or need medical aid will be normothermic and the challenge may be to maintain the normal core temperature[2].

Hyperthermic EAC can include EHS and requires immediate cooling measures. Runners with hyperthermic collapse should be moved to a cool or shaded area, any excess clothing must be removed, and active cooling strategies should be initiated for runners with rectal temperatures >40.5 °C (105 °F). Continued muscle contractions like shivering or seizure, that can produce intrinsic heat and slow core cooling, can be controlled with diazepam, magnesium sulphate or dantolene sodium (off label indications). Rectal temperature should be monitored every five to 10 minutes to assess the efficacy of treatment and avoid overcooling.

Hypothermic EAC casualties rarely have core temperatures <32 °C (90 °F)[2]. These casualties should be moved to a warm area, have wet clothing removed, have the skin dried and the body insulated with blankets (prewarmed if a portable clothes dryer, microwave or heating duct is available). The best field warming method is the use of a Barc Hugger™ external warmer, which circulates warmed fluid through a plumbed blanket that can be wrapped around the runner for heat exchange. Warm packs placed in the neck, axilla and groin using hot water bottles or warmed iv bags can also add heat to the body. Runners with rectal temperatures >35 °C (95 °F) can walk to generate intrinsic heat and raise the core temperature. External heating can be augmented with warmed, humidified air from a Bennett or Bird respirator. From our clinical experience in the medical treatment area at the Twin Cities marathon, some hypothermic runners respond with a faster warming rate after an infusion of iv dextrose 50% in water.

Discharge the runner from the race

The decision to transfer or discharge the EAC casualty is the final step in the care of the runner. Transfer to an emergency facility is the logical choice for a casualty not responding as expected to the usual treatment protocol, or for severe casualties who are not responding rapidly to medical intervention. In races where EHS is a common occurrence and the medical team is accustomed to treating it in athletes, the runners are often discharged if they meet predetermined criteria[33]. Races that rarely treat EHS may elect to have runners evaluated in an emergency facility after cooling therapy is completed on site. EAC casualties can be discharged from the race medical facility if they are clinically stable and normothermic, and they are instructed in fluid and

Table 3 *Number of Twin Cities marathon EAC casualties by temperature, classification and severity from 1983 to 1994*

	Mild (male/female)	Moderate (male/female)	Severe (male/female)	Total (% male/% female)*
No temperature recorded	*506 (405/101)*	*32 (21/11)*	*1 (1/0)*	*539 (38%/39%)*
Normothermic	192 (143/49)	59 (50/9)	3 (2/1)	254 (17%/19%)
Hypothermic	28 (16 /10)	16 (15/1)	2 (2/0)	46 (3%/3%)
Hyperthermic	6 (3/3)	7 (4/3)	10 (7/2)**	23 (1%/3%)

* % of injured male and female runners
** Gender not specified for one casualty

energy replacement and in re-evaluation criteria for a change in medical status. It is prudent to recommend a follow-up examination for severe casualties discharged from the race medical facility.

Data on EAC casualties in the Twin Cities marathon are summarized in Table 3[46]. In the first 13 years of the race, there were 81,277 entrants, 60,757 finishers, 1,459 medical encounters, 112 iv starts, 30 emergency room transfers, no hospital admission and one death. After medical evaluation and treatment, 98% of the finish line casualties walked away from the medical area[46]. Since 1994, there have been several severe hyperthermic collapses in two races with start temperatures >14 °C (55 °F). The most life-threatening form of EAC is the severe hyperthermic class, and onsite recognition and management will decrease morbidity and mortality.

Conclusions

EHS, exertional hyperthermia and exercise exhaustion can be prevented or lessened in most runners by applying the environment modifications stated in Table 1. Scheduling races at an appropriate time of the year, starting races early in the morning in warmer climates, providing fluids for hydration during the race, acclimatization of athletes before the race, and educating athletes and race volunteers about conditions that increase EHS risk will help prevent these disorders[2,23,47]. The EAC classification and management system will enhance the provision of care for runners in the finish area. It is best to treat runners with EAC and EHS on-site, transferring those who do not respond rapidly to the usual treatment protocols to an emergency facility. Recognition of EHS is important to the final outcome and should, therefore, be suspected in all collapsed runners. The race medical team should be aware of hyponatraemia as a cause of collapse, especially in slower runners who complete the marathon in more than four hours. The medical team should either be equipped to measure serum sodium on-site or be prepared to transfer the runners who may have the clinical presentation of hyponatraemia and do not respond to on-site treatment.

The future care of collapsed athletes will be enhanced by the technological advances in portable and easily used equipment that can withstand the rigors of field use bringing laboratory and intensive care capabilties to the race medical site. Computerized race timing and medical records will augment the ability to track injured runners in the medical system and to use the data for improved medical care and race safety.

References

1 Maron B, Poliac LC, Roberts WO. Risk for sudden death associated with marathon running. *J Am Coll Cardiol* 1996; **28**: 428–31.

2 American College of Sports Medicine. Position statement on heat and cold illnesses during distance running. *Med Sci Sports Exerc* 1996; **28**: I–vii.

3 Roberts WO. Assessing core temperature in collapsed athletes. *Phys Sportsmed* 1994; **22**: 49–55.

4 Brengelman GL. The dilemma of body temperature measurement. In: Shiraki K, Yousef MK, eds. *Man in stressful environments: thermal and work physiology*. Springfield: Thomas, 1987.

5 Deschamps A, Levy RD, Cosio MG *et al*. Tympanic temperature should not be used to assess exercise induced hyperthermia. *Clin J Sports Med* 1992; **2**: 27–32.

6 Benzinger TH. On physical heat regulation and the sense of temperature in man. *Proc Nat Acad Sci US* 1959; **45**: 645–59.

7 Benzinger TH. The human thermostat. *Sci Am* 1961; **204**: 134–47 *[is this the correct journal name?]*.

8 Benzinger TH. Clinical temperature. *JAMA* 1969; **209**: 1200–6.

9 Cooper KE, Cranston WI, Snell ES. Temperature in the external auditory meatus as an index of central temperature changes. *J Appl Physiol* 1964; **19**: 1032–5.

10 McCaffrey TV, McCook RD, Wurster RD. Effect of head skin temperature on tympanic and oral temperature in man. *J Appl Physiol* 1975; **39**: 114–8.

11 Shiraki K, Sagawa S, Tajima F *et al*. Independence of brain and tympanic temperatures in an unanesthetized human. *J Appl Physiol* 1988; **65**: 482–6.

12 Armstrong LE, Maresh CM, Crago AE *et al*. Interpretation of aural temperatures during exercise, hyperthermia, and cooling therapy. *Med Exerc Nut Health* 1994; **3**: 9–16.

13 Noakes TD, Myburgh KH, du Pliessis J *et al*. Metabolic rate, not percent dehydration, predicts rectal temperature in marathon runners. *Med Sci Sports Exerc* 1991; **23**: 443–9.

14 McCann DJ, Adams WC. Wet bulb globe temperature index and performance in competitive distance runners. *Med Sci Sports Exerc* 1997; **29**: 955–61.

15 Nadel ER. Recent advances in temperature regulation during exercise in humans. *Fed Proc* 1985; **44**: 2286–92.

16 Hubbard RW, Matthew CB, Durkot MJ, Francesconi RP. Novel approaches to the pathophysiology of heatstroke: The energy depletion model. *Ann Emerg Med* 1987; **16**: 1066–75.

17 Sawka MN, Young AJ, Latzka WA *et al*. Human tolerance to heat strain during exercise: influence of hydration. *J Appl Physiol* 1992; **73**: 368–75.

18 Coyle EF, Montain SJ. Benefits of fluid replacement with carbohydrate during exercise. *Med Sci Sports Exerc* 1992; **24**(suppl 9): S324–30.

19 Booth J, Marino F, Ward JJ. Improved running performance in hot humid conditions following whole body precooling. *Med Sci Sports Exerc* 1997; **29**: 943–9.

20 Crouse B, Beattie K. Marathon medical services: strategies to reduce runner morbidity. *Med Sci Sports Exerc* 1996; **28**: 1093–6.

21 Armstrong LE, Maresh CM. The induction and decay of heat acclimatisation in trained athletes. *Sports Med* 1991; **12**: 302–12.

22 Roberts WO. Environmental Concerns. In: Kibler WB, ed. *ACSM's handbook for the team physician*. Baltimore: Williams and Wilkins, 1996.

23 Barthel HJ. Exertion-induced heat stroke in a military setting. *Milit Med* 1990; **155**: 116–9.

24 Gardner JW, Kark JA, Karnei K *et al*. Risk factors predicting exertional heat illness in Marine Corps recruits. *Med Sci Sports Exerc* 1996; **28**: 939–44.

25 Knochel JP. Heat stroke and related heat stress disorders. *Disease-a-Month* 1989; May: 305–75.

26 Vassallo SU, Delaney KA. Pharmacologic effects on thermoregulation: mechanisms of drug related heatstroke. *Clin Toxicology* 1989; **27**: 199–224.

27 Armstrong LE, Crago AE, Adams R *et al*. Whole-body cooling of hyperthermic runners: comparison of two field therapies. *Am J Emerg Med* 1996; **14**: 355–8.

28 Lin JJ, Chang MK, Sheu YD *et al*. Permanent neurologic deficits in heat stroke. *Chin Med J (Taipei)* 1991; **47**: 133–8.

29 Armstrong LE, De Luca JP, Hubbard RW. Time course of recovery and heat acclimation ability of prior exertional heatstroke patients. *Med Sci Sports Exerc* 1990; **22**: 36-48.

30 Hunter SL, Rosenberg H, Tuttle GH *et al*. Malignant hyperthermia in a college football player. *Phys Sportsmed* 1987; **15**: 77–81.

31 Ogletree JW, Antognini JF, Gronert GA. Postexercise muscle cramping associated with positive malignant hyperthermia contracture testing. *Am J Sports Med* 1996; **24**: 49–51.

32 Costrini AM. Emergency treatment of exertional heat stroke and comparison of whole body cooling techniques. *Med Sci Sports Exerc* 1990; **22**: 15–8.

33 Brodeur VB, Dennett, SR, Griffin LS. Exertional hyperthermia, ice baths, and emergency care at The Falmouth Road Race. *J Emerg Nurs* 1989; **15**: 304-12.

34 Noakes TD. Dehydration during exercise: What are the real dangers? *Clin J Sport Med* 1995; **5**: 123–8.

35 O'Toole ML, Douglas PS, Laird RH, Hiller WDB. Fluid and electrolyte status in athletes receiving medical care at an ultradistance triathlon. *Clin J Sport Med* 1995; **5**: 116–22.

36 Seraj ME, Channa AB, Al Harti SS *et al*. Are heat stroke patients fluid depleted? Importance of monitoring central venous pressure as a simple guideline for fluid therapy. *Resuscitation* 1991; **21**: 33–9.

37 Laird RH. Medical care at ultra endurance triathlons. *Med Sci Sports Exerc* 1989; **21**(suppl 5): S222-5.

38 Bouchama A, Cafege A, Devol EB *et al*. Ineffectiveness of dantrolene sodium in the treatment of heatstroke. *Crit Care Med* 1991; **19**: 176–80.

39 Channa AB, Seraj MA, Saddique AA *et al*. Is dantrolene effective in heat stroke patients? *Crit Care Med* 1990; **18**: 290–2.

40 Roberts WO. Managing heatstroke: on-site cooling. *Phys Sportsmed* 1992; **20**: 17–28.

41 Roberts WO. Exercise associated collapse in endurance events: a classification system. *Phys Sportsmed* 1989; **17**: 49–55.

42 Holtzhausen LM, Noakes TD, Kroning B *et al*. Clinical and biochemical characteristics of collapsed ultramarathon runners. *Med Sci Sports Exerc* 1994; **26**: 1095–101.

43 Holtzhausen LM, Noakes TD. Collapsed ultraendurance athlete: proposed mechanisms and an approach to management. *Clin J Sport Med* 1997; **7**: 247–51.

44 Moore GE, Blair-Holbein ME, Knochel JP. Exercise associated collapse in cyclists is unrelated to endotoxemia. *Med Sci Sports Exerc* 1995; **27**: 1238–42.

45 Shearer S. Dehydration and serum electrolyte changes in South African gold miners with heat disorders. *Am J Ind Med* 1990; **17**: 225–39.

46 Roberts WO. A twelve year profile of medical injury and illness for the Twin Cities Marathon. *Med Sci Sports Exerc* 2000; **32**: 1549–55.

47 American College of Sports Medicine. Position statement on exercise and fluid replacement. *Med Sci Sports Exerc* 1996; **28**: i–vii.

Exercise in extreme environments

DR MICHAEL STROUD

SENIOR LECTURER IN MEDICINE & NUTRITION, CONSULTANT GASTROENTEROLOGIST,
INSTITUTE OF HUMAN NUTRITION, SOUTHAMPTON UNIVERSITY HOSPITALS TRUST,
SOUTHAMPTON, UK

Extreme environmental conditions can limit exercise performance, change fluid and nutrient needs, and lead to illness or injury. Despite this, increasing numbers of people are involved in athletic events or physically demanding expeditions in the hottest, coldest and highest places on earth. Table 1 shows examples of long-distance running events held under extreme environmental conditions, along with a few potential associated problems. This chapter will discuss the effect of extreme conditions on exercise, focusing on extremes of cold and altitude.

Extremes of heat

Two annual running events illustrate the capacity for men and women to run under conditions of extreme heat.

Table 1 *Examples of athletic events held in extreme environment*

Organized event	Environmental extreme	Nature of problems
Marathon of the Sands (Moroccan Sahara)	Temperatures up to 35 °C	Impaired exercise performance Dehydration Hyponatraemia
Badwater marathon (Death Valley, US)	Temperatures up to 50 °C	Heat exhaustion Heat stroke Sunburn
Antarctic marathon	Temperatures as low as −20 °C +/− strong winds	Impaired exercise performance Increased energy demands Altered substrate metabolism
Karrimor Mountain marathon (UK)	Temperatures as low as 0 °C +/− wind and rain	Frost injuries Nonfreezing cold injuries Hypothermia
Everest marathon	Starting altitude of 5,184 m Temperatures down to −10 °C	Impaired exercise performance Decreased oxygen availability Anorexia Pulmonary oedema Cerebral oedema

Marathon of the Sands

This is an annual race held in the Moroccan Sahara Desert during April. Temperatures range from 0 °C at night to a maximum daytime shade temperature of 30 °C; intense solar radiation adds to this heat stress. The race is run over a period of seven days and covers a distance of approximately 210 km in stages of between 20 and 86 km/day. Runners carry their own food supplies and camping equipment for the whole week, along with regularly replenished supplies of water of up to four litres at any time.

Clearly, in an event such as this, the problems of hyperthermia seen in more conventional marathon running are extreme. In general, they are countered in the same way as for normal events with additional care to ensure full pre-acclimatization. Since frequent drinks points are not available and, indeed, may be as far as 30 km apart, the risk of dehydration is very high. This is especially true on the longer days which may take many hours to complete. Most runners, therefore, carry pack-integrated systems that permit sips of fluid to be taken constantly while on the run in order to maximize absorption rates while minimizing gastric discomfort. Sunburn is another problem posed by the prolonged desert runs and many competitors choose to wear long, loose clothing rather than conventional running kit. Others rely on high factor sunscreens although even they wear hats with peaks and neck shades. Despite these measures, however, some runners still get sunburned, which puts them at additional risk of hyperthermia since areas of sun-damaged skin have defective sweating capability.

Studies on four runners revealed an average daily energy intake of 14.6 MJ consisting of 10% protein, 71% carbohydrate and 19% fat. Just over one-third of the total energy intake was derived from 5% carbohydrate 'sports' drinks used during running, or 6% carbohydrate drinks used for post-run rehydration/glycogen repletion. Both drinks had a sodium content of 25 mmol/l but additional 150 mmol sodium daily supplements were taken. Mean daily energy expenditures of the four subjects over the seven-day period, measured using double isotope-labelled water, ranged from 22.0 to 32.5 MJ while mean daily fluid intakes were 13.5 l, although this masked considerable inter-subject/inter-day variation. On the longest day, for example, one individual consumed 18.0 l in 24 hours and passed 2.4 l urine, whereas another consumed only 8.0 l and passed 1.8 l urine. The latter subject fell victim to heat stroke towards the end of the event. As all subjects had undergone training and an artificial acclimatization programme together, this suggests that variation in an individual's maximal sweating capacity may lead to unusual susceptibility to heat. Case reports of heat illness in members of the UK armed forces, when exercising at only modest levels within the UK, also indicate that some individuals are more prone to heat-related problems than others.

Badwater marathon

This is another hot climate, ultra-distance event, which is held annually in Death Valley, US, and attracts a field of more than 70 runners. The race covers a continuous 135 miles and the July summer temperatures can exceed 50 °C, with a minimum of 30 °C. It also ascends more than 4,500 m from the valley floor to a mountain peak.

Extremes of cold

Early humans and their predecessors dwelt exclusively in warm or hot climates until 5,000–10,000 years ago. Since then, humans have generally adapted poorly to cold, and vasoconstrictive responses to cooling may be inappropriate[1] as this leads to severe peripheral cooling, impairment of handgrip, and dangers of freezing or non-freezing cold injury. Hypothermia may also occur in relatively modest conditions, especially if wind and rain are added to environmental cooling power[2]. A wind speed of 40 km/h, for example, will make a still air temperature of 5 °C seem like –50 °C in terms of cooling power. Sensible behaviour, clothing and heat-generating hard work, however, allow people to undertake expeditions to the coldest of Polar and mountain environments. Marathons have also been held in Antarctica.

Thermoregulation in the cold

Under normal conditions, our thermoregulatory system aims to maintain resting core temperatures within circadian limits of 36 °C to 37.5 °C, and exercising core temperatures of up to 39 °C or even 40 °C. This regulation is achieved by a combination of behavioural and physiological changes that respond to both conscious assessment of the environment and sub-conscious hypothalamic monitoring[3].

Behavioural changes to cold include alterations in voluntary physical activity which may increase heat production from a resting 100 W to 1–2 kW. As a result, although it takes highly specialized (>5 clo) insulative clothing to keep warm when stationary at 5 °C, modest work levels will allow normal core temperatures to be maintained at –20 °C by clothing equivalent to normal office dress (1 clo). High levels of heat production with exertion also mean that stronger marathon runners are unlikely to suffer from hypothermia during the event itself, even when running in very cold conditions. Nevertheless, after cessation of exercise they may be at considerable risk in conventional marathon environments. During events held in more extreme circumstances, weaker runners may run into hypothermic difficulties while still running — this is likely to occur if they slow down later in the race. In events such as the Karrimor Mountain marathon, where threats from adverse weather are complicated by difficult terrain and problems of route-finding, the best of athletes may have to slow down or stop and all competitors are at risk of hypothermia out on the course.

When significant generalized cooling does occur, a number of physiological responses influence exercise performance and metabolism, resulting in overall impairment of function. A falling skin temperature causes an early increase in peripheral vasoconstriction, induced by both increased sympathetic adrenergic tone and direct cooling effects on peripheral arterioles[4]. The consequent decrease in skin blood flow reduces surface heat losses from conduction, convection and radiation, and maximizes the insulative value of skin and subcutaneous tissues including the outer layers of underlying muscle[5]. Unfortunately, these vasoconstrictive responses can also lead to limited circulation of blood to the hands and feet and consequent peripheral cooling with pain, loss of function and the risks of peripheral cold injury. This may be the limiting factor in an athlete's capacity for coping with exercise under cold conditions.

A cold environment also stimulates increased heat production from shivering, primarily triggered by decreases in skin temperature, although a fall in core temperature releases resting hypothalamic inhibition[5]. In contrast to voluntary muscular activity, shivering can only increase resting metabolic rate by about 500 W, but this will contribute to higher oxygen demands and some evidence suggests that severe cooling may influence substrate use in other ways (see below).

Exercise metabolism in cold environments

Exceptionally high levels of energy expenditure have been reported in studies of men on Polar expeditions in which cross-country skiing was combined with pulling heavy sledge loads. In 1992/93, two men attempted to ski across the Antarctica on a self-sustained expedition, each one towing a sledge with a starting weight of 222 kg. Exercise was performed for >10 h each day for 95 days in temperatures ranging from –10 °C to 55 °C. The men had planned a 23.5 MJ/day diet, but this was not always consumed for a variety of reasons. The final intake provided an average over the whole journey of 21.3 MJ/day, of which 56.7% was derived from fat, 35.5% from carbohydrate and 7.8% from protein. Although these intakes were high, both men lost more than 25% of their starting body weights. The losses led to marked debilitation towards the end of the journey[6].

During the expedition, energy expenditures were measured using both energy balance (EB) and isotope-labelled water ($^2H_2{}^{18}O$); isotope doses were taken on day 0 and day 50. For the first 50 days, both methods provided reasonable agreement with energy expenditures of 28.6 (EB) and 29.1($^2H_2{}^{18}O$) MJ/day in one subject and 38.3 (EB) and 35.5 ($^2H_2{}^{18}O$) MJ/day in the other. However, these average values masked exceptional levels for days 20 to 30 when the isotope data gave daily expenditures of 48.7 MJ and 44.6 MJ in respective individuals. Estimates of energy expenditure for the second part of the expedition were found to be much lower by both techniques[6].

These significantly high energy expenditures, sustained over such a long period, are unusual. They may simply be due to the increased levels of motivation involved in such expeditions; even the highest levels recorded between days 20 and 30 are credible since they correspond to the period when the heavy sledges were dragged uphill to the Antarctic plateau. They also fall short of the theoretical energy expenditure ceiling of 58.5 MJ/day that it has been calculated could be attained by ultra-long distance runners[7]. Nevertheless, it seems possible that they may be partly explained by thermoregulatory or other metabolic responses to cold.

Many studies of men working in the cold have concluded that heat production from the exercise is nearly always adequate to prevent need for any thermoregulatory additions; they have also shown that the observed 5–15% increases in the energy cost of tasks can be ascribed to the restrictive effect of Polar protective gear or the increased workloads entailed when walking or running on snow. However, some studies suggest that exposure to cold affects metabolic efficiency. For example, O'Hara et al reported that fat losses in men on an Arctic military exercise were much higher than anticipated[8] and were accompanied by persistent ketonuria. This could have been explained by a cold-induced switch from carbohydrate to fat utilization with some energy lost as ketones on the breath and in the urine. The same group followed up their observations with a study that demonstrated similar excessive fat losses for men living and exercising for 10 days in a cold chamber[9]. Interestingly, however, the excess fat losses observed took place despite normal subject core temperatures and only minimal falls in skin temperatures and, although not proposed by O'Hara et al, it seems possible that the findings of higher than anticipated energy use might reflect changes in exercise metabolism due to cooling of the face which is not so easily protected.

Riggs et al found slightly raised levels of oxygen consumption and lower respiratory exchange ratios (RERs) in men exercising with their faces exposed to a 6.5 m/s wind at 10 °C[10]. This is only moderate facial cooling compared to that of the Polar regions. Stroud examined exercise metabolism during more intense facial cooling[11], where men exercised on cycle ergometers at increasing work loads (0, 75, 100, 125 and 150 W) with and without the face exposed to a –20 °C wind. Although this resulted in significant decreases in facial temperatures, only small increases in oxygen consumption were reported, with the mean for all levels of exertion rising from 0.82 l/min to 0.86 l/min. There were, however, more marked changes in exercising RER which fell with facial cooling from 0.94 to 0.85. This indicates that intense facial cooling in isolation to whole body cooling may cause a switch in metabolism towards the utilization of fat, but even during extreme events, it is unlikely that lightly clad marathon runners will face such marked facial heat loss in the absence of more generalized chilling; under such circumstances, other studies suggest that a cold-induced switch towards carbohydrate metabolism is more likely.

Weller et al demonstrated such changes in a study in which subjects walked on a treadmill in either cold or thermoneutral conditions at exercise intensities of 60% maximal oxygen uptake (VO_{2max}) for two hours followed by 30% VO_{2max} for four hours[12]. With the higher rate of exercise, cooling caused lower skin temperatures but had no effect on core temperatures, heart rates, oxygen consumption, RER or lactate levels. However, during the lower rates of exercise, when levels of work were inadequate to provide sufficient spare heat, both skin and core temperatures were lower under cold conditions and there was an associated increase in both oxygen consumption and RER. Striking lactate accumulation also occurred under the cold conditions at exercise intensities, which would normally be considered to be much lower than the lactate threshold (Figure 1).

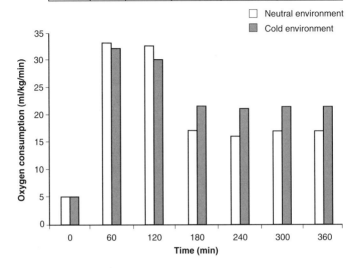

	High intensity			Low intensity	
	RER	Lactate		RER	Lactate
Neutral	0.9	1.2	Neutral	0.75	0.8
Cold	0.9	1.2	Cold	0.8	2.0

Figure 1

Changes in oxygen consumption, RER and lactate levels during higher (60% VO$_{2max}$) and lower (30% VO$_{2max}$) intensity exercise in normal or cold, wet and windy environments[12]

Other studies have demonstrated similar results[13,14] and it seems likely that these can be attributed to shivering occurring simultaneously with exercise during work in the cold, although there is considerable debate about substrate use by shivering muscle. Young *et al* reported that nutritional carbohydrate deprivation and consequent depletion of resting muscle glycogen levels does not affect shivering capacity in resting individuals, and hence argued that free fatty acids (FFAs) must be the most important substrates for shivering muscles[15]. He further supported this argument by highlighting that even violent shivering is equivalent to a work at a level of around only 30% VO$_{2max}$ and so the muscle use of FFAs would be analogous to the predominant use of these substrates during low-intensity exercise. Conversely, Martineau and Jacobs reported that glycogen depletion leads to a decline in shivering heat production at rest and argued that, since shivering does not involve all muscle units equally, some may be working at very high fractions of VO$_{2max}$ even if whole body oxygen consumption is only 30% of maximal[16]. Glycogen would therefore be expected to be the chief substrate in actively shivering units. The most likely explanation for these apparently opposing reports would be that Martineau and Jacobs' subjects were markedly thinner than those used by Young *et al* and hence were exposed to more intense cooling. As with exercise, low-intensity shivering probably uses fat predominantly, while higher intensities will use carbohydrate.

These findings suggest that endurance-type exercise in cold weather can lead to premature depletion of glycogen that could contribute to the onset of a fatigue/exhaustion/hypothermia cycle. Patton and Vogel reported a 40% decline in cycling time to exhaustion after subjects spent two days living and then exercising at –20 °C compared to 20 °C[14], and Bergh and Ekblom have shown a reduction in mean maximal aerobic capacity from 4.43 l/min at a normal exercising core temperature of 38.4 °C, to 4.33 l/min at 37.7 °C, 3.9 l/min at 35.8 °C and 3.75 l/min at 34.9 °C[17]. They also demonstrated a decline in dynamic muscular strength and peak muscle power output with pre-cooling[18]. Furthermore, marathon runners are usually lightly clad and are often thin individuals who will cool easily due to their increased surface to volume ratios, their reduced subcutaneous insulation, and the relatively low mass of their heat-producing muscle. Glycogen depletion may also contribute to the onset of hypothermia through an increased risk of hypoglycaemia that is known to impair the normal vascular and shivering responses to cold. This impairment is thought to be due to a central neuroglypenic effect on the hypothalamus[19].

Hypothermic illness

A progressive decline in function has been reported following the onset of hypothermia[20]. At 34–6 °C, hypothermic individuals are conscious of feeling cold and try to move around, add clothing or seek shelter to keep warm. Simultaneously, physiological defences are activated. Further temperature reductions are related to an increase in mental and physical problems, with some individuals becoming withdrawn while others exhibit aggression or disinhibition. Once temperatures fall to 33–4 °C, victims often stagger and become confused or drowsy. At this stage, 'paradoxical undressing' may also occur. This phenomenon is well described and is thought to be due to hypothalamic dysfunction with alteration of set-point temperature. Victims, therefore, think they are hot and appropriate behavioural and physiological responses disappear. Coma will ensue at temperatures varying between 26 °C and 32 °C, and cardiac output becomes inadequate to sustain life for prolonged periods between 17–26 °C. The risk of ventricular fibrillation is also high, but successful resuscitations of victims with core temperatures <15 °C have been reported[21].

General management of the hypothermic casualty is similar to that for a comatose or semi-comatose individual. Abnormalities in blood gases, pH, electrolytes and glucose are common, and pancreatitis or rhabdomyolysis are recognized complications. Accurate measurement of core temperature is surprisingly difficult and axillary, tympanic and oral temperatures can all be misleading; a low-reading rectal thermometer is best. Several re-warming methods are available. For example, warm blankets and hot drinks will suffice in many cases — although used widely in post-marathon events, metallized 'space blankets' are of no proven benefit. Warmed intravenous fluids are helpful and, in extreme cases, peritoneal warmed fluids or cardiac bypass can be used. Specialized equipment providing heated, humidified air also allows core re-warming. Hot baths are effective but may not always be safe since a paradoxical fall in temperature can occur as blood flow is rapidly restored to cold limbs. In general, if cooling was prolonged in onset or duration, re-warming must be undertaken with extreme caution and careful monitoring is vital. Blood volumes are often low due to early cold-induced diuresis followed by the inability of hypothermic kidneys to retain salt and water. Warming cell membranes are also extremely unstable and uncontrollable fluxes in potassium and other electrolytes may occur, although care must be taken in interpreting biochemical results from cold peripheral blood sampling. In critical cases, where rapid re-warming is needed, full resuscitation facilities must be available; safe defibrillation in the presence of water is impossible.

Non-freezing cold injury

Local temperatures of <12 °C prevent normal membrane pumping and paralyse nerve and muscle conduction[22]. This may result in permanent damage if such cooling is prolonged. Immersion in cold water is particularly likely to cause this type of damage and is, therefore, unlikely to occur in runners, although there have been reports of such damage from events held on snow and from orienteering type events where runners cross mountain and marsh. Long-term damage is likely whenever an anaesthetic, paralysed, cold region becomes hot, red, painful and swollen after re-warming and this change may take several days. Degeneration of nerve and muscle can then follow leading to prolonged anaesthesia, muscle contractures or inappropriate peripheral vascular control with intolerance to local heat or cold. There may be slow improvement over months or years.

Frostbite

Human tissues freeze at about –2 °C. Ice forms outside cells but the remaining extracellular fluid becomes hyperosmolar and severe intracellular dehydration occurs, which causes protein denaturation. Vascular endothelial cells are particularly vulnerable and, following re-warming of small blood vessels, may secrete plasma and become blocked by a red blood cell clot. Additional ischaemic necrosis is then superimposed on the frost damage[22].

Frozen tissues appear hard and white and are anaesthetic. Re-warming leads to pain and swelling often accompanied by blistering. Deep freezing results in irreversible necrosis but appearances can be misleading and early amputation of digits should be avoided. If still frozen, re-warming is best achieved rapidly by immersion in water at 40–2 °C, although any thawing should be avoided if refreezing is likely. Once thawed, treatment is similar to that used for burns with prevention of infection paramount. Generous analgesia is required.

Extremes of altitude

Every two years, runners participate in the Everest marathon which starts at 5,184 m near the Mount Everest base camp and descends to finish at Namche Bazaar at 3,446 m.

This race is preceded by an 18-day trek that allows time for altitude acclimatization — this is an essential feature because atmospheric oxygen concentration at the starting point is only 50% that at sea level. There is a risk of high altitude pulmonary or cerebral oedema, and extreme breathlessness is an inevitable problem for all runners. Most runners complete the course in twice the time usually taken for an event of the same distance but performed under more conventional circumstances. Competitors also face the threat of cold, local infective gastrointestinal tract upsets, and trauma to knees and feet from the difficult downhill terrain. All medical events are made more worrying by the isolation from proper facilities. The medical team even carries Gamow bags in which patients with severe acute mountain sickness can be manually repressurized[23].

A survey carried out in 1999 revealed that, among the 70 prospective runners, 65 consultations were reported for gastrointestinal upset before the race and 19 for cough, most of which were probably due to high altitude-related resetting of cough receptors [Buckler, personal communication]. Six runners suffered from altitude sickness before the race — five with symptoms of headache and nausea, and one with severe truncal ataxia and declining conscious level — but two were able to start the race after spending a few days at a lower altitude. One of the sufferers had onset of rapid atrial fibrillation, possibly related to the use of acetazolamide in treatment, and another withdrew for personal reasons. Two failed to complete the race due to exhaustion and, thus, there was an overall 90% success rate. Interestingly, resting pulse oximetry on 25 contestants measured a day before the race showed a mean oxygen saturation of 79% (range 73–87%).

References

1 Stroud MA. Heart of darkness. In: *Survival of the fittest*. London: Jonathan Cape, 1998: 122–50.

2 Pugh LGC. Accidental hypothermia in walkers, climbers and campers: report to the medical commission on accident prevention. *BMJ* 1966; **1**: 123–9.

3 Stroud MA. Environmental temperature and physiological function. In: Ulijaszek SJ, Strickland SS, eds. *Seasonality and human ecology*. Cambridge University Press, 1993: 38–53.

4 Keatinge WR, Harman C. *Local mechanisms controlling blood vessels*. San Diego: Academic Press, 1980: 37, Chapter 8.

5 Toner MM, McArdle WD. Physiological adjustments of man to the cold. In: Pandolf KB, Sawka MN, Gonzalez RR, eds. *Human performance physiology and environmental medicine at terrestrial extremes*. Benchmark Press, 1988: 361–99.

6 Stroud MA, Coward W, Sawyer M. Measurements of energy expenditure using isotope-labelled water during an Antarctic expedition. *Eur J Appl Physiol* 1993; **67**: 375–9.

7 Davies CTM, Thompson D. Aerobic performance of female marathon and male ultramarathon athletes. *Eur J Appl Physiol* 1979; **41**: 223–45.

8 O'Hara WJ, Allen C, Shepard RJ, Allen G. Loss of body fat during an Arctic winter expedition. *Can J Physiol Pharm* 1977; **55**: 1235–41.

9 O'Hara WJ, Allen C, Shepard RJ, Allen G. Fat loss in the cold — a controlled study. *J Appl Physiol* 1979; **46**: 872–7.

10 Riggs CE, Johnson DJ, Kilgour RD, Konopka RD. Metabolic effects of facial cooling in exercise. *Aviat Space Environ Med* 1983; **54**: 22–6.

11 Stroud MA. Effects on energy expenditure of facial cooling during exercise. *Eur J Appl Physiol* 1991; **63**: 376–80.

12 Weller AS, Millard CM, Stroud MA *et al*. Physiological responses to a cold, wet, and windy environment during prolonged intermittent walking. *Am J Physiol* 1997; **272**: R226–33.

13 Jacobs I, Romet TT, Kerrigan-Brown D. Muscle glycogen depletion during exercise at 9 °C and 21 °C. *Eur J Appl Physiol* 1985; **54**: 35–9.

14 Patton JF, Vogel JA. Effects of acute cold exposure on submaximal endurance performance. *Med Sci Sports Exerc* 1984; **16**: 494–7.

15 Young AJ, Sawka MN, Neufer PD *et al*. Thermoregulation during cold water immersion is unimpaired by low muscle glycogen levels. *J Appl Physiol* 1989; **66**: 1809–16.

16 Martineau L, Jacobs I. Muscle glycogen availability and temperature regulation in humans. *J Appl Physiol* 1989; **66**: 72–8.

17 Bergh U, Ekblom B. Physical performance and peak aerobic power at different body temperatures. *J Appl Physiol* 1979; **46**: 885–9.

18 Bergh U, Ekblom B. Influence of muscle temperature on maximal muscle strength and power output in human skeletal muscles. *Acta Physiol Scand* 1979; **107**: 33–7.

19 Gale EAM, Bennett T, Green JH, MacDonald IA. Hypoglycaemia, hypothermia and shivering man. *Clin Sci (Colch)* 1981; **61**: 463–9.

20 Hamlet MP. Human cold injuries. In: Pandolf KB, Sawka MN, Gonzalez R, eds. *Human performance physiology and environmental medicine at terrestrial extremes*. Indianapolis: Benchmark Press 1988: 435–66.

21 Southwick FS, Dalglish PH Jr. Recovery after prolonged asystolic cardiac arrest in profound hypothermia. A case report and literature review. *JAMA* 1980; **243**: 1250–3.

22 Granberg PO. Cold injury. In: Chant ADB, Barros D'Sa AA, eds. *Emergency vascular practice*. London: Arnold, 1997: 119–34.

23 Buckler D. Three miles high and one hundred miles from the nearest road. *Br J Sports Med* 1998; **3**: 262–3.

DISCUSSION

Dr Dan Tunstall Pedoe: A problem we have noticed in the London marathon is that runners stand inadequately clothed after the finish becoming extremely cold, even hypothermic, without apparently reacting by shivering. I gather there is some evidence that sub-clinical hypoglycaemia can prevent shivering?

Dr Michael Stroud: Ian Macdonald in Nottingham showed that if insulin is used to slowly reduce blood sugar, individuals can no longer shiver and thermoregulation fails. Of course, the symptoms of hypoglycaemia are very much identical to those of hypothermia, and I think hypoglycaemia is a significant factor in the development of hypothermia in some individuals. I even wonder whether it is a significant factor in the sort of hill-walking deaths sometimes seen in the UK, where people are thought to have died of cold alone but may have become hypoglycaemic after they had continued beyond fatigue and so become prone to hypothermia through their low blood sugars.

Dr William Roberts: Our experience at marathons in the US is similar. Runners finish and become hypothermic while standing around after the race. Our experience is that when their body temperatures are low, and we give iv dextrose 50 ml of 50% for a quick glucose load, they often recover quickly. We have tried to measure blood glucose with the home glucose monitors and give glucose to those with low glucose levels. That has helped speed the recovery process. On the other hand, we have also had runners who have become very hyperglycaemic after the finish, and do not recover quickly. By changing the iv solution to normal saline they recover faster. I think low blood sugar affects recovery and which came first, the hypothermia or the hypoglycaemia, is a difficult question.

Professor Ron Maughan: What is the situation at London? How quickly can you move people on after the finish and get them to their dry clothing rather than have them stand about and get cold?

Dr Dan Tunstall Pedoe: The biggest catastrophe that can happen to a marathon is for the finish to get clogged and dammed back so that people cannot reach the finish line and obtain their finishing time accurately; there are therefore lots of people moving the runners along. Runners go through the finish chutes and have about 400 or 500 yards before they reach the baggage buses. We used to have a problem when the finish was at County Hall — people used to sit for some time on the County Hall steps and chat with each other before they reached the baggage buses, and so we had to use loud speakers to tell them to move on and get their warm, dry clothing. They seemed to think that it was normal to sit around in a vest and pants in London weather, when 90% of the year that is not a normal thing to do because it is much too cold. We have less of a problem now with the finish in the Mall, but they still seem to take a long time to put their clothes on even after they have got them from the baggage area.

Sir Roger Bannister: In the Persian Gulf in the army just post-Suez, I saw a few cases in which there was sudden sweating failure and this was not recognized then as one of the variants of heat illness. Of course, once you have stopped sweating in that environment you are only minutes away from heat stroke. Can you comment on whether you have seen this in your studies at the end of marathons, and if you have what you think the cause is? One cause could be a viral, bacterial or other infection that was almost sub-clinical except under these circumstances, but it could also be physiological in some way due to derangement of the hypothalamic control.

Dr William Roberts: I think that once sweating ceases, the runner experiences problems and has moved beyond exertional heat stroke into a classic heat stroke with hypothalamic shut down. Does exertional heat stroke exist the way I defined it? I think it does. The reason I use that definition is so runners undergo treatment more quickly than occurs if you wait for them to stop sweating. I use this classification to speed the initiation of treatment to enable runners to reach normal core temperature as quickly as possible. Of the number of people I have seen with exertional heat stroke, only two had stopped sweating and fit the definition of classic heat stroke. I think, as you said, once you quit sweating you are very close to the more serious morbidity and mortality that occurs with classic heat stroke. So the key point for medical providers is to treat quickly and do not wait for sweating to cease. I also think the term 'heat exhaustion' is a misnomer, because athletes collapse in all environments with the same symptoms described for heat exhaustion. I prefer the term 'exercise exhaustion' as it seems to be the duration and intensity of exercise rather than the heat that causes the symptoms. I do not think that exercise exhaustion occurs more frequently in hot conditions due to the extra energy cost of cooling the body in the heat. The usual race environments that I work in are different and a lot less severe than in Saudi Arabia or that which Dr Stroud deals with in his challenges in the dessert.

Dr Michael Stroud: I am more than happy with the classification of exertional heat exhaustion, exertional heat stroke and classic heat stroke. I am sure heat stroke with cessation of sweating is caused by catastrophic failure of hypothalamic function probably at temperatures of 42 °C, but the temperature is probably variable in different individuals.

Dr William Roberts: I think also that once the brain starts to malfunction, its regions shut down at different rates — the hypothalamus shut-down in particular causes problems. We have had people measured at 44 °C (110 °F) who are still sweating but they do not know who they are, where they are or what they are doing. They need treatment quickly to decrease the risk of severe sequelae.

Professor Peter Raven: The living high, training low studies that Drs Levine and Stray-Gundersen performed demonstrated that most of the non-adaptors or non-responders to the altitude and training regimen were due to an iron deficiency, and specifically the women were less responsive to the adaptation process. Is there a dietary need which is gender-specific.

Professor Bengt Saltin: If you want to expand your total amount of haemoglobin, I would suggest the use of iron supplements.

Professor Ron Maughan: Would you recommend that even without assessing iron status and irrespective of starting iron?

Professor Bengt Saltin: Yes. I went to Bolivia, 5,260 m in the summer of 1998, where there were 16 Danish lowlanders. There was only normal elevation in haemotocrit and haemoglobin in those taking iron supplementation and they were well-fed Danes.

Dr Roger Wolman: Can anyone develop exertional heat stroke or does it only affect genetically susceptible individuals, such as those who get malignant hyperthermia with anaesthetic?

Dr William Roberts: I think people susceptible to malignant hyperthermia are so on a genetic basis, but anybody running hard enough in the right conditions can develop exertional heat stroke. I think there are probably individual variations in how susceptible an athlete is to heat stroke. Larry Armstrong's work shows people who have had exertional heat stroke, are re-stressed, but does not recur in about 80%. Finding those people who repeat and keeping them out of the races is probably the key. We have had runners at Falmouth Road race and at Twin Cities marathon with exertional heat stroke, who come back year after year to run. They automatically turn into the medical tent and get checked after each race and then they are fine. A young man ran as a bandit at Falmouth in one of the early years of the race and had a post-race temperature of >108 °F. He has been back almost every year without any problems. Falmouth is a short race, and I think there is a difference between the shorter races and the prolonged exertion in the army training or marathon racing. There is probably less heat stroke risk for people in longer, less intense events.

Morbidity and mortality in the London marathon

DR DAN TUNSTALL PEDOE

MEDICAL DIRECTOR OF THE LONDON MARATHON,
CONSULTANT CARDIOLOGIST, ST BARTHOLOMEW'S & HOMERTON HOSPITALS, LONDON, UK

The London marathon has been a major participant event since it was first run by 6,500 mainly novices in 1981 — it now has 32,000 finishers. Christopher Brasher ran in New York in 1979 and was so impressed by the New York marathon that he transferred the concept of a people's marathon (rather than a traditional British athletic club event that only attracted <200 athletic club members) to London and founded the event. This chapter will discuss various aspects of the London marathon, including entry, pre-participation medical advice and medical services provided on the day, but will focus on the related morbidity and mortality over the past 20 years.

Marathon entry

Entry for the current London marathon is open to anyone over 18 years of age and is not dependent on a certificate of medical fitness to compete. Entry can be by one of four routes.

- Entry is guaranteed for a specific number of elite athletes and some entries are allocated to athletic clubs and other institutions, such as the police force, which help with the organization. These guaranteed entries are about 3,000 in number.
- Charities can buy a 'golden bond' guaranteeing entries for a fixed number of runners prepared to raise money for the charity. These now comprise about 12,000 entries.
- Open entry selected by lottery — about 65,000 apply and 14,000 obtain places.
- Foreign entries and travel tour operators' entries comprise the rest.

There are associated wheel chair events and a children's three-mile mini-marathon.

Since 1981, the charity element has expanded significantly — many participants are not traditional runners but aim to complete the course as they have been sponsored by friends and colleagues to raise money for charity. A survey of runners and charities has revealed that 75% of participants in the 2000 race were raising money for charity and, between them, raised £20 m ($30 m) [Press statement released by David Bedford of the London marathon].

Table 1 London marathon advice sheet

MARATHON MEDICAL ADVICE FROM THE MEDICAL DIRECTOR

MEDICAL PROBLEMS

Discuss any medical problems with your general practitioner (GP). This advice supplements anything he or she says. See your GP if you have a problem that makes it a risk to run in a marathon. We are happy for people with serious medical conditions to run, but only with your GP's agreement and if you send me details of your condition and the treatment you are undergoing. Please send these to me and quote your running number when you know it. Address the envelope to me, mark it 'Confidential' and send it to: Flora London Marathon office, PO Box 1234, London SE1 8RZ.

If you have a medical problem that may lead to you having a blackout, such as fits or diabetes, put a cross on the front of your number and write the details, especially your medication, on the reverse of the number.

CARDIAC EVENTS AND SCREENING

Over the past 20 years, >430,000 runners have successfully completed the London marathon, but we have experienced five fatalities from heart disease (four from severe coronary heart disease) in runners apparently unaware that they had a problem. Their condition would have been detected if medical advice had been sought and relevant tests carried out. A 'fitness test' is not sufficient to detect these problems.

If you have a family history of heart disease or sudden death, or you have symptoms of heart disease ie chest pain or discomfort on exertion, sudden shortness of breath or rapid palpitations, see your GP who can arrange for you to have a proper cardiac assessment. As a cardiologist, I am aware that such an assessment may not be instantly available, but continuing to run with these symptoms may shorten your running career catastrophically!

TRAINING

Muscular aches and pains occur most commonly after an increase in training. Training should be increased gradually so that you do not suffer prolonged exhaustion and in-

Carbo loading

Do not change your normal diet drastically in the last week before the marathon, but decrease your intake of protein (meat and increase your intake of carbohydrate (pasta, bread, potatoes, cereals, rice and sweet things), especially for the last three days when you should also be markedly reducing your training. This loads the muscle with glycogen. Unless you reduce your protein intake you will not eat enough carbohydrate. (Not all runners are helped by first depleting carbohydrate with a long run and low carbo diet and then loading — this can make your muscles very heavy.)

CLOTHING

When training in the dark, be seen. Wear white clothing and reflective flashes or bandoliers.

In a recent London marathon, at least 50 people sought medical treatment for blisters at the start. They had either been training too hard in the final two weeks with ill-fitting shoes, or they had worn a new pair of shoes for the last long training run.

Use shoes you know from experience will *not* give you blisters.

ON THE DAY

Do not run if you feel unwell or have just been unwell, even if you are raising money for charity. Most medical emergencies occur in people who have been unwell but do not wish to miss the event. If you feel feverish, have been vomiting, have had severe diarrhoea or any chest pains, or otherwise feel unwell, it is unfair to you, your family, your sponsoring charity and the marathon support staff to risk serious illness and become a medical emergency. You are unlikely to do yourself justice. There are many other marathons.

Wear appropriate clothes for the weather. On a cold, wet day you can become very cold if you reduce your running pace or walk. A hat and gloves will prevent heat loss and are easily carried. If it is hot, wear loose mesh clothing, start slowly and, if possible, run in the shade.

tersperse days of heavy mileage with one or two days of lighter training, so that your body can replace its fuel (muscle glycogen). Rest days are also important.

If you have 'flu, a feverish cold or a tummy bug, do not train until you have fully recovered. Then start gently and build up gradually. Do not attempt to catch up on lost mileage after illness or injury — this may cause further damage or illness. To reduce injury risk, train on soft surfaces when you can, especially on easy training days. Vary routes; do not always use the same shoes and run on differing cambers, hills, etc. Always face oncoming traffic, especially in the dark.

Note: if you cannot run 15 miles comfortably one month before the marathon, you will not manage it in safety or enjoy it. Please do not run on this occasion.

FLUIDS

Fluids lost in sweat must be replaced otherwise your body becomes dehydrated and less efficient. Alcoholic drinks are dehydrating. A pint of beer produces more than a pint of urine; spirits have a worse effect. Take plenty of non-alcoholic drinks, especially before the race and in hot weather. Thirst is a poor guide to how much you need. Drink enough to keep your urine copious and a pale straw colour. Drink plenty of liquids after training, especially long runs, and drink during races, especially in the first half of a marathon. Practice drinking during longer training runs. Drink plenty of fluids and reduce alcohol intake in the two days before the race.

DIET

Eat what suits you! Large doses of supplementary vitamins and minerals (such as iron) are not essential and produce no benefit if you are on a good mixed diet, but additional vitamin C in small doses is reasonable when fresh fruit and vegetables are in short supply.

Training helps you to sustain a high level of muscle glycogen if you eat a lot of carbohydrate. If you can, eat within two hours of your long runs and the marathon. This helps replace the muscle glycogen quickly and speeds recovery.

Do not be greedy and pour bottles of drinking water over yourself; you may be depriving slower runners of much needed drinks. If it is hot, extra water will be provided and showers set up on the course — use these to cool yourself.

Start the race well hydrated (urine looks pale) and drink whenever you can, especially in the first half of the race when you may not feel thirsty, as you lose a lot of fluid 'insensibly'. This will help you feel better late in the race and may prevent cramp. Cramp is most common in runners who have not trained sufficiently or are dehydrated. Do not gulp large volumes of liquid during or after the race. It is possible to become ill from drinking too much, too quickly.

AT THE FINISH

Do not stand about getting cold. Keep walking, especially if you feel dizzy, and drinking to replace lost liquid. Go to the baggage area as soon as you can, use the baggage system, change into warm, dry clothing, and then go to the reunion area. Foil blankets will not stop you from becoming cold. Keep on drinking and have something to eat. Some runners feel faint more than half-an-hour after finishing the race, often because they have taken insufficient fluid at the finish and/or not eaten anything.

FINALLY

Train sensibly. Follow this simple advice and you will probably not need medical aid. St John medical aid posts are located about 50–100 m past the drink stations and after the finish line. If you drop out, go to an aid station or to the nearest underground station — you can travel free to the finish if you show your running number.

Keep this advice and refer to it nearer the day and on marathon eve.

Dr Dan Tunstall Pedoe FRCP DPhil
Race medical director

Medical advice sheet

Entrants are sent a medical advice sheet[1] which gives them the responsibility of being fit and well on the day of the race. It suggests that they discuss with their general practitioner any medical problems that may make it hazardous for them to run, and that they do not participate if they have such a problem without their agreement. It also suggests that they surrender their entry if they cannot run 15 miles (24 km) comfortably one month before the event. Runners who take advantage of this facility for the 'sick, lame and lazy' are guaranteed entry the following year. The medical advice sheet has been widely copied by other races and has been refined. The most recent version is shown in Table 1.

Organization of medical services

The St John Ambulance Brigade — a voluntary, primarily first aid organization — arranges, in association with the race medical director and the London marathon administration, >40 first aid posts along the route and at the finish, and two field hospitals at the finish. One of these hospitals has an 'intensive care unit' for more serious collapses, but intravenous fluids may be given at other sites if necessary.

There is a much larger first aid post in the Isle of Dogs, which is two-thirds of the way around the course. There are also cardiac units at the finish and automatic electric defibrillators (AEDs) along the course and at the finish, with >1,000 St John Ambulance first aid workers, nurses, doctors and paramedics who all volunteer for a long day's work. In addition to St John Ambulance staff, non-St John doctors, physiotherapists and podiatrists with an interest in sports medicine are recruited for the day by the race medical director, chief physiotherapist and chief podiatrist, and work closely with St John, principally at the finish.

Communications

The staff is divided into 15 geographical sectors and is able to communicate and liaise with senior staff at designated receiving hospitals by radio and mobile and land line telephone. These hospitals are pre-warned about the race and receive written advice from the race medical director during the preceding week of the race, and have St John race liaison officers posted to their accident and emergency departments on the day.

Collection of medical statistics

A runner who makes contact with the aid facilities during the race is logged as a 'casualty contact' and a marathon casualty card, using the runner's race number, is completed for subsequent analysis. Diagnosis is made by the first aid staff unless the condition receives medical, physiotherapy or podiatric treatment, in which case the card is completed by the relevant practitioner. Each first aid station reports the numbers of casualties and the primary diagnosis.

Types of casualty

To minimize newspaper headlines such as 'One in five runners casualties in marathon' when many of the problems were trivial, a small working party suggested a classification of race day contacts which made the seriousness of each condition more evident[1]. The classification divides casualty contacts into:

- social contacts — who stop and ask for, eg, a drink, shoelace, dressing, or petroleum jelly to treat themselves
- musculoskeletal contacts — with cramps or painful joints, bones or muscles
- topical contacts — with blisters, abrasions, runner's nipple, groin or axillary skin chafing, or subungual haematomas
- constitutional contacts — who collapse, have chest or abdominal pain, diarrhoea, fits, or vomit etc.

The St John Ambulance reports are supplemented by enquiries to the designated receiving hospitals, which are requested to flag up all marathon accident and emergency cases and record their race numbers.

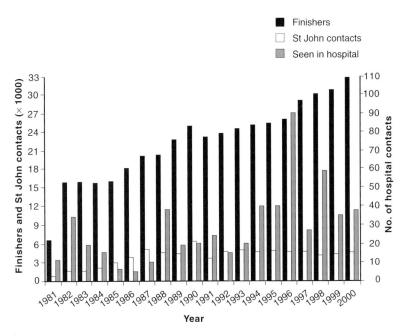

Figure 1

Number of people who completed the London marathon, and St John and hospital accident and emergency contacts (1981–2000)

Morbidity and mortality statistics

In 2000, 32,600 runners completed the race, and 4,633 St John Ambulance and 38 hospital contacts were recorded (Figure 1). In comparison, 19,970 runners completed the race in 1987, when there were 4,984 St John Ambulance contacts and 10 hospital contacts. Totals for the 20 years show a casualty contact rate of 0.13% (one in 787). Hospital admissions are roughly one in 10 of the hospital contacts, but are increasingly difficult to define as runners may spend some hours in accident and emergency. A breakdown of the diagnoses for 1987 classification contacts is shown in Figure 2a, with the constitutional casualties subdivided into their St John Ambulance diagnoses (Figure 2b). In 1991, 24 hospital cases were reported, of whom one was admitted (Figure 3).

Only those deaths or collapses leading to death that occur during the marathon or within the finish area of the race are considered marathon deaths. Five cardiac deaths have been reported in the London marathon, four from severe coronary heart disease (in 1991, 1994, 1995 and 1997) and one with hypertrophic cardiomyopathy (HCM) in a 39-year-old man (in 1990) [personal communication]. Five successful cardiac resuscitations have taken place (in 1983, 1988, 1990, 1997 and 1998); all patients had coronary heart disease and were subsequently discharged from hospital [personal communication].

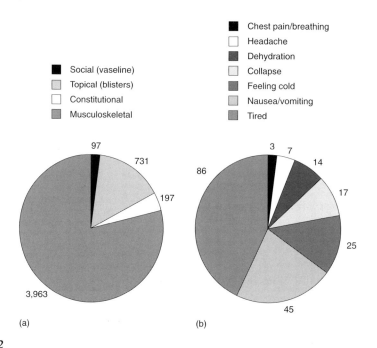

Figure 2

(a) Breakdown of diagnoses for classification contacts in the 1987 London marathon

(b) Breakdown of constitutional casualties for 1987 diagnoses

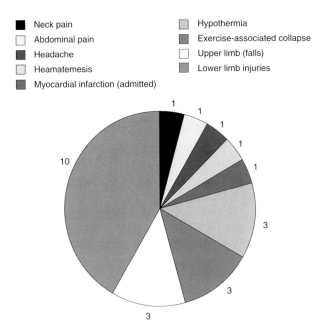

Neck pain
☐ Abdominal pain
■ Headache
☐ Heamatemesis
■ Myocardial infarction (admitted)

☐ Hypothermia
■ Exercise-associated collapse
☐ Upper limb (falls)
■ Lower limb injuries

Figure 3

Hospital accident and emergency contacts (24 with one admission) in the 1991 London marathon

In the millennium race, a young man collapsed at the finish complaining of neck pain and rapidly developed severe pulmonary oedema. He was intubated and ventilated, and evacuated to hospital where he had a computed tomography (CT) brain scan which was interpreted as showing a subarachnoid haemorrhage. He died the following day after withdrawal of ventilatory support. The overall mortality rate from the 20 years is one in 74,140 or roughly one death for each two million miles run.

Discussion on these figures

The medical director of the race is updated on the casualty contact numbers and the numbers taken to hospital by the St John Ambulance Brigade. The director can check the more serious medical problems at hospitals designated to receive casualties from the race. However, unless specifically notified, he will not be aware of casualties who bypass the race casualty control system and go to other hospitals, or of those who arrive at the designated hospitals later in the day without wearing running clothes and a race number and, thus, not being recorded as race casualties.

The more attractive, obvious and frequent the aid points are in a marathon, the more likely a tired, cramping, blistered runner will make a 'pit stop' and become a marathon medical statistic. Some races offer psychotherapists at the start and massage therapists at the finish, which increases the potential for collecting casualty numbers. Definition of an injury and the numbers are, therefore, contentious. Most runners suffer from minor injuries such as cramps, blisters, skin chafing and subungual hae-matomas. The medical staff may be unaware of many of these injuries, especially as the successful runners are euphoric, anxious to go home, and probably convinced that they can handle the problems themselves. The staff loses contact with participants immediately after the race as the runners disperse across the UK and to several other countries, taking their non-immediate medical problems to a multiplicity of doctors and physiotherapists. This makes a survey of the impact of the marathon on medical providers even more difficult than that for a questionnaire to runners.

The sports medicine definition of an injury as something that prevents training for a defined number of days is impossible to apply when severe muscle stiffness is almost universal and full training may not be part of the runner's post-race agenda. Aches and pains and severe delayed onset muscle stiffness are common after a marathon, and may only be appreciated as significant injuries if they fail to subside in the follow-ing two weeks. Some runners may experience severe pain for days after a marathon race when walking up or down stairs.

Deaths occurring during or shortly after a marathon are naturally blamed on the event, particularly by the media, but may in fact be random and possibly unrelated. For ex-ample, a known epileptic ran the London marathon, went home, suffered a fit in his bath while nobody was in the house, and drowned. If the fit was an unlikely event, precipitated by running the marathon, it could legitimately be blamed on the race; however, without knowing the frequency of the fits, whether or not the man had taken his medication and other factors, the culpability of the marathon is indirect.

Another runner died in his sleep 36 hours after completing the marathon. He had told his wife how well he had felt during and after the marathon. He went swimming the next day, but his wife was awakened by him having a terminal anoxic fit that night. He was found to have HCM at post mortem. A claim was made in the press that the marathon caused his death, and it is conceivable that a lingering biochemical or endocrine effect of prolonged exertion precipitated a fatal cardiac arrhythmia. This raises many questions, eg for how long after a marathon can the run itself be blamed for death in the presence of a lethal condition that can kill at any time? Deaths in HCM can occur at any time and an infrequent or unusual event may be blamed as the cause. Epileptic fits may occur in close proximity to running the marathon, and a statistical analysis of fit frequency and the total number of epileptics running the marathon would be needed to draw sound conclusions. If HCM has an incidence of 1 in 500[2], and people with this condition are not inhibited from running, it can be calculated that about 1,000 runners with this condition have run the London mara-thon and only one has died during the race.

Use of questionnaires

Questionnaires have been used to assess marathon morbidity in locally based mara-thons but cannot be applied to major international races. They have a notoriously poor return. For example, a small survey of British doctors running the London marathon in 1996 showed that <20% returned a questionnaire after the race, making invalid the finding of a low percentage reporting upper respiratory tract infections in the week after the marathon [personal communication]. The anticlimax and fatigue following completion of a marathon appeared to militate against completing and returning a questionnaire.

Qualifying remarks on statistics

The statistics (eg total number of runners, number of St John Ambulance contacts, and diagnoses) included in this chapter are based on data collected at the time of each marathon, show some discrepancies and are open to question.

Total participant numbers

The number of runners actually participating in a race of this size (≤34,000) is not easily verified. There are accepted entries, registrants, and people who start and finish. The entries outnumber the total people accepted; 25% follow the medical advice sheet and, having developed a medical problem, decide not to run. They have the inducement of guaranteed entry for next year's race and, thus, do not need to subject themselves to the lottery which only selects about 25–50% of entries. Many runners who register in the week before the race do not attend on race day. Of those who do reach the start point on race day, a few drop out along the route. This varies from 2–5% of the people who start.

In addition to the genuine race entrants, there are a certain number of 'bandits' who may have excellent replicas of the official race number. Runners in most of the London marathons have the bar code on their race number that is read at the beginning and end of the race. Unfortunately, this is not infallible. In the past three races, electronic chips have been attached to the runners' shoes, which should provide an accurate record of starters and finishers of the race. However, the width of unencumbered road surfaces over which they can be read makes their use at the start problematic.

The numbers of runners included in this chapter are usually those declared as finishing the race to the press on the evening of the marathon. The race organizers subsequently correct this figure after verification of the finishers and disqualification of runners with false numbers and the few who have taken short cuts, but this is only a minor correction and does not influence the statistics significantly.

St John Ambulance casualty contacts

These totals are the numbers declared the day after the marathon, once St John Ambulance has had returns (hopefully) from all station crews who disperse over much of southern England after the race. This number is sometimes subsequently corrected and discrepancies may occur when spectators are included in some returns and not in others. The total number of runners who make contact with the medical first aid posts may, if they outnumber the first aid provision, be under-reported as treatment may take priority over reporting if a first aid post becomes swamped.

Accurate reporting of race casualties also becomes a problem where, like geriatric patients, the fallen runner may have more than one diagnosis, eg exercise-associated collapse, plus blisters, plus subungual haematoma, plus groin chafing, but is only reported under the presenting complaint of collapse. A further complication is that the same runner may make contact with more than one aid station, making pit stops for 'repairs' at several and being counted as a fresh casualty or contact at each point. The multiple reporting error was assessed in one marathon and found to be a minor source of error in the grand total.

Hospital cases

Collection of information concerning runners seen in hospital is complicated by patient confidentiality. Press enquiries, sometimes masquerading as relatives or medical personnel, have made some hospitals wary about enquiries even from the marathon medical director. A further study is being mounted of hospital contacts and admissions.

Diagnoses

Casualties are assessed rapidly by first aiders and only very few are seen by trained diagnosticians. The diagnoses are, therefore, anatomical rather than accurate, where pain is the prime complaint. A painful shin may be a fatigue fracture, but there is usually no easy follow-up. Exercise-associated collapse (EAC) may be registered under a variety of names, eg hypothermia, dehydration, hyperthermia, collapse, and severe fatigue even in hospital cases.

Conclusions

The London marathon is a mass marathon with open entry, not requiring medical certification. Medical support is provided mainly by the St John Ambulance Brigade which mans >40 aid posts, but is supplemented by volunteer doctors, physiotherapists, podiatrists and designated hospitals.

Marathon medical statistics are based on data collected on the day of the race by the St John Ambulance and returns from the hospitals designated by the London ambulance service to receive marathon casualties. Race day statistics include many trivial problems such as blisters and muscle cramps, which are probably under-reported but even so give a high contact rate compared with other marathons[3]. More serious constitutional problems are accurately reported provided they become apparent during the race or within the confines of the finish area. The approximate overall risks of running the London marathon are contact with St John, one in six, with a hospital accident and emergency deparment one in 800, hospital admission one in 10,000, and death one in 74,000. The risk of death is comparable to many daily activities (see Dr Tunstall Pedoe's chapter on *Marathon myths and marathon medicine*)[4].

References

1 Tunstall Pedoe DS, ed. Popular marathons, half marathons and other long distance runs; recommendations for medical support. *BMJ* 1984; **288**: 1355–9.

2 Maron BJ, Gardin JM, Flack JM *et al.* Assessment of the prevalence of hypertrophic cardiomyopathy in a general population of young adults. Echocardiographic analysis of 4,111 subjects in the CARDIA study. Coronary artery risk development in (young) adults. *Circulation* 1995; **92**: 785–9.

3 Roberts WO. A 12 year profile of medical injury and illness for the Twin Cities marathon. *Med Sci Sports Exerc* 2000; **32**: 1549–55.

4 Tunstall Pedoe DS. Sudden cardiac death in sport-spectre or preventable risk. *Br J Sports Med* 2000; **34**: 137–40.

Sudden death in sports and the marathon

DR BARRY MARON

DIRECTOR, HYPERTROPHIC CARDIOMYOPATHY CENTER,
MINNEAPOLIS HEART INSTITUTE FOUNDATION, MINNEAPOLIS, MINNESOTA, USA

Sudden deaths of competitive athletes are personal tragedies with great impact on the lay and medical communities[1] — they are mainly due to a variety of usually unsuspected cardiovascular diseases[2-19] and occasionally low-energy chest blows[20]. Such events often assume a high public profile because of the widely held perception that trained athletes constitute the healthiest segment of society and that cardiovascular fitness suggests the absence of cardiac disease; the occasional deaths of well-known elite athletes have exaggerated this visibility[1,21]. These athletic field catastrophes have also increased interest in the role and efficacy of pre-participation screening for the detection of cardiovascular disease in young athletes[22].

Road racing and marathon running have become popular competitive sports activities in many parts of the world, including the US and UK, and involve many older individuals. The high participation levels have raised questions and concerns about the causes and frequency of sudden cardiac death during these sporting events. There has been much interest regarding sports in general, and distance running in particular, as well as the recent public health initiatives on physical activity and exercise[23]. This chapter will discuss the causes of sudden deaths in athletes, focusing on marathon runners.

Definitions and general considerations

The competitive athlete can be defined as one who participates in an organized team or individual sport requiring systematic training and regular competition against others, while placing a high premium on athletic excellence and achievement[19].

Eligibility/disqualification guidelines for competitive athletes are predicated on the probability that intense athletic training is likely to increase the risk for sudden cardiac death (or disease progression) in trained athletes with clinically important and underlying structural cardiovascular disease, although it is currently not possible to quantify the risk with precision. Sudden death in young athletes most commonly occurs during athletic training or competition[2-6]. These observations support the proposition that physical exertion is an important trigger for sudden death, given the presence of certain underlying cardiovascular diseases. The early detection of clinically significant cardiovascular disease through pre-participation screening can, in many instances, allow timely therapeutic interventions that may prolong life[24].

208

Table 1 *Cardiovascular abnormalities in 134 young competitive athletes with sudden death*

Primary cardiovascular lesions	Number of athletes	% of athletes	Median range
Hypertrophic cardiomyopathy (HCM)	48	36	17 (13–28)
Unexplained increase in cardiac mass ('possible HCM')	14	10	17 (14–24)
Anomalous coronary arteries	17*	13	15 (12–23)
Other coronary anomalies	8	6	17 (14–40)
Ruptured aortic aneurysm	6**	5	17 (16–31)
Tunnelled LAD	6	5	17 (14–20)
Aortic valve stenosis	5	4	14 (14–17)
Consistent with myocarditis	4	3	15 (13–16)
Idiopathic dilated cardiomyopathy	4	3	18 (18–21)
ARVC	4	3	16 (15–17)
Idiopathic myocardial scarring	4	3	20 (14–27)
Mitral valve prolapse	3	2	16 (15–23)
Coronary artery disease	3	2	19 (14–28)
Other congenital heart abnormalities	2	1.5	13 (12–15)
Long QT syndrome	1***	0.5	–
Sarcoidosis	1	0.5	–
Sickle-cell trait[†]	1	0.5	–
'Normal' heart	3[††]	2	18 (16–21)

* including anomalous origin of: left main coronary artery from right sinus of Valsalva, right coronary artery from left sinus of Valsalva, left main coronary artery with acute-angled take-off, and LAD coronary artery from pulmonary trunk

** the Marfan syndrome was present in three athletes with ruptured aortic aneurysm and in one athlete with mitral valve prolapse
LAD=left anterior descending coronary artery; ARVC=arrhythmogenic right ventricular cardiomyopathy

*** also had anomalous origin of right coronary artery from left sinus of Valsalva

† judged to be the probable cause of death in the absence of any identifiable structural cardiovascular abnormality

†† absence of structural heart disease on standard autopsy examination

Causes of sudden death in young athletes

A variety of cardiovascular abnormalities represent the most common causes of sudden death in competitive athletes[2–19]. The precise lesions responsible differ greatly with age. For example, in youthful athletes (<35 years old), most lesions are due to a number of congenital cardiac malformations (Table 1)[2–14]. Virtually any disease capable of causing sudden death in young people may potentially do so in young competitive athletes. It should be emphasized that, although these cardiovascular diseases may be relatively common among young athletes dying suddenly, they are uncommon in the general population. Also, lesions responsible for sudden death do not occur with the same frequency, with most responsible for ≤5% (Figure 1). In the US, such deaths occur most commonly in intense team sports, such as basketball and football, which also have high levels of participation.

Hypertrophic cardiomyopathy

The most common cardiovascular abnormality among the causes of sudden death in young athletes is hypertrophic cardiomyopathy (HCM), usually in the non-obstructive

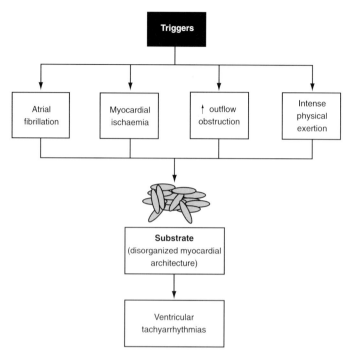

Figure 1

Proposed mechanism by which sudden cardiac death may occur in athletes with hypertrophic cardio-myopathy

form[3–5,8,11,12,14,25–8] and accounting for about 35% of athletic field deaths (Table 1)[3]. It is a primary and familial cardiac disease, characterized morphologically by a hyper-trophied and non-dilated left ventricle, but with heterogeneous expression[29], com-plex pathophysiology and diverse clinical course. More than 100 disease-causing mutations in nine genes encoding proteins of the cardiac sarcomere have been reported[28,30–5], including in β-myosin heavy chain, cardiac troponin-T and troponin-I, α-tropomyosin, essential and regulatory light chains of myosin, actin, and cardiac myosin-binding protein C and titin. HCM is a relatively uncommon malformation occurring in about 0.2% of the general population[36].

It is not uncommon for HCM to be responsible for sudden cardiac death in young and asymptomatic individuals, and it has been shown to occur frequently during moderate or severe exertion[3,4,21–3,31] — the stress of intense training and competition (and associated changes in blood volume, hydration and electrolytes) undoubtedly increases the risk to some degree[23]. Strenuous physical activity, in particular, may act as a trigger mechanism in HCM for generating potentially lethal ventricular tachyar-rhythmias (Figure 1), given the underlying electrophysiologically unstable myocar-dial substrate comprised of replacement fibrosis (which is probably the consequence of ischaemia) and disorganized cardiac muscle cell arrangement (Figure 1).

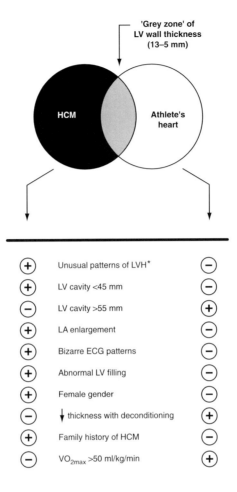

Figure 2

Chart showing criteria used to distinguish HCM from athlete's heart when the left ventricular (LV) wall thickness is within the shaded grey zone of overlap, consistent with both diagnoses

Redrawn and reproduced with permission[40].

* May involve a variety of abnormalities, including heterogeneous distribution of left ventricular hypertrophy (LVH) in which asymmetry is prominent, and adjacent regions may be of different thicknesses, with sharp transitions evident between segments. Also, patterns in which the anterior ventricular septum is spared from the hypertrophic process and the region of predominant thickening may be in the posterior portion of septum or anterolateral or posterior free wall, or apex.

Disease variables that may identify individuals at high risk of HCM include[30,31,37,38]:

- previous aborted cardiac arrest or sustained ventricular tachycardia
- family history of a sudden or other premature HCM-related death (or identification of a high-risk genotype)
- multiple repetitive or prolonged non-sustained ventricular tachycardia on ambulatory Holter electrocardiogram recordings
- exertional syncope, particularly when recurrent and related to exertion in the young

- massive degrees of left ventricular hypertrophy (≥30 mm for maximum wall thickness)
- hypotensive blood pressure response to exercise.

HCM patients predicted to be at high risk for sudden death should be considered for primary prevention of sudden death with prophylactic cardioverter-defibrillator implants[39]. One recent study showed a 5% annual discharge rate in high-risk HCM patients receiving implantable defibrillators for the primary prevention of sudden cardiac death[39].

Although HCM may be suspected during pre-participation sports evaluations by the previous occurrence of exertion-related syncope, family history of HCM or premature cardiac death, or presence of a heart murmur, these features are relatively uncommon among all individuals affected by the disease[22]. Consequently, screening procedures limited to customary history and physical examination cannot be expected to identify HCM reliably and consistently. Findings from 10% of hearts from young athletes dying suddenly are reminiscent, but not diagnostic, of HCM. In these cases the heart weight and left ventricular wall thicknesses are increased and the ventricular cavities non-dilated, but there are no other clinical or morphological features consistent with HCM (or other specific forms of heart disease). Thus, the disease responsible for death in these athletes remains unresolved.

HCM and the athlete's heart

It may be difficult to distinguish young athletes with segmental ventricular septal thickening (13–5 mm), consistent with a relatively mild morphological expression of HCM, from those with the physiological and benign form of left ventricular hypertrophy that represents an adaptation to athletic training (ie 'athlete's heart')[40]. Athletes within this morphological 'grey zone' represent an important and not uncommon clinical problem in which differential diagnosis between HCM and athlete's heart can often be resolved by non-invasive testing (Figure 2)[40]. This distinction may have particularly important implications, given that young athletes with an unequivocal diagnosis of HCM are discouraged from participating in most competitive sports to minimize risk, with the exception of those sports considered to be of low intensity, such as golf[41]. Conversely, the improper diagnosis of cardiac disease in an athlete may lead to unnecessary withdrawal from athletics, thereby depriving that individual of the varied benefits of sports.

Congenital coronary anomalies

Several congenital coronary anomalies cause sudden death in young athletes, mainly those of wrong aortic sinus origin, which account for about 20% of deaths[3]. The most common of these lesions appear to be anomalous origin of the left main coronary artery from the right (anterior) sinus of Valsalva (Figure 3)[42–4]. The mirror image malformation, anomalous right coronary artery from the left aortic sinus, has also been incriminated in these catastrophes[43]. Such malformations are difficult to recognize clinically because they are not usually associated with symptoms (eg exertional

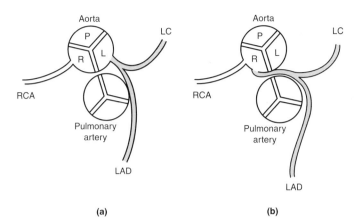

Figure 3

Congenital coronary artery anomalies capable of causing sudden death in young athletes: (a) normal anatomy; (b)anomalous origin of the left main coronary artery from the right (anterior) sinus of Valsalva. The left coronary artery may have a separate ostium from or common ostium with the right coronary artery (RCA), which also arises from the right (R) sinus of Valsalva. Note the acute leftward bend of the left main coronary artery at its origin and it posterior course between the aorta and pulmonary trunk. LAD=left anterior descending coronary artery; LC=left circumflex coronary artery; P=posterior (noncoronary) cusp; L=left

syncope or chest pain) or changes in the 12-lead or exercise electrocardiogram[44]; consequently, clinical diagnosis requires a high index of suspicion that may be raised with two-dimensional echocardiography[44-7]. Individuals with these coronary malformations should be excluded from intense competitive sports in order to reduce the potential risk of a cardiac event[23]. Wrong sinus anomalies are amenable to surgical correction with bypass grafting, which is the most common approach to restore distal coronary flow[43,44,46]. However, congenital coronary artery malformations cannot be reliably identified by standard screening for participation in athletics.

Myocardial ischaemia in young people with coronary artery anomalies involving wrong sinus origin probably occurs in infrequent bursts, cumulative with time, and ultimately resulting in patchy myocardial necrosis and fibrosis[44]. This process could predispose to lethal ventricular tachyarrhythmias by creating an electrically unstable myocardial substrate. Potential mechanisms that have been advanced include acute angled take-off and kinking or flap-like closure at the aortic origin of the coronary artery, or compression of the anomalous artery between aorta and pulmonary trunk during exercise. Furthermore, the proximal portion of the artery may lie intramural (ie within the aortic tunica media), which could further aggravate coronary obstruction, particularly with the aortic expansion during exercise.

Other very uncommon coronary anomalies relevant to sudden death in young athletes include: hypoplasia of the right coronary and left circumflex arteries; left anterior descending or right coronary artery origin from pulmonary trunk; virtual absence of the left coronary artery; spontaneous coronary arterial intersusception; and coronary artery dissection[3–5,14].

Coronary artery disease

Atherosclerotic coronary artery disease may be responsible for sudden death during physical exertion in youthful athletes[2,5–8,14,48,49], and may be associated with acute plaque rupture[49]. Corrado *et al* have emphasized the occurrence of premature athero-sclerotic coronary disease as a prominent cause of sudden death in young people (including some competitive athletes) in the Veneto region of north-eastern Italy[48]. The disease is usually confined to the left anterior descending coronary artery and is due to obstructive fibrous and smooth muscle cell plaques in the absence of acute thrombus. Atherosclerotic coronary artery disease, as well as HCM, was found to be the leading causes of death in a study of sports-related sudden deaths not limited to competitive athletes[2].

Myocarditis

Myocarditis is an acknowledged cause of sudden death in young athletes, even with-out previous symptoms; however, definitive diagnosis may be difficult clinically, par-ticularly in the healed phase[41]. The importance of myocarditis as an aetiology for sudden death in the young may have been exaggerated in the past due to either over-interpretation of histological data[50] or the lack of standardized morphological crite-ria[51]; others have suggested that this diagnosis is now probably underestimated[52]. Myocarditis can be missed at routine autopsy examination; however, diagnosis can now be verified by direct analysis of the viral genome[53]. In a large autopsy based series of 134 competitive athletes, only 6% showed areas of myocardium with acute inflammatory changes consistent with acute myocarditis[3], or areas of idiopathic myo-cardial scarring possibly representing healed myocarditis. The inflammatory process of myocarditis is usually triggered by several viral agents, often enterovirus but also adenovirus[54]; chronic cocaine use may provoke a similar clinical and pathological profile[55].

Myocarditis does not necessarily require permanent withdrawal from competitive ath-letics. Athletes should, however, undergo a prudent convalescent period of about six months after the onset of clinical manifestations, and should be allowed to return to competition when ventricular function and cardiac dimensions have returned to nor-mal and when clinically relevant arrhythmias are absent on ambulatory monitoring and stress testing[41].

Intramural coronary arteries

It remains unresolved whether or not the presence of short (1–3 cm) segments of the left anterior descending coronary artery, tunnelled and surrounded by left ventricular myocardium (ie myocardial 'bridges'), constitute a potentially lethal anatomical variant responsible for sudden and unexpected death in otherwise healthy young individuals during exertion[56,57]. Some believe muscle bridges produce critical systolic arterial narrowing and residual diastolic compression, resulting in myocardial ischaemia; in one report, this abnormality even increased the risk for cardiac arrest in young patients with HCM[57]. Short-acting β-blockers may alleviate anginal symptoms and ischaemia by increasing the luminal diameter of tunnelled coronary segments and normalizing flow velocities — this suggests myocardial bridges may have pathophysiological significance[58]. Nevertheless, coronary blood flow occurs mainly during diastole. Furthermore, necropsy studies have frequently documented tunnelled coronary arteries in patients who had not died suddenly, or had died of chronic non-cardiac diseases[3].

Aortic rupture and Marfan's syndrome

Young athletes may die suddenly due to rupture of the aorta[2–5,14], some also with the physical stigmata of Marfan's syndrome, in whom disruption of the aortic media with reduced numbers of elastic fibres is usually evident at autopsy (ie cystic medial necrosis). Certain individuals with Marfan's syndrome may participate successfully in strenuous competitive sports for many years without experiencing a catastrophic event, presumably before aortic dilatation becomes significantly marked and predisposition for dissection or rupture increases critically. Aortic dilatation is the primary determinant of whether or not athletes with Marfan's syndrome should be judged medically ineligible for competition[23].

Valvular heart disease

Aortic valvular stenosis is not a particularly common cause for sudden death in young athletes[2–6,14], although older hospital-based studies suggest that it causes sudden unexpected death frequently in children and young asymptomatic adults[50]. This may be due to the fact that aortic stenosis is likely to be identified early in life, even during pre-participation screening, by the characteristically loud heart murmur, thereby leading to disqualification from competitive sports[22,23]. Despite its relative frequency within the general population (probably 2–4%)[59], mitral valve prolapse appears to be a particularly uncommon cause of morbidity or sudden death in young competitive athletes[23,59,60].

Cardiac conduction system abnormalities

A spectrum of congenital or acquired abnormalities confined to the cardiac conduction system (in the absence of other structural cardiac abnormalities) has been regarded as the occasional cause of sudden death, presumably by producing heart block and bradyarrhythmias[61–3]. These include malformations of the atrioventricular conduction tissue, such as accessory atrioventricular pathways, or morphologically abnormal small intramural arteries of the sinoatrial node or atrioventricular nodes with thickened vessel walls and narrowed lumen. Such vascular abnormalities have been incriminated as determinants of sudden death and myocardial ischaemia as a result of tissue degeneration, scarring and haemorrhage in surrounding conducting tissue.

Arrhythmogenic right ventricular cardiomyopathy

Arrhythmogenic right ventricular cardiomyopathy (ARVC) is an unusual, often familial, condition that may be associated with important ventricular or supraventricular arrhythmias, and has been cited as a cause of sudden death in young people, including athletes[6,64–6]. It is characterized morphologically by myocyte death in the right ventricular wall and replacement by fibrous or adipose tissue as part of a repair process, often associated with myocarditis and evidence of programmed cell death. This disease process may be segmental or may diffusely involve the right ventricle. In several autopsy studies of sudden death in young athletes, ARVC is shown to be uncommon[2–5,11–4]. One exception is reports from the Veneto region of Italy where ARVC is the most common cause of sudden death in young competitive athletes[6,24]; this may be due to either a unique genetic substrate or the long-standing Italian national screening programme for competitive athletes[67] which has probably identified and disqualified more athletes with HCM than with ARVC[24].

Dilated cardiomyopathy

A small number of athletic field deaths in young athletes have been attributable to the dilated form of cardiomyopathy, with marked ventricular cavity enlargement. These unusual cases appear to have been completely sub-clinical before the sudden and unexpected death. Such events have raised concern that the particularly marked physiological ventricular cavity enlargement observed in some highly trained athletes (left ventricular end-diastolic dimension $\geqslant 60$ mm in about 15%)[68] may ultimately have deleterious consequences and predispose in some way to a premature cardiac event. At present, however, there is no definitive evidence to support such a scenerio. On the other hand, preliminary findings from deconditioning studies in former highly trained elite athletes demonstrate a substantial (although incomplete) decrease in cavity size after several years of detraining. The fact that these cavity dimensions often fail to return to the normal range leaves open the question of whether or not training induced ventricular cavity enlargement is a completely physiological and benign clinical finding.

Apparently normal hearts

Occasionally, no evidence is found of structural cardiovascular disease in athletes dying suddenly, even after careful examination of the heart. These cases account for about 2% of athletic field deaths[3], and it may not be possible to definitely exclude non-cardiac factors, such as substance abuse[55,69]. Such deaths may also be due to occult conduction system disease[9,61–3], clinically unidentified Wolff-Parkinson-White syndrome, or rare conditions in which structural cardiac abnormalities are characteristically lacking at necropsy ie idiopathic ventricular fibrillation[70] and long QT[28,71], Brugada syndromes[72], or unrecognized segmental ARVC[65].

General considerations for older athletes

Older athletes (>35 years of age) may also harbour occult cardiac disease and die suddenly and unexpectedly while participating in intense, often competitive, athletic activities. Unlike youthful athletes, the cause of death in older conditioned athletes is usually atherosclerotic coronary artery disease. Occasionally these deaths may also be due to diseases unrelated to atherosclerosis, ie HCM or valvular heart disease[11,41,73].

Older trained athletes who have died suddenly of coronary heart disease, reported in several necropsy based investigations, comprise a heterogeneous athletic population including competitive runners and recreational joggers, as well as participants in sports such as rugby, squash and golf[11,15–8,49,74–6]. Most of these deaths occur during or immediately after physical activity. In contrast to young competitive athletes, many older athletes who have died of coronary heart disease had known risk factors, cardiovascular symptoms or previous myocardial infarction, with severe coronary artery involvement (atherosclerotic narrowing of two or three major extramural coronary arteries) and myocardial scarring.

Prevalence of sudden death

The frequency of sudden unexpected death due to cardiovascular disease in young athletes during competitive sports appears to be low, occurring in about one in 200,000 individual student athletes per academic year[77,78] and in one in 70,000 over a three-year high school career[77]. In comparison, older athletes have higher rates of exercise-related sudden death, reported to be one in 50,000 marathon competitors[76] and about one in 15,000 joggers per year[16]. Considering such a relatively low prevalence, the intense public interest in sudden deaths in athletes is perhaps disproportionate to the actual numerical impact as a public health problem. However, the emotional and social impact of athletic field catastrophes remains high because the competitive athlete, to much of the lay public and physician community, intuitively represents the healthiest element of society[1,78–80].

Demographics of sudden death

Data from broad-based US populations have provided a profile of young competitive athletes who died suddenly[2–5,11,14]. These athletes had participated in many sports, the most frequent of which was basketball and American football, probably reflecting the relatively high participation level in these team sports as well as their intensity; in Italian studies, the most common sport associated with sudden death is football (soccer)[6,63]. About 90% of athletic field deaths occurred in men, mainly of high school age[3,4]; however, others had achieved collegiate or even professional levels of competition.

Most athletes who incur sudden death, regardless of their underlying disease, are free of symptoms during their lives, with their underlying cardiovascular disease completely unsuspected. Sudden collapse has been linked to exercise occurring on the athletic field, mainly in the late afternoon and early evening hours corresponding to the peak periods of competition and training, particularly for organized team sports[3]. These observations confirm that, in the presence of certain structural cardiovascular diseases, physical activity represents a trigger and an important precipitating factor for sudden death on the athletic field[3,78].

Risk of sudden death associated with the marathon

Road racing of 5 km and 10 km distances and the marathon have become immensely popular sporting activities, particularly in North America and western Europe. A growing proportion of the general public takes part in long-distance running, which often includes thousands of competitors on a given day. There is a wide age range of marathon participants; in some races, >50% of runners are 40 years or older. Marathon racing can, thus, be regarded as an organized master's level sporting activity[81]. However, as a result of the nature of the sport and the large number of participants, there is generally little in the way of systematic pre-participation screening for cardiovascular disease available for marathon competitors.

Few data are available on the frequency of cardiovascular events and sudden deaths directly attributable to participation in the marathon. One study assessed the prevalence of sudden cardiac death in athletes competing in two long-standing annual events — the Marine Corps (Washington DC, 1976–94) and Twin Cities (Minneapolis, MN, 1982–94) marathons — held over a cumulative 30-year period[76]. A total of 215,413 runners completed the two races; this represented about 75% of the starters. The average age of participants was 37 years, and 82% were men. Four exercise-related sudden deaths occurred, each due to unsuspected structural cardiovascular disease and all without warning (Figure 4). Three of these deaths occurred during the race at 15–24 miles, and the other took place 15 minutes after completion of the race; the latter athlete had experienced chest pain after running 20 miles but, nevertheless, completed the race. Three sudden deaths were due to atherosclerotic coronary artery disease with >50% narrowing of the cross-sectional luminal area of two to three major extramural arteries; all athletes were male, aged 32, 40 and 58 years. This is consistent with the findings of other studies showing coronary artery disease to be the main cause of sudden death in older athletes[11]. The fourth death was of a 19-year-old girl with anomalous origin of the left main coronary artery from the right sinus of Valsalva. None of these four runners had previous history of structural heart disease or experienced prodromal cardiac symptoms during training or before competitions; two had previously completed three marathon races each and two were competing in their first marathon. All had trained intensively before the race, running 40–100 miles/week.

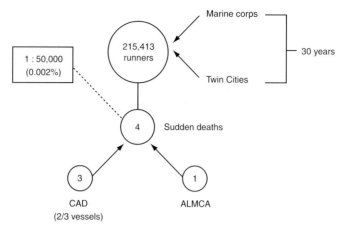

Figure 4

Flow diagram showing outcome of two US marathon events (Marine Corps, Washington, DC, and Twin Cities, Minneapolis) encompassing 215,413 runners over a cumulative period of 30 years). (ALMCA=anomalous left main coronary artery, CAD=atherosclerotic coronary artery disease)

The overall prevalence of sudden cardiac death associated with the marathon population in the US was 0.002%, (1:50,000)[76], much lower than that of other variables of risk for premature death calculated in the general US population (Table 2). The risk of sudden death for a single marathon race was estimated at about one-hundredth of the annual overall risk associated with living, with or without heart disease. The only activity associated with a lower risk than marathon racing was commercial airline travel. These figures for sudden cardiac death are similar to those informally reported for the London and New York marathons (eight deaths in 850,000 runners) which are extremely large public events with thousands of participants at various levels of expertise[80]. It has been estimated that running the London marathon, which has about 30,000 runners annually (over a four-hour period) conveys a risk equivalent to riding a motorcycle for two hours, cycling for 10 hours, or riding in a car or on a scheduled

Table 2 *Relative risks for sudden cardiac death in the US (one-year duration)*

	%	per 100,000
Overall mortality — all causes	0.23	230
(general risk of living 15–54 years old)		
Cardiac-related	0.04	40
Accidents	0.03	30
Motor vehicle	0.02	20
Homicide	0.01	10
Marathon (race/y)	*0.002*	*2*
Commercial airline travel	0.00005	0.05
(no. of departures)		

219

airline flight for 28 hours (discussed in Dr Tunstall Pedoe's chapter *Marathon myths and marathon medicine*)[80].

Thus, although highly trained athletes such as marathon runners may harbour underlying and potentially lethal cardiovascular disease, the risk for sudden cardiac death is exceedingly small. This low risk in long-distance runners suggests that routine pre-participation screening for cardiovascular disease in such athletic populations may not be justified.

Future perspectives

It will be advantageous to assemble additional data to better define the prevalence and causes of sudden death in older competitive athletes, particularly those participating in road racing and marathon events. The overall frequency of these catastrophes during the marathon may now be even lower than the reported 1:50,000[76], given the perceived reduction in deaths due to structural heart disease at these events coupled with the increasing level of participation.

Prevention of sudden death will be of increasing importance over the next 10–20 years. It is difficult, however, to envision a strategy that will make pre-participation screening for detection of cardiovascular abnormalities mandatory for all participants in marathon and other road racing events. Nevertheless, the dissemination of information and the concerted efforts at educating the public about the risks and benefits associated with sports, and the warning signs of coronary artery disease, by the news media, American Heart Association and other agencies and institutions may have had a positive effect by reducing cardiovascular catastrophes during competitive long-distance running. These possible trends and relationships, however, need to be documented in future studies.

In addition, efforts to prevent sudden death in the next decade will require greater availability and use of the automated external defibrillator (AED)[82] at large sporting events, including marathon races. Such devices can be operated by non-physicians with little formal training, and have been shown to be life-saving at athletic events, casinos, airports, and on commercial aircraft[83,84].

Mechanisms of sudden death and resuscitation

Although the precise mechanism responsible for sudden death in athletes depends on the particular disease state involved, cardiac arrest resulting from electrical instability and ventricular tachyarrhythmias occurs in most cases, including atherosclerotic coronary artery disease. In the case of HCM, disorganized cardiac muscle cells distributed widely throughout the left ventricular wall probably represent the substrate for ventricular tachycardia/fibrillation when associated with a number of potential clinical triggers (including intense physical activity) (Figure 1)[39]. A notable exception to this model is Marfan's syndrome, in which sudden death is due to aortic rupture. Regardless of the underlying mechanism, few athletes with cardiovascular disease who collapse on the athletic field are successfully resuscitated by bystanders with cardiopulmonary resuscitation (although there was, in fact, a 50% success rate in the London marathon (see Dr Tunstall Pedoe's chapter, *Morbidity and mortality in the London marathon*).

The routine presence of AED, and public access defibrillation, at athletic events may lead to the survival of greater numbers of such athletes[82]. However, the great infrequency with which these events occur ultimately represents an obstacle to efficient resuscitation practice on the rare occasion of such an occurrence. Therefore, it would appear equally important to emphasize the early detection of potentially lethal cardiovascular abnormalities through pre-participation screening[22] with the withdrawal of such athletes from intense training and competition[23].

Criteria for eligibility and disqualification

When a previously unsuspected cardiovascular abnormality is identified in a competitive athlete, by standard screening or by other means, the following must be considered:

- the magnitude of risk for sudden cardiac death associated with continued participation in competitive sports
- the criteria to be implemented for determining whether or not the athlete would benefit from disqualification from athletics.

The 26th Bethesda Conference sponsored by the American College of Cardiology[23] offers prospective and consensus recommendations for athletic eligibility or disqualification, taking into account the severity of the cardiovascular abnormality as well as the nature of sports training and competition. These recommendations are predicated on the likelihood that intense athletic training will increase the risk for sudden cardiac, or disease, progression in trained athletes with clinically important underlying structural heart disease, although it is not presently possible to quantify that risk precisely for individual participants. Nevertheless, it is presumed that the temporary or permanent withdrawal of selected athletes from participation in certain intense sports is prudent and will diminish the perceived risk. The Bethesda Conference report provides clear benchmarks for the expected standard of care that may be used to resolve future medicolegal disputes, and has been cited by a US Appellate Court as consensus expert guidelines that team physicians should rely on in formulating appropriate decisions regarding the eligibility of competitive athletes with cardiovascular disease[79].

References

1 Maron BJ. Sudden death in young athletes: lessons from the Hank Gathers affair. *N Engl J Med* 1993; **329**: 55–7.

2 Burke AP, Farb V, Virmani R *et al*. Sports-related and non-sports-related sudden cardiac death in young adults. *Am Heart J* 1991; **121**: 568–75.

3 Maron BJ, Shirani J, Poliac LC *et al*. Sudden death in young competitive athletes: clinical, demographic and pathological profiles. *JAMA* 1996; **276**: 199–204.

4 van Camp SP, Bloor CM, Mueller FO *et al*. Nontraumatic sports death in high school and college athletes. *Med Sci Sports Exerc* 1995; **27**: 641–7.

5 Maron BJ, Roberts WC, McAllister HA *et al*. Sudden death in young athletes. *Circulation* 1980; **62**: 218–29.

6 Corrado D, Thiene G, Nava A *et al*. Sudden death in young competitive athletes: clinicopathologic correlations in 22 cases. *Am J Med* 1990; **89**: 588–96.

7 Thiene G, Nava A, Corrado D *et al*. Right ventricular cardiomyopathy and sudden death in young people. *N Engl J Med* 1988; **318**: 129–33.

8 Tsung SH, Huang TY, Chang HH. Sudden death in young athletes. *Arch Pathol Lab Med* 1982; **106**: 168–70.

9 James TN, Froggatt P, Marshall TK. Sudden death in young athletes. *Ann Intern Med* 1967; **67**: 1013–21.

10 Furlanello F, Bettini R, Cozzi F *et al*. Ventricular arrhythmias and sudden death in athletes. *Ann N Y Acad Sci* 1984; **427**: 253–79.

11 Maron BJ, Epstein SE, Roberts WC. Causes of sudden death in competitive athletes. *J Am Coll Cardiol* 1986; **7**: 204–14.23

12 Drory Y, Turetz Y, Hiss Y *et al*. Sudden unexpected death in persons <40 years of age. *Am J Cardiol* 1991; **68**: 1388–92.

13 Driscoll DJ, Edwards W. Sudden unexpected death in children and adolescents. *J Am Coll Cardiol* 1985; **5**(suppl B): 118B–22B.

14 Liberthson RR. Sudden death from cardiac causes in children and young adults. *N Engl J Med* 1996; **334**: 1039–44.

15 Thompson PD, Stern MP, Williams P *et al*. Death during jogging or running. A study of 18 cases. *JAMA* 1979; **242**: 1265–67.

16 Thompson PD, Funk EJ, Carleton RA *et al*. Incidence of death during jogging in Rhode Island from 1975 through 1980. *JAMA* 1982; **247**: 2535–8.

17 Waller BF, Roberts WC. Sudden death while running in conditioned runners aged 40 years or over. *Am J Cardiol* 1980; **45**: 1292–300.

18 Virmani R, Robinowitz M, McAllister HA Jr. Nontraumatic death in joggers: a series of 30 patients at autopsy. *Am J Med* 1982; **72**: 874–82.

19 Maron BJ, Mitchell JH. Revised eligibility recommendations for competitive athletes with cardiovascular abnormalities. *J Am Coll Cardiol* 1994; **24**: 848–50.

20 Maron BJ, Poliac L, Kaplan JA *et al*. Blunt impact to the chest leading to sudden death from cardiac arrest during sports activities. *N Engl J Med* 1995; **333**: 337–42.

21 Maron BJ, Garson A. Arrhythmias and sudden cardiac death in elite athletes. *Cardiol Rev* 1994; **2**: 26–32.

22 Maron BJ, Thompson PD, Puffer JC *et al*. Cardiovascular preparticipation screening of competitive athletes. *Circulation* 1996; **94**: 850–6.

23 Maron BJ, Mitchell JH. 26th Bethesda Conference: Recommendations for determining eligibility for competition in athletes with cardiovascular abnormalities. *J Am Coll Cardiol* 1994; **24**: 845–99.

24 Corrado D, Basso C, Schiavon M *et al*. Screening for hypertrophic cardiomyopathy in young athletes. *N Engl J Med* 1998; **339**: 364–9.

25 Wigle ED, Sasson Z, Henderson MA *et al*. Hypertrophic cardiomyopathy: The importance of the site and extent of hypertrophy — a review. *Prog Cardiovasc Dis* 1985; **28**: 1–83.

26 Maron BJ, Bonow RO, Cannon RO *et al*. Hypertrophic cardiomyopathy. Interrelation of clinical manifestations, pathophysiology, and therapy (I). *N Engl J Med* 1987; **316**: 780–9.

27 Maron BJ, Bonow RO, Cannon RO *et al*. Hypertrophic cardiomyopathy. Interrelation of clinical manifestations, pathophysiology, and therapy (II). *N Engl J Med* 1987; **316**: 844–52.

28 Maron BJ, Moller JH, Seidman CE *et al*. Impact of laboratory molecular diagnosis on contemporary diagnostic criteria for genetically transmitted cardiovascular diseases. Hypertrophic cardiomyopathy, long-QT syndrome, and Marfan syndrome. *Circulation* 1998; **98**: 1460–71.

29 Klues HG, Schiffers A, Maron BJ. Phenotypic spectrum and patterns of left ventricular hypertrophy in hypertrophic cardiomyopathy. Morphologic observations and significance as assessed by two-dimensional echocardiography in 600 patients. *J Am Coll Cardiol* 1995; **26**: 1699–708.

30 Spirito P, Seidman CE, McKenna WJ, Maron BJ. Management of hypertrophic cardiomyopathy. *N Engl J Med* 1997; **336**: 775–85.

31 Maron BJ. Hypertrophic cardiomyopathy. *Lancet* 1997; **3350**: 127–33.

32 Thierfelder L, Watkins H, MacRae C *et al*. **a**-tropomyosin and cardiac troponin T mutations cause familial hypertrophic cardiomyopathy: A disease of the sarcomere. *Cell* 1994; **77**: 701–12.

33 Niimura H, Bachinski LL, Sangwatanaroj S *et al*. Mutations in the gene for human cardiac myosin-binding protein C and late-onset familial hypertrophic cardiomyopathy. *N Engl J Med* 1998; **338**: 1248–57.

34 Schwartz K, Carrier L, Guicheney P *et al*. Molecular basis of familial cardiomyopathies. *Circulation* 1995; **91**: 532–40.

35 Marian AJ, Roberts R. Recent advances in the molecular genetics of hypertrophic cardiomyopathy. *Circulation* 1995; **91**: 532–40.

36 Maron BJ, Gardin JM, Flack JM *et al*. Assessment of the prevalence of hypertrophic cardiomyopathy in a general population of young adults: Echocardiographic analysis of 4,111 subjects in the CARDIA Study. *Circulation* 1995; **92**: 785–9.

37 Sadoul N, Prasas K, Elliott PM *et al*. Prospective prognostic assessment of blood pressure response during exercise in patients with hypertrophic cardiomyopathy. *Circulation* 1997; **96**: 2987–91.

38 Olivotto I, Maron BJ, Montereggi A *et al*. Prognostic value of systemic blood pressure response during exercise in a community-based patient population with hypertrophic cardiomyopathy. *J Am Coll Cardiol* 1999; **33**: 2044–51.

39 Maron BJ, Shen W-K, Link MS *et al*. Efficacy of implantable cardioverter-defibrillators for the prevention of sudden death in patients with hypertrophic cardiomyopathy. *N Engl J Med* 2000; **342**: 365–73.

40 Maron BJ, Pelliccia A, Spirito P. Cardiac disease in young trained athletes. Insights into methods for distinguishing athlete's heart from structural heart disease with particular emphasis on hypertrophic cardiomyopathy. *Circulation* 1995; **91**: 1596–601.

41 Maron BJ, Isner JM, McKenna WJ. 26th Bethesda Conference: recommendations for determining eligibility for competition in athletes with cardiovascular abnormalities. Task Force 3: hypertrophic cardiomyopathy, myocarditis and other myopericardial diseases, and mitral valve prolapse. *J Am Coll Cardiol* 1994; **24**: 880–5.

42 Cheitlin MD, De Castro CM, McAllister HA. Sudden death as a complication of anomalous left coronary origin from the anterior sinus of Valsalva. A not-so-minor congenital anomaly. *Circulation* 1974; **50**: 780–7.

43 Roberts WC. Congenital coronary arterial anomalies unassociated with major anomalies of the heart or great vessels. In: *Adult congenital heart disease*. Philadelphia: FA Davis Co, 1987: 583.

44 Basso C, Maron BJ, Corrado D, Thiene G. Clinical profile of congenital coronary artery anomalies with origin from the wrong aortic sinus leading to sudden death in young competitive athletes. *J Am Coll Cardiol* 2000; **35**: 1493–501.

45 Gaither NS, Rogan KM, Stajduhar K *et al*. Anomalous origin and course of coronary arteries in adults. Identification and improved imaging utilizing transesophageal echocardiography. *Am Heart J* 1991; **122**: 69–75.

46 Maron BJ, Leon BJ, Swain JA. Prospective identification by two-dimensional echocardiography of anomalous origin of the left main coronary artery from the right sinus of Valsalva. *Am J Cardiol* 1991; **68**: 140–2.

47 Jureidini SB, Eaton C, Williams J *et al*. Transthoracic two-dimensional and color flow echocardiographic diagnosis of aberrant left coronary artery. *Am Heart J* 1994; **127**: 438–40.

48 Corrado D, Basso C, Poletti A *et al*. Sudden death in the young. Is acute coronary thrombosis the major precipitating factor? *Circulation* 1994; **90**: 2315–23.

49 Burke AP, Farb A, Malcom GT *et al*. Plaque rupture and sudden death related to exertion in men with coronary artery disease. *JAMA* 1999; **281**: 921–6.

50 Lambert EC, Menon VA, Wagner HR *et al*. Sudden unexpected death from cardiovascular disease in children. A cooperative international study. *Am J Cardiol* 1974; **34**: 89–96.

51 Aretz HT, Billingham ME, Edwards WD *et al*. Myocarditis: a histopathologic definition and classification. *Am J Cardiovasc Pathol* 1986; **1**: 3–14.

52 Zeppilli P, Santini C, Palmieri V *et al*. Role of myocarditis in athletes with minor arrhythmias and/or echocardiographic abnormalities. *Chest* 1994; **106**: 373–80.

53 Martin AB, Webber S, Fricker FJ *et al*. Acute myocarditis. Rapid diagnosis by PCR in children. *Circulation* 1994; **90**: 330–9.

54 Pauschinger M, Bowles NE, Fuentes-Garcia FJ *et al*. Detection of adenoviral genome in the myocardium of adult patients with idiopathic left ventricular dysfunction. *Circulation* 1999; **99**: 1348–54.

55 Isner JM, Estes NAM III, Thompson PD *et al*. Acute cardiac events temporally related to cocaine abuse. *N Engl J Med* 1986; **315**: 1438–43.

56 Morales AR, Romanelli R, Boucek RJ. The mural left anterior descending coronary artery, strenuous exercise and sudden death. *Circulation* 1980; **62**: 230–7

57 Yetman AJ, McCrindle BW, MacDonald C *et al*. Myocardial bridging in children with hypertrophic cardiomyopathy — a risk factor for sudden death. *N Engl J Med* 1998; **339**: 1201–9.

58 Schwarz ER, Klues HG, vom Dahl J. Functional, angiographic and intracoronary Doppler flow characteristics in symptomatic patients with myocardial bridging: Effect of short-term intravenous beta-blocker medication. *J Am Coll Cardiol* 1996; **27**: 1637–45.

59 Freed LA, Levy D, Levine RA *et al*. Prevalence and clinical outcome of mitral valve prolapse. *N Engl J Med* 1999; **341**: 1–7.

60 Dollar AL, Roberts WC. Morphologic comparison of patients with mitral valve prolapse who died suddenly with patients who died from severe valvular dysfunction or other conditions. *J Am Coll Cardiol* 1991; **17**: 921–31.

61 Bharti S, Lev M. Congenital abnormalities of the conduction system in sudden death in young adults. *J Am Coll Cardiol* 1986; **8**: 1096–104.

62 Burke AP, Subramanian R, Smialek J *et al*. Nonatherosclerotic narrowing of the atrioventricular node artery and sudden death. *J Am Coll Cardiol* 1993; **21**: 117–22.

63 Thiene G, Nava A, Corrado D *et al*. Right ventricular cardiomyopathy and sudden death in young people. *N Engl J Med* 1988; **318**: 129–33.

64 Marcus FI, Fontaine GH, Guiraudon G *et al*. Right ventricular dysplasia: a report of 24 adult cases. *Circulation* 1982; **65**: 384–98.

65 Corrado D, Basso C, Thiene G *et al*. Spectrum of clinicopathologic manifestations of arrhythmogenic right ventricular cardiomyopathy/dysplasia: a multicenter study. *J Am Coll Cardiol* 1997; **30**: 1512–20.

66 McKenna WJ, Thiene G, Nava A *et al*. Diagnosis of arrhythmogenic right ventricular dysplasia/cardiomyopathy. *Br Heart J* 1994; **71**: 215–8.

67 Pelliccia A, Maron BJ. Preparticipation cardiovascular evaluation of the competitive athlete: perspectives from the 30 year Italian experience. *Am J Cardiol* 1995; **75**: 827–8.

68 Pelliccia A, Culasso F, Di Paolo F, Maron BJ. Physiologic left ventricular cavity dilatation in elite athletes. *Ann Intern Med* 1999; **130**: 23–31.

69 Kloner RA, Hale S, Alker K, Rezkalla S. The effects of acute and chronic cocaine use on the heart. *Circulation* 1992; **85**: 407–19.

70 Survivors of out-of-hospital cardiac arrest with apparently normal heart. Need for definition and standardized clinical evaluation. *Circulation* 1997; **95**: 265–72.

71 Vincent GM, Timothy KW, Leppert M, Keating M. The spectrum of symptoms and QT intervals in carriers of the gene for the long-QT syndrome. *N Engl J Med* 1992; **327**: 846–52.

72 Brugada P, Brugada J. Right bundle-branch block; persistent ST segment elevation and sudden cardiac death: a distinct clinical and electrocardiographic syndrome. A multicenter report. *J Am Coll Cardiol* 1992; **20**: 1391–6.

73 Noakes TD, Rose AG, Opie LH. Hypertrophic cardiomyopathy associated with sudden death during marathon racing. *Br Heart J* 1979; **41**: 624–7.

74 Siscovick DS, Weiss NS, Fletcher RH *et al*. The incidence of primary cardiac arrest during vigorous exercise. *N Engl J Med* 1984; **311**: 874–7

75 Northcote RJ, Evans ADB, Ballantyne D. Sudden death in squash players. *Lancet* 1984; **21**: 148–51.

76 Maron BJ, Poliac LC, Roberts WO. Risk for sudden cardiac death associated with marathon running. *J Am Coll Cardiol* 1996; **28**: 428–31.

77 Maron BJ, Gohman TE, Aeppli D. Prevalence of sudden cardiac death during competitive sports activities in Minnesota high school athletes. *J Am Coll Cardiol* 1998; **32**: 1881–4.

78 Maron BJ. Cardiovascular risks to young persons on the athletic field. *Ann Intern Med* 1998; **129**: 379–86.

79 Maron BJ, Mitten MJ, Quandt EK *et al*. Competitive athletes with cardiovascular disease — the case of Nicholas Knapp. *N Engl J Med* 1998; **339**: 1632–5.

80 Tunstall Pedoe D. Sudden cardiac death in sport — spectre or preventable risk? *Br J Sports Med* 2000; **34**: 137–40.

81 Maron BJ, Araújo CGS, Thompson PD *et al*. Recommendations for preparticipation screening and the assessment of cardiovascular disease in Master's athletes. *Circulation* 2001; **103**: 327–34.

82 Kerber RE, Becker LB, Bourland JD *et al*. Automatic external defibrillators for public access defibrillation. Recommendations for specifying and reporting arrhythmia analysis algorithm performance, incorporating new waveforms, and enhancing safety. *Circulation* 1997; **95**: 1677–82.

83 Valenzuela TD, Roe DJ, Nichol G *et al*. Outcomes of rapid defibrillation by security officers after cardiac arrest in casinos. *N Engl J Med* 2000; **343**: 1206–9.

84 Page RL, Joglar JA, Kowal RC *et al*. Use of automated external defibrillators by a US airline. *N Engl J Med* 2000; **343**: 1210–6.

DISCUSSION

Attendee: Dr Maron, are some deaths in sports related to cocaine use?

Dr Barry Maron: Cocaine is a dangerous drug for athletes, but we do not have data because of the conditions, political correctness, as well as confidentiality, and other problems such as athletes not telling the truth. However, we think there is a chance that in both the Lewis and Gathers high-profile cases that there could have been cocaine cardiomyopathy. Cocaine can scar the heart — their hearts were very scarred with no other cause. It is a myocarditis with scarring but probably not due to a virus.

Attendee: Can the difference in hypertrophic cardiomyopathy deaths in male and female athletes be related to testosterone?

Dr Barry Maron: It may be, but that is speculative as there is still a huge preponderance of male athletes — one would expect the death rates to be higher.

The female athlete triad: disordered eating, amenorrhoea and osteoporosis

DR ROGER WOLMAN

THE ROYAL NATIONAL ORTHOPAEDIC HOSPITAL, LONDON, UK

Menstruation begins at the time of puberty (the menarche) and continues until the menopause. Amenorrhoea is defined as the absence of menstruation for at least three months during this time period. It can be a normal/physiological response as seen during pregnancy and lactation, but it may occur as a result of an underlying medical disorder.

Amenorrhoea in athletes was first recognized in the late 1970s. Before this, it was unusual for women athletes to exercise and train sufficiently hard to develop the problem. Since 1980, however, women have participated increasingly in aerobic sports and there has also been an increase in the number of endurance competitions for women; for instance, the first Olympic marathon for women was held in 1984 and the first Olympic 10,000 m race in 1988.

In the early 1980s, high training intensity was thought to be the main underlying aetiological factor for amenorrhoea. However, studies carried out in the mid-1980s indicated that many of these amenorrhoeic athletes had disordered eating habits, in particular low calorie intake in the diet relative to the amount of exercise being undertaken. A combination of disordered eating and intense endurance exercise was emerging as important in the cause of amenorrhoea.

Amenorrhoea is usually a reflection of low oestrogen production in the body. As oestrogen is important in maintaining bone strength, amenorrhoea and low oestrogen usually result in reduced bone strength. Exercise is known to have a protective effect on bone and, therefore, it was initially thought that this would protect amenorrhoeic athletes from getting osteoporosis. However, studies from 1984 have shown that amenorrhoeic athletes do have low bone density[1] and are thus at risk of osteoporosis. Collectively, these interrelated components of disordered eating, amenorrhoea and osteoporosis form a syndrome, which is now referred to as the female athlete triad. This chapter will outline the aetiology and pathophysiology of the triad, and its effects on bone density. Treatment strategies for the management of the syndrome will also be discussed.

Incidence and aetiology

The female athlete triad is associated with endurance sports. The incidence of amenorrhoea varies in different sports and reflects the requirements for that particular activity in terms of training intensity, calorie restriction and age (Figure 1)[2].

Training intensity can be difficult to quantify in certain sporting events, but is relatively easy in runners as the number of miles run per week provides an accurate estimate. Studies have shown that the incidence of amenorrhoea increases as weekly training mileage increases[3], occurring in about 50% of those running >80 miles/week.

Disordered eating is common in female athletes and may occur in >60% of competitors in some sports, such as gymnastics[4,5]. In many cases, disordered eating is the result of external pressure to maintain a prescribed body weight and appearance. This may come from the athletes' peer group, their coach and sometimes the parents. The eventual outcome in some of these cases may be an overt eating disorder and anorexia nervosa. Restricted eating patterns may lead to deficiency of several nutrients but the two of greatest relevance to the female athlete triad are calorie and calcium deficiency.

The relevance of calorie restriction is seen in rowers, where the incidence of amenorrhoea is significantly higher among the lightweight competitors (who must weigh <59 kg in order to compete) compared to their heavyweight counterparts[2]. Both groups have similar training regimens but the lightweights frequently follow a restricted diet

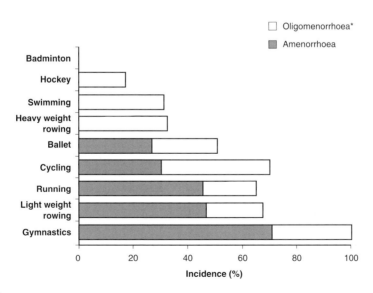

Figure 1

Incidence of amenorrhoea among elite athletes in different sports[2]

* Oligomenorrhoea = three to nine menstrual cycles in one year.

so they can comply with the weight regulation for competition. Furthermore, nutritional studies on runners show that those with amenorrhoea have lower daily calorie intake than their eumenorrhoeic (normally menstruating) counterparts[1,6].

Athletes in their late teens are more vulnerable to menstrual irregularity than those in their 20s. In activities such as gymnastics and ballet, where there are many teenage performers, there is a high incidence of both primary and secondary amenorrhoea[7,8].

Pathophysiology

Endurance exercise training causes a spectrum of menstrual disorders. At relatively low levels of training, a shortened luteal phase of the menstrual cycle may occur. This is usually associated with reduced progesterone levels. Menstrual cycles may also become anovulatory. These abnormalities become more frequent as training intensity increases. With further increases in training, menstrual cycles may eventually become irregular and infrequent (oligomenorrhoea) or absent (amenorrhoea).

The menarche, the onset of menstruation, is often delayed in athletes performing sports in which training begins before puberty. This is typically seen in gymnastics and ballet where, on average, it is delayed by one year[9]. Primary amenorrhoea may result and, in some cases, athletes may even reach their 20s before menstruation begins. Sports such as ballet and gymnastics attract people with low body weight (and body fat) and the delayed menarche may be the result of this selection bias rather than due to the high level of training.

There are many similarities between the female athlete triad and anorexia nervosa, so much so that many believe they are part of the same spectrum of ill health. Both involve disordered eating, energy imbalance and low body weight. The psychological profiling of patients with these two disorders is very similar[10] while a significant proportion of those with the female athlete triad have had a previous history of anorexia nervosa[4].

The aetiology of amenorrhoea is also similar[11]. There is impaired hypothalamic function with a functional decline of the gonadotrophin-releasing hormone (GnRH) pulse generator in terms of both amplitude and frequency; this leads to a reversible hypogonadotrophic hypogonadism with severe impairment of oestrogen production. The gonadotrophin release seems to revert to a pre-pubertal pattern.

Over the past 15 years, there has been much focus on investigating the factors responsible for suppressing the GnRH pulse generator in female athletes. Several hypotheses exist, including endorphin release, central 'stress' and energy deprivation. Each of these hypotheses involves the release of specific hormones that may influence hypothalamic function. Such hormones include endorphins, cortisol, insulin-like growth factor binding protein-1 (IGFBP-1) and leptin[11].

The inhibitory action of opioids on the GnRH pulse generator is now well established[11]. However, although endorphin levels increase with acute aerobic training (which may account for the so-called 'runner's high' (refer to Dr Morgan's chapter)), there is much less evidence that they remain elevated with regular exercise[11]. Thus, endorphin release alone is unlikely to account for the gonadal suppression observed in athletes.

Serum cortisol levels are higher in amenorrhoeic athletes than their eumenorrhoeic counterparts. This represents central 'stress' and occurs as a result of central activation of corticotrophin-releasing hormone (CRH). CRH increases GnRH sensitivity to opioid inhibition and, thus, in combination with endorphin release, provides a possible mechanism for amenorrhoea. The raised cortisol may also adversely affect bone density (discussed overleaf).

An alternative hypothesis is that amenorrhoea occurs as a result of energy deprivation (Figure 2)[12,13]. Several independent studies have demonstrated that the energy

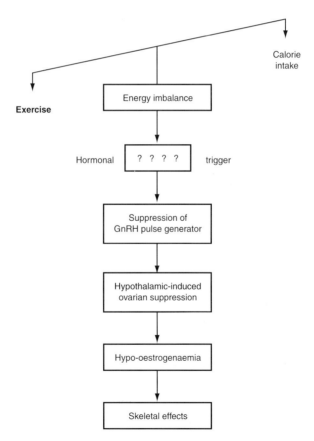

Figure 2

Energy deprivation hypothesis for the female athlete triad

(calorie) intake of amenorrhoeic athletes is significantly lower than their eumenorrhoeic counterparts, even when matched for exercise intensity. This produces an energy imbalance — ie low energy intake from the diet compared with a high energy output in the form of exercise — that results in weight loss. Amenorrhoeic athletes, similar to those with anorexia nervosa, have low body fat (often <18%) and a low body mass index (often <19). Furthermore, they have a lower resting metabolic rate and reduced levels of insulin, insulin-like growth factor I (IGF-1) and tri-iodothyronine. These changes are seen in situations of energy deprivation. It is uncertain whether or not any of these three hormones can act as a metabolic signal influencing the release of GnRH.

Two other possible candidates that may influence hypothalamic function are IGFBP-1 and leptin. IGFBP-1 is directly regulated by insulin such that their levels are inversely related. Amenorrhoeic athletes have elevated levels of IGFBP-1[11]. Serum leptin concentrations are related to body fat and are reduced in anorexia nervosa and probably in the female athlete triad. Further work is needed to determine whether or not either hormone has a direct effect on the GnRH pulse generator.

Skeletal effects

Bone density

Osteoporosis is a condition where the calcium content of bone is reduced, making the bone more vulnerable to fracture. The calcium concentration in bone, known as the bone mineral density (BMD), can be accurately measured in several ways. Over the past 12 years, dual energy X-ray absorptiometry (DEXA) has become the method of choice in clinical practice. This produces a highly reproducible measure of BMD using a very thin X-ray beam. It exposes the patient to a very low dose of radiation making the technique extremely safe. Although DEXA will provide an absolute figure for the calcium concentration, the computer also gives a result in reference to the BMD of the average level seen in someone of the same sex at their peak level of bone density (usually in the late 20s). This provides a score in terms of a percentage or a standard deviation above or below the mean. This is known as the T-score. Current convention defines osteoporosis as a T-score of <–2.5 (ie lower than 2.5 standard deviations below the mean).

Amenorrhoeic athletes have reduced bone densities[1]. Although this is seen most obviously in the spine, where there is a high proportion of trabecular bone, other sites such as the proximal femur and wrist may also be affected. The fall in bone density is mainly due to the low oestrogen levels, but it does not always improve when oestrogen replacement is given. This suggests that other factors may also be important in maintaining bone density. Two worth consideration are IGF-1 and cortisol. The former is reduced while the latter is increased in the female athlete triad (see

Pathophysiology section). While IGF-1 has important anabolic effects on the skeleton, cortisol has a catabolic action so that either hormonal change could enhance the decline in bone density.

The stress loading effect of exercise will partially prevent the reduction in bone density caused by amenorrhoea. Amenorrhoeic athletes have higher bone density levels than amenorrhoeic non-athletes. However, the extent of bone density protection also depends on the type of exercise undertaken. For example, amenorrhoeic rowers have greater spinal bone density than amenorrhoeic runners[14]. This is presumably due to intense exercise involving the trunk. Amenorrhoeic gymnasts have higher spinal and femoral neck bone density than amenorrhoeic runners[15], probably due to the weight training and jumping activity that is involved in gymnastic training.

During short (six to 12 months) episodes of amenorrhoea, the reduction in bone density can be reversed once normal menstruation is restored. With longer episodes, however, the changes may become irreversible and bone density remains persistently low. Occasionally, the bone loss may be very severe with BMD levels similar to the levels in postmenopausal women — the risk of osteoporotic fracture in this subgroup is significantly increased[1,16]. More commonly, bone density reduction is less extreme and the risk is of premature (10–15 years early) osteoporosis.

Other skeletal effects

Bone adapts to stress when it is exposed to it. With time, bone remodelling takes place and the bone becomes stronger. Stress fractures occur when the remodelling process has not been effective, often because the athlete has increased his or her training too rapidly, not giving time for effective remodelling to occur. They are commonly seen in runners and occur most frequently in the shin and foot but can also be present in the femur. These stress injuries produce a defect in the cortex of the bone. If the athlete continues to train despite the associated pain, the small defect may extend across the bone leading to a full fracture.

Stress fractures occur more frequently in amenorrhoeic athletes[17,18]. This may be related to low bone density. It may also be due to impaired bone remodelling. Oestrogen and IGF-1 have anabolic effects on the bone cells responsible for remodelling. Both are reduced in amenorrhoeic athletes, which may impair the remodelling process.

Athletes with delayed menarche and primary amenorrhoea may have delayed skeletal maturation, including delayed epiphyseal closure. Until the epiphysis fuses, it remains a site of potential weakness and is at increased risk of injury. Epiphyseal injuries may therefore occur more commonly in athletes with delayed menarche, although no study has so far addressed this relationship.

Diagnosis and management strategies

When investigating an athlete with menstrual abnormalities it is important to exclude the other causes of amenorrhoea before making a diagnosis of the female athlete triad. This will include taking an accurate history from the athlete regarding the relationship between training and menstrual abnormalities, and risk factors for other causes of amenorrhoea. A blood test should include investigations to exclude other causes and a serum tri-iodothyronine, which is likely to be low in the female athlete triad. In addition, a nutritional assessment to determine calorie and calcium intake is helpful, and bone density should be measured. The key points to note when investigating for this syndrome are summarized in Table 1.

Once the diagnosis of the triad has been made[19], the most effective treatment is to re-establish natural menstruation. This can be achieved by a combination of reducing training intensity and increasing calorie intake (Table 2). It is important to educate athletes about both the short- and long-term risks of remaining amenorrhoeic otherwise many will not accept this type of intervention. Psychological intervention may be necessary in athletes with an apparent eating disorder.

Athletes who remain amenorrhoeic despite attempts to adjust training and diet should be offered oestrogen replacement. Both the oral contraceptive and hormone replacement therapy provide sufficient oestrogen for this. Unfortunately, many athletes have difficulty tolerating either due to the side-effects, which include fluid retention, breast tenderness and pre-menstrual symptoms. Furthermore, anecdotal experience suggests that oestrogen replacement is not always effective. This is presumably because it fails to address the other associated hormonal abnormalities (mentioned earlier). Calcium supplements should also be considered, especially in those with low intakes, as should vitamin D supplements. Experience with bisphosphonates and raloxifene in teenagers and those in their 20s is too limited to offer clear advice; more research is needed with these newer drugs.

The effectiveness of treatment should be monitored with bone densitometry. The progressive decline in bone density or recurrent injuries will force athletes who remain amenorrhoeic to eventually change their lifestyle in terms of training and nutrition. By this time, however, it may be too late to reverse the effects. Thus, there needs to be an emphasis on education at an early stage.

Table 1 *Investigation of the female athlete triad*

- Exclude other causes of amenorrhoea
- Measure serum tri-iodothyronine levels
- Nutritional assessment for energy and calcium
- Measure bone mineral density

Table 2 *Treatment of the female athlete triad*

- Reduce the intensity and frequency of exercise (with the help of the coach)
- Increase energy intake (with the help of a dietician)
- Consider psychological intervention
- Oestrogen replacement: hormone replacement therapy or oral contraceptive
- Calcium and vitamin D supplements
- ? Bisphosphonates
- ? Raloxifene

Conclusions

Since the female athlete triad was first recognized >15 years ago, there has been continuing progress in our understanding of the aetiologies of amenorrhoea and osteoporosis and the factors that link these two conditions. It is now clear that prolonged amenorrhoea is detrimental to the bone health of a female runner. The cause of the amenorrhoea should be established and appropriate treatment should be given. Ideally, natural menstruation should be restored, but if this is not possible oestrogen replacement should be considered. Education and counselling of the athlete is an important aspect of the overall management.

References

1 Drinkwater BL, Nilson K, Chesnut CH *et al.* Bone mineral content of amenorrhoeic and eumenorrhoeic athletes. *N Engl J Med* 1984; **311**: 277–81.

2 Wolman RL, Harries MG. Menstrual abnormalities in elite athletes. *Clin Sports Med* 1989; **1**: 95-100.

3 Feicht CB, Johnson TS, Martin BJ *et al.* Secondary amenorrhoea in athletes. *Lancet* 1978; **2**: 1145–6.

4 Rosen LW, McKeag DB *et al.* Pathogenic weight-control behaviour in female athletes. *Physician Sports Med* 1986; **14**: 79–86.

5 Yates A, Leehey K, Shisslak CM. Running an analogue of anorexia? *New Engl J Med* 1983; **308**: 251–5.

6 Marcus R, Cann C, Madvig P *et al.* Menstrual function and bone mass in elite women distance runners: endocrine and metabolic features. *Ann Intern Med* 1985; **102**: 158–63.

7 Lutter JM, Cushman S. Menstrual patterns in female runners. *Physician Sports Med* 1982; **10**: 60–72.

8 Malina RM. Menarche in athletes: a synthesis and hypothesis. *Ann Hum Biol* 1983; **10**: 1–24.

9 Frisch RE, Gotz-Webergen AV *et al.* Delayed menarche and amenorrhoea of college athletes in relation to age of onset of training. *JAMA* 1981; **246**: 1559–63.

10 Gadpaille WJ, Sanborn CF, Wagner WW. Athletic amenorrhea, major affective disorders and eating disorders. *Am J Psychiatry* 1987; **144**: 939–42.

11 Jenkins PJ, Grossman A. The control of the gonadotrophin-releasing hormone pulse generator in relation to opioid and nutritional cues. *Hum Reprod* 1993; **8**: 154–61.

12 Loucks AB, Vaitukaitis J, Cameron JL *et al.* The reproductive system and exercise in women. *Med Sci Sports Exerc* 1992; **24**: S288–93.

13 Zanker CL, Swaine IL. The relationship between serum oestradiol concentration and energy balance in young women distance runners. *Int J Sports Med* 1998; **19**: 104–8.

14 Wolman RL, Clark P, McNally E *et al.* Menstrual state and exercise as determinants of spinal trabecular bone density in female athletes. *BMJ* 1990; **301**: 516-8.

15 Robinson TL, Snow-Harter C, Taaffe DR *et al*. Gymnasts exhibit higher bone mass than runners despite similar prevalence of amenorrhoea and oligomenorrhoea. *J Bone Miner Res* 1995; **10**: 26–35.

16 Wilson J, Wolman RL. Osteoporosis and fracture complications in an amenorrhoeic athlete. *Br J Rheumatol* 1994; **33**: 480–1.

17 Myburgh KH, Hutchins J *et al*. Low bone density is an aetiological factor for stress fractures in athletes. *Ann Intern Med* 1990; **113**: 754–9.

18 Barrow GW, Saha S. Menstrual irregularity and stress fractures in collegiate female distance runners. *J Am Sports Med* 1988; **16**: 209–16.

19 Otis CL, Drinkwater B, Johnson M *et al*. American College of Sports Medicine position stand. The female athlete triad. *Med Sci Sports Exerc* 1997; 29: 1–9.

DISCUSSION

Attendee: What effect does the female athlete triad have on the fertility of athletes and what happens to their ovaries?

Dr Roger Wolman: Ultrasound scans on these athletes show an above average incidence of polycystic ovaries. In terms of their fertility, I have seen several examples of amenorrhoeic athletes thinking they were safe from a contraceptive point of view and becoming pregnant, having not menstruated for two to three years — thus, athletes are still ovulating in some situations. Once they stop training or increase their calorie intake they return to normal menstrual patterns and are still potentially fertile.

Attendee: Similar to athletes, swimmers also train extensively. Why is there a difference in the incidence of amenorrhoea between swimmers and young runners?

Dr Roger Wolman: There are at least two theories to explain this. The first recognizes the adverse effect extremes of body temperature has on hypothalamic function. Prolonged exertion in water (eg swimming) allows better control of body temperature, so there may be less effect on the hypothalamus. Second, in order to become a quality swimmer you possibly need to have an inherently high level of body fat. This may protect against developing amenorrhoea. Having said that, there has been at least one study from the early 1990s showing that swimmers may experience menstrual problems but not for the same reasons as athletes; this was due to excessive amounts of androgens which were suppressing the hypothalamic–pituitary–ovarian axis. It was unclear whether or not this was due to external androgens or something inherent within a top-quality female swimmer.

Attendee: At what stage would you start to treat an amenorrhoeic athlete? Would you wait until the dual energy X-ray absorptiometry (DEXA) scan showed bone density to be lower than normal?

Dr Roger Wolman: Persistent amenorrhoea in an athlete will almost always produce a progressive fall in bone density and therefore intervention will be needed at some point. However, some female athletes may initially have a high level of bone density and it is helpful to know this. Clearly if an amenorrhoeic athlete has a low bone density at the first visit, you will need to start treatment quicker than in someone whose bone density is normal or high. In the later situation you have more time to give the athlete an opportunity to re-establish natural menstruation before needing to resort to hormone replacement.

Air pollution — acute and chronic effects

DR LAWRENCE FOLINSBEE & PROFESSOR PETER RAVEN

ENVIRONMENTAL MEDIA ASSESSMENT BRANCH, NATIONAL CENTER FOR ENVIRONMENTAL
ASSESSMENT, US ENVIRONMENTAL PROTECTION AGENCY, RESEARCH TRIANGLE PARK, NC, USA
& DEPARTMENT OF INTEGRATIVE PHYSIOLOGY,
UNIVERSITY OF NORTH TEXAS HEALTH SCIENCE CENTER, FORT WORTH, TEXAS, USA

When discussing endurance performance of participants in major popular endurance events such as the London and New York marathons, the age-related decrement of functional reserves that each individual faces must be taken into account. The absolute functional reserves of an individual are dependent on age, fitness and underlying disease. For example, the maximal difference in pulmonary transfer factor (DLCO) per litre functional residual capacity (FRC) from rest to maximal exercise is 2 ml/min/mmHg at birth, 13 ml/min/mmHg at 25 years and 7 ml/min/mmHg at 52 years[1]. This confirms that we begin and end our lives with small cardiopulmonary reserves. It follows that, when extrapolating data obtained from young, healthy subjects, the reduction in reserves due to the age of the individual and the degree of exposure of the particular environmental stressor must be considered.

Ambient air surrounding large metropolitan cities contains small amounts (parts per million (ppm)) of gases and particulates other than its normal constituents. During times of air stagnation and temperature inversion, many air pollutants reach concentrations that produce significant detrimental effects on functional performance[2–7], morbidity[8–12] and subjective feelings[13]. Of the most common atmospheric pollutants, oxidants (mainly ozone (O_3)), sulphur oxides and particulate matter have been found to be harmful to the cardiopulmonary system. In addition carbon monoxide (CO) has been demonstrated to interfere with cardiovascular function at low concentrations of exposure. This chapter will discuss the effects of these air pollutants on humans.

Ozone

Individuals who have had the unpleasant experience of exercising in ambient air polluted with high concentrations of O_3 have been subjectively convinced that their ability to function was or would be significantly reduced. Complaints of substernal pain, chest tightness, dyspnoea, coughing and, on some occasions, a feeling of nausea have been reported; eye irritation has also been documented although this is not due to O_3 but peroxyacetyl nitrates present in the photochemical smog mixture.

The main targets of O_3 action are the lungs and the respiratory tract[14–25]. The effects of pollutant gases are related to the quantity (dose) delivered to the target tissue, such that increased ventilation (by increased O_3 concentration, increased overall ventilation particularly through exercise, and increased exposure duration) increases the quantity of O_3 inhaled and, hence, its effect on the lungs. A dose-response relationship, therefore, exists between lung function and symptom responses, and O_3. Decrements in lung vital capacity and expiratory flow rates have been observed during acute exposures of O_3[16,21–5]. Although increased airway resistance has been measured, bronchoconstriction is not a main feature of the response in non-asthmatic individuals. Some bronchoconstriction does occur, however, and this effect has been shown to be cholinergically mediated via vagal pathways[26]. Changes in lung function measures may take place even at rest if exposure to higher O_3 concentrations, such as 0.2–0.5 ppm, occurs for many hours. Exposure on a chronic basis (eg many hours in a day, or for weeks and months during the 'ozone season') becomes a reason for concern for people, especially children, who live, work and play in such environments. Studies have shown that chronic exposure to O_3 causes some 'adaptations' and the lung function decrements observed with acute exposure become attenuated. There are also data suggesting that lung growth and development may become impaired in people living in oxidant atmospheres while maturing.

The relationship between endurance exercise and the effects of O_3 is a consequence of the interaction between delivered O_3 and the resulting lung function decrements and symptoms. Ozone concentrations multiplied by the level of ventilation and time of exposure are predictive of lung function decrement[27–30]. This decrease in exercise performance was thought to be due to respiratory symptoms such as cough, irritation and chest pain that severely limited pulmonary capacity. It was also noted that O_3 exposure alters the ventilatory modality — for a given oxygen (O_2) uptake (workload), the O_3-exposed subject decreases his or her tidal volume and increases his or her respiratory rate with no appreciable change in total ventilation.

Studies investigating the exposure of lower O_3 concentrations while performing light to moderate exercise for one hour or more showed that 0.3 ppm O_3 produced decrements in function[31–5]. Several other investigations have explicitly examined endurance performance of highly trained cyclists in O_3 polluted environments ranging from 0.0, 0.08, 0.16 and 0.24 ppm[32,36,37]; many cyclists were unable to complete one hour of heavy exercise (90–120 l/min ventilation). Exposures to 0.12 ppm and 0.24 ppm O_3 produced clinically significant decrements in forced vital capacity (FVC) and forced expiratory volume ($FEV_{1.0}$), and increases in reported symptoms of difficulty in breathing and substernal pain. Depending on length of exposure, O_3 concentration and exercise intensity, these endpoints of respiratory discomfort were associated with marked reductions in performance time (16–30%) and maximal O_2 uptake (VO_{2max}) (6–16%). The causal mechanisms responsible for these decrements, however, have not yet been determined.

In their recent study, Folinsbee *et al* asked individuals to perform six bouts of 50 minutes of mild to moderate exercise (35–45 l/min ventilation) over a six-hour period of

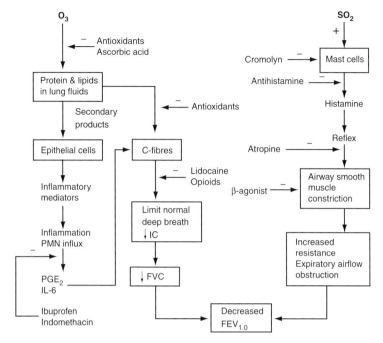

Figure 1

Comparison of response mechanisms leading to a decrease in FEV$_{1.0}$ in asthmatics and non-asthmatics exposed to SO$_2$ and O$_3$ respectively. O$_3$ interacts with surface fluids and associated compounds to produce secondary reaction products; these initiate a cascade of events resulting in limitation of taking a deep breath. SO$_2$ induces release of histamine from mast cells and may also act directly to cause a cholinergically medicated reflex stimulation of airway smooth muscle; this results in airway narrowing, increased airway resistance and obstruction of expired air flow. Both gases cause a reduction in expired flow: SO$_2$ by airway narrowing and O$_3$ via inhibition of taking of a deep breath[38]

IC = inspiratory capacity.

exposure to air with 0.08 and 0.10 ppm O$_3$. Significant reductions in FVC and FEV$_{1.0}$ were observed after two hours. However, no investigations of the effect of such exposures on exercise performance were included.

Figure 1 summarizes the proposed mechanisms of O$_3$ action for changes in lung function. General exposure to O$_3$ in susceptible individuals causes physical symptoms of pain and discomfort, inflammation, alteration in lung volumes and reduced expiratory flow. However, the individual variability in response, and degree of response, identifies the effects of O$_3$ to be a consequence of multiple factors.

As the O$_3$-induced increases in airway resistance are blocked by atropine pre-treatment, it is believed that vagally mediated cholinergic reflex bronchoconstriction must be involved[39]. However, O$_3$ response increases the responsiveness of the airway smooth muscles and results in an increased bronchoconstriction response in asthmatics[40]. A β-agonist relieves the bronchoconstriction of asthmatics but does not reduce it for non-asthmatics[39,41].

O_3 exposure increases breathing rate and reduces tidal volume — this change in breathing pattern is a physiological response to pain and irritation[35,42-4]. Evidence from repeated exposure studies indicates that this response may also become behavioural to reduce the sensation of pain. It has been revealed that, when stimulated, non-myelinated bronchial C-fibres play a role in the reflex mechanism for making breathing more rapid and more shallow[45-7]. This physiological mechanism may explain the O_3-induced changes in breathing patterns. As bronchial C-fibres are stimulated by lung autocoids, such as prostaglandin E_2[48-50] and interleukin-6, some investigators have demonstrated that pre-treatment with the cyclo-oxygenase inhibitor indomethacin (and ibuprofen) abolishes O_3-induced pulmonary function decrements[51-3]. In addition, antioxidant supplements limit the detrimental effects of O_3, possibly by the reduction in formation of lipoperoxides, ozonides and oxidation products.

Sulphur dioxide

Sulphur dioxide (SO_2) in the ambient air results from the combustion of fossil fuels and from industrial processes such as metal refining, cement manufacturing, and pulp and paper production. It is the main pollutant involved in the formation of acidic aerosols. In developed countries, technological requirements by regulatory agencies have reduced SO_2 and acid aerosol concentrations to less than the levels that would significantly affect lung function or exercise performance in healthy individuals. Although this is not the case in developing countries, especially in Asia, healthy endurance athletes are unlikely to experience problems associated with SO_2 inhalation. Patients with asthma, however, are nearly 10-fold more sensitive to SO_2 than non-asthmatics, and can develop bronchoconstriction following exposure during exercise.

SO_2 is a highly soluble gas that is removed from the inspired air stream by the moist surfaces of the upper airways, especially the nose. During resting breathing, SO_2 may be almost completely absorbed before reaching the trachea. However, since the resistance of the nasal airways is reduced markedly during exercise[54], the amount of air breathed through the mouth (oral breathing) generally increases as exercise intensity increases. The mouth has a limited SO_2 absorbing capacity, thus the increased inspired flow rate leads to a greater penetration of SO_2 to the intrathoracic airways. The prevalence of asthma in the general US population is currently about 4–5%, but this figure is expected to increase. It is greatest in children and adolescents, males, Puerto Rican Hispanics and African Americans. The prevalence rate for Australia, home for the 2000 Olympics, has been reported to be 10%[55]. As asthmatics generally suffer from exercise-induced bronchospasm, the prevalence of asthma among the US athletic population may be as high as 10–2%[56].

SO_2 causes exacerbation of asthma symptoms and decrements in lung function in exercising asthmatics exposed to $\geqslant 0.25$ ppm concentrations for two to 10 minutes; there is a 50–60% decrease in $FEV_{1.0}$ in the most responsive individuals. Exercising in SO_2 polluted environments causes wheezing, chest tightness, dyspnoea and, in many cases, requires the use of a bronchodilator to alleviate the symptoms. Cold dry air and mouth breathing exacerbate these symptoms. Specific effects of SO_2 on endurance performance in asthmatics have not been tested.

All symptoms and lung function changes associated with exercising in SO_2 atmosphere can be rapidly reversed by β_2-adrenergic agonist medication, eg salbutamol and terbutaline; cromolyn sodium or β-agonists have been used prophylactically. Not all asthma medications are effective in counteracting SO_2 symptoms. Theophylline or inhaled steroids, for instance, do not significantly reduce the effects of SO_2 in asthmatics[57]. Following SO_2 inhalation, asthmatics are refractory for about three to four hours, during which time the airway response to SO_2 is blunted.

In an environment where significant SO_2 exposure may occur, preventive treatment with cromolyn sodium or β-sympathomimetics will probably limit any potential effects on endurance performance. The probability of exposure to SO_2 concentrations sufficient to induce symptomatic bronchoconstriction is relatively low in developed countries due to the effective regulation of SO_2 emissions. The likelihood of significant exposure (ie asthmatics exercising in a high concentration of SO_2) is about 2–5% annually in the general asthmatic population, although it may be higher in asthmatic endurance athletes because of their greater frequency and duration of exercise and increased time spent outdoors.

Figure 1 provides a schematic summary of the mechanism of SO_2 action. SO_2 stimulates the release of histamine from the mast cells in the respiratory tract tissues; this produces airway smooth muscle contraction and increased resistance to expiratory airflow. FVC and $FEV_{1.0}$ measurements reflect the reflex vasoconstriction. Cromolyn sodium will block histamine release and, therefore, stop the interaction of the broncho-constriction. Atropine probably blocks the vagal efferent nerves and a β-agonist will produce airway smooth muscle relaxation.

Carbon monoxide

CO is a gas that is not easily detected by human senses, but is readily absorbed from inhaled air (when present in low quantities) and combines with haemoglobin to interfere with tissue oxygenation. Without this strong attraction for CO, the haemoglobin molecule would be unable to scavenge the endogenously produced CO (from the breakdown of red blood cells) and, in competition with the high partial pressures of O_2, would be unable to transport and excrete it through the lungs thereby limiting CO build-up. Unfortunately, when CO is present in the ambient air (eg from cigarette smoking, air pollution and vehicle exhaust fumes), its excretion is compromised and dependent on the equilibrium pressures between pulmonary venous blood ($P_V CO$) and the alveoli ($P_A CO$); a significant increase in blood carboxyhaemoglobin (COHb) concentrations may result. Although theoretical predictions of resultant COHb levels in the blood, based on physical and physiological data, have been verified by several experiments[58–63], these have concentrated primarily on relating COHb levels to decrements in cognitive function.

Another issue that has not yet been experimentally investigated is whether or not an increase in blood COHb alters the transfer of O_2 from haemoglobin, via the myoglobin molecule, to the cell mitochondria. If, for example, O_2 is displaced from haemoglobin onto myoglobin in a muscle that is contaminated with small amounts of CO, then the transfer of O_2 may be impaired due to differences in the O_2 diffusion gradient and transfer kinetics. In addition, there will be a CO-induced leftward shift in the relationship between the O_2 partial pressure and percentage of oxyhaemoglobin saturation as a result of difficulty in unloading O_2 from haemoglobin at normal tissue O_2 pressures.

Early studies have shown that VO_{2max} in healthy men decreases linearly with increased blood COHb levels (Figure 2)[64–74]. VO_{2max} reduction was not statistically significant until COHb concentrations of >4.3% were obtained[72]; however, 2.7% COHb has been shown to significantly decrease maximal performance time on the treadmill[69–71]. Another question that needs to be investigated is whether or not such low concentrations of circulating COHb affect anaerobic metabolism.

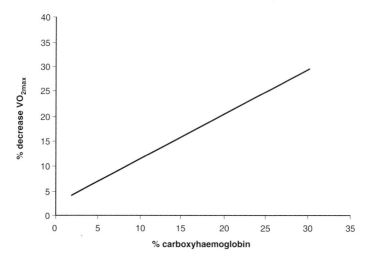

Figure 2

Linear relationship between increasing levels of carboxyhaemoglobin and the decrement in maximal aerobic power (VO_{2max})[25]

During submaximal work of short duration at 40–60% VO_{2max}, 15% COHb was shown to have little effect on energy production and ventilation in healthy individuals, but the submaximal heart rate was significantly increased[65–7]. Muscular exercise efficiency was, therefore, not affected below 15% COHb. However, the lowered O_2-carrying capacity resulting from the increased COHb concentration was overcome by a hyperkinetic circulation. As work intensity expanded, ventilation volume was increased by means of a faster respiratory rate — similar to the changes observed during altitude hypoxia[66,67]. During more prolonged work (three-and-a-half to four hours) at approximately 35% VO_{2max} with exposure to 50 ppm CO resulting in COHb levels of 4.6–6.8%, only heart rate was increased above that observed during filtered-air exposures[75]. Additional exposures to concentrations of 75 ppm and 100 ppm in the expired air for four hours and at 35% VO_{2max} of exercise resulted in COHb concentrations of 10.7% and 13.2% and failed to alter the cardiopulmonary response significantly[75]. In summary, in the healthy, non-cardiovascularly compromised individual, ambient CO concentrations resulting in COHb below 15% do not alter physiological responses to low intensity work (35–60% VO_{2max}). In view of the physiological requirements during aerobic training and endurance performance, the reduction in the cardiopulmonary reserves incurred by CO loading will be detrimental to the elite performer and most certainly will affect the individual exercising with compromised reserves.

In a series of unique experiments involving patients with exertional angina pectoris, Aronow *et al* exposed patients to ambient air pollutants while driving in heavy traffic and during controlled environmental laboratory responses[76–9]. There was a significant decrease in the exercise time to angina when the patients breathed the traffic ambient air (COHb=3.9%), 50 ppm CO (COHb=2.7%) and 100 ppm CO (COHb = 4.5%). Another investigation found that 10% of clinically healthy individuals exhibit ST segment depression >1.00 mm when COHb exceeded 4.0%[80]. Debias *et al* exposed monkeys to 100 ppm CO for six hours (COHb=9.3%) and found their myocardiums to be more susceptible to fibrillation than the non-CO exposed monkeys[81]. Furthermore, monkeys post-infarction and exposed to the same duration and concentration of CO were more susceptible to fibrillation than the healthy CO exposed animal. These findings confirm that cardiac-impaired patients are exposed to additional risks of cardiac events if exercising in ambient environments >2% COHb.

Conclusions

Combustion-related pollutants, including O_3 and CO, affect exercise performance detrimentally[82,83]. O_3 produces substantial pain on deep inspiration. The pain appears to reduce pulmonary function performance and affects the psychobiology of the exercising human, while O_3 may physiologically alter the breathing pattern. Prophylactic use of antioxidants and non-steroidal anti-inflammatory drugs may be of benefit.

Acidic pollutants, mainly SO_2, may selectively affect bronchoconstriction in asthmatic individuals. Prophylactic use of common asthma medications, such as cromolyn sodium and β-agonists, can prevent or alleviate the bronchoconstriction.

CO binds to haemoglobin and reduces the O_2-carrying capacity of the haemoglobin molecule. This reduces VO_{2max}, which causes the relative intensity of a given exercise load to be greater than when exercising in non-polluted atmospheres.

References

1 Bjure J, Grimbey G, Nellson MJ. Pulmonary gas exchange during submaximal and maximal exercise in healthy middle-aged men. In: Sherrer M, ed. *Pulmonary diffusing capacity on exercise*. Bern: Hans Huber, 1970: 107–22.

2 Bouhuys A. *Air pollution in breathing: physiology, environment and lung disease*. New York: Grune & Stratton, 1974: 385–415.

3 Bates DV, Macklem PT, Christie RV. Response to chemical and physical irritants. In: *Respiratory function in disease*. Philadelphia: Saunders, 1971: 361–400.

4 *Proceedings of the conference on health effects of air pollutants. National Academy of Sciences and the National Research Council, October 3–5, 1973.* Washington: Government Printing Office, 1973.

5 Stokinger HE. Toxicity of airborne chemicals: air quality standards — a national and international view. *Annu Rev Pharmacol* 1972; **12**: 407–22.

6 Wayne WS, Wehle PA, Carroll RE. Oxidant air pollution and athletic performance. *JAMA* 1967; **199**: 151–4.

7 Jaffe LS. The biological effects of photochemical air pollutants on man and animals. *Am J Public Health* 1967; **57**: 1269–77.

8 Becker WH, Schilling FD, Verma MP. The effect on health of the 1966 Eastern Seaboard air pollution episode. *Arch Environ Health* 1968; **16**: 414–9.

9 Greenburg L, Field F, Read JI *et al*. Air pollution and morbidity in New York City. *JAMA* 1962; **182**: 161–8.

10 Greenburg L, Jacobs MB, Dobette BM *et al*. Report of an air pollution incident in New York City, November 1963. *Public Health Rep* 1962; **77**: 7–16.

11 Logan WPD. Mortality in the London Fog Incident 1952. *Lancet* 1968; **1**: 336–8.

12 Schrenk HH, Heinann HH, Clayton GD *et al*. Air pollution in Donora, Pennsylvania. US Public Health Bull 1949, 306:1–173.

13 Hammer DI, Hasselblad V, Protnoy B *et al*. Los Angeles Student Nurse Study. *Arch Environ Health* 1974; **28**: 255–60.

14 Stokinger HE. Effect of air pollution on animals. In: Stern A, ed. *Air pollution*. Volume 1. New York: Academic Press, 1962: 282–334.

15 Stokinger HE. Pollutant gases. In: Fenn FO, Rahn H, ed. *Handbook of physiology*. Volume 2, section 3. Washington: American Physiological Society, 1965: 1067–86.

16 Stokinger HE. Evaluation of acute hazards of ozone and oxides of nitrogen. *AMA Arch Indust Health* 1957; **15**: 181–90.

17 Scheel LD, Dobrogorski J, Mountain JT *et al*. Physiologic, biochemical, immunologic, and pathologic changes following ozone exposure. *J Appl Physiol* 1959; **14**: 67–80.

18 Trucke R. Toxicity of ozone. *Arch Maladies Professionnelles: Hygiene Toxicol Industrielles* 1951; **12**: 55–8.

19 Vaughan TR, Jennelle LF, Lewis TR. Long-term exposure to low levels of air pollutants. *Arch Environ Health* 1969; **19**: 45–50.

20 Griswold SS, Chambers LA, Motley HL. Report of a case of exposure to high ozone concentrations for two hours. *AMA Arch Indust Health* 1957; **15**: 108–18.

21 Bennett G. Contamination of high altitude aircraft cabins. *Aerospace Med* 1972; **33**: 969–73.

22 Goldsmith JR, Nadel JA. Experimental exposure of human subjects to ozone. *J Air Pollut Control Assoc* 1969; **19**: 329–30.

23 Hallett WY. Effect of ozone and cigarette smoke on lung function. *Arch Environ Health* 1965; **10**: 295–302.

24 Young WA, Shaw DB, Bates DV. Effect of low concentrations of ozone on pulmonary function. *J Appl Physiol* 1964; **19**: 765–8.

25 Bates DV, Bell GM, Burham CD *et al*. Short-term effects of ozone on the lung. *J Appl Physiol* 1972; **32**: 176–81.

26 Lee LY, Bleecker ER, Nadel JA. Effect of ozone on bronchomotor response to inhaled histamine aerosol in dogs. *J Appl Physiol* 1977; **43**: 626–31.

27 Bates DV, Hazucha M. The short-term efects of ozone on the human lung. In: *Proceedings of the conference on health effects of air pollutants. National Academy of Sciences and the National Research Council, October 3–5 1973.* Washington: Government Printing Office, 1973: 507–40.

28 Hazucha M, Silverman F, Parent C *et al*. Pulmonary function in man after short-term exposure to ozone. *Arch Environ Health* 1973; **27**: 183–8.

29 Folinsbee LJ, Silverman F, Shephard RJ. Exercise responses following ozone exposure. *J Appl Physiol* 1975; **38**: 996–1001.

30 Silverman F, Folinsbee LJ, Shephard RJ. Pulmonary function changes following ozone exposure — interaction ventilation and concentration. *J Appl Physiol* 1976; **41**: 859–64.

31 Avol EL, Linn WS, Venet TG *et al*. Comparative respiratory effects of ozone and ambient oxidant pollution exposure during heavy exercise. *J Air Pollut Cont Assoc* 1984; **34**: 804–9.

32 Gong H, Bradley PW, Simmons MS, Tashkin DP. Impaired exercise performance and pulmonary function in elite cyclists during low-level ozone exposure in a hot environment. *Am Rev Resp Dis* 1986; **134**: 726–33.

33 Schelegle ES, Adams WC. Reduced exercise time in competitive simulations consequent to low level ozone exposure. *Med Sci Sports Exerc* 1986; **18**: 408–14.

34 Folinsbee LJ, Silverman F, Shephard RJ. Decrease of maximum work performance following ozone exposure. *J Appl Physiol* 1977; **42**: 531–6.

35 Folinsbee LJ, Drinkwater BL, Bedi JF, Horvath SM. The influence of exercise on the pulmonary function changes due to exposure to low concentrations of ozone. In: Folinsbee LJ, Wagner JA, Borgia JF *et al*, eds. *Environmental stress: individual human adaptations*. New York: Academic Press, 1978: 125–45.

36 Folinsbee LJ, Bedi JF, Horvath SM. Pulmonary function changes after 1 h continuous heavy exercise in 0.21 ppm ozone. *J Appl Physiol* 1984; **57**: 984–8.

37 Foxcroft WJ, Adams WC. Effects of ozone exposure on four consecutive days on work performance and VO_{2max}. *J Appl Physiol* 1986; **61**: 960–6.

38 Folinsbee LJ. Chapter 20. In: Garrett WE Jr, Kirkendahl D, eds. *Effect of air pollutants on exercise: basic and applied science.* Page 294.

39 Beckett WS, McDonnell WF, Horstman DH, House, DE. Role of the parasympathetic nervous system in acute lung response to ozone. *J Appl Physiol* 1985; **59**: 1879–85.

40 Holtzman MJ, Cunningham JH, Sheller JR *et al*. Effect of ozone on bronchial reactivity in atopic and nonatopic subjects. *Am Rev Resp Dis* 1979; **120**: 1059–67.

41 Gong H Jr, Bedi JF, Horvath SM. Inhaled albuterol does not protect against ozone toxicity in nonasthmatic athletes. *Arch Environ Health* 1988; **43**: 46–53.

42 Adams WC, Savin WM, Christo AE. Detection of ozone toxicity during continuous exercise via the effective dose concept. *J Appl Physiol* 1981; **51**: 415–22.

43 McDonnell WF, Horstman DH, Hazucha MJ *et al*. Pulmonary effects of ozone exposure during exercise: dose-response characteristics. *J Appl Physiol* 1983; **54**: 1345–52.

44 Kulle TJ, Sauder LR, Hebel JR, Chatham MD. Ozone response relationships in healthy nonsmokers. *Am Rev Respir Dis* 1985; **132**: 36–41.

45 Lee LY, Dumont C, Djokic TD *et al*. Mechanism of rapid shallow breathing after ozone exposure in conscious dogs. *J Appl Physiol* 1979; **46**: 1108–14.

46 Coleridge JCG, Coleridge HM, Schelegle ES, Green JF. Acute inhalation of ozone stimulates bronchial C-fibers and rapidly adapting receptors in dogs. *J Appl Physiol* 1993; **74**: 2345–52.

47 Schelegle ES, Carl ML, Coleridge HM *et al*. Contribution of vagal afferents to respiratory reflexes evoked by acute inhalation of ozone in dogs. *J Appl Physiol* 1993; **74**: 2338–44.

48 Coleridge HM, Coleridge JCG, Baker DG *et al*. Comparison of the effects of histamine and prostaglandin on afferent C-fiber endings and irritant receptors in the intrapulmonary airways. *Adv Exp Med Biol* 1978; **99**: 291–305.

49 Schelegle ES, Adams WC, Siefkin AD. Indomethacin pretreatment reduces ozone-induced pulmonary function decrements in human subjects. *Am Rev Respir Dis* 1987; **136**: 1350–4.

50 McDonnell W, Koren H, Devlin R *et al*. Biochemical and cellular correlates of changes in pulmonary functions and symptoms in humans exposed to ozone. *Am Rev Respir Dis* 1990; **141**: A72.

51 Eschenbacher WL, Ying RL, Kreit JW, Gross KB. Ozone-induced lung function changes in normal and asthmatic subjects and the effect of indomethacin. In: Schneider T, Lee SD, Wolters GJR, Grant LD, eds. *Atmospheric ozone research and its policy implications. Proceedings of the 3rd US–Dutch international symposium, May 1988, Nijmegen, The Netherlands*. Amsterdam: Elsevier Science Publishers, 1989: 493–9.

52 Ying RL, Gross KB, Terzo TS, Eschenbacher WL. Indomethacin does not inhibit the ozone-induced increase in bronchial responsiveness in human subjects. *Am Rev Respir Dis* 1990; **142**: 817–21.

53 Hazucha MJ, Bates DV, Bromberg PA. Mechanism of action of ozone on the human lung. *J Appl Physiol* 1989; **67**: 1535–41.

54 Forsyth RD, Cole P, Shephard RJ. Exercise and nasal patency. *J Appl Physiol* 1983; **55**: 860–5.

55 Bates DV. Observations on asthma. *Environ Health Perspect* 1995; **103**(suppl 6): 243–7.

56 Voy RO. The US Olympic Committee experience with exercise-induced bronchospasm. *Med Sci Sports Exerc* 1984; **18**: 328–30.

57 Folinsbee LJ. Sulfur oxides: controlled human exposure studies. In: Lee SD, Schneider T, eds. *Comparative risk analysis and priority setting for air pollution issues. Proceedings of the 4th US–Dutch international symposium, June 1993, Keystone, CO*. Pittsburgh: Air & Waste Management Association: 326–34.

58 Forbes WH, Sargent F, Roughton FJW. The rate of carbon monoxide uptake by normal men. *Am J Physiol* 1945; **143**: 594–608.

59 Stewart RD, Petersen JE, Baretta ED *et al*. Experimental human exposure to carbon monoxide. *Arch Environ Health* 1970; **21**: 154–64.

60 Petersen JE, Stewart RD. Absorption and elimination of carbon monoxide by inactive young men. *Arch Environ Health* 1970; **21**: 176–81.

61 Stewart RD. The effect of carbon monoxide on humans. *Annu Rev Pharmacol* 1975; 409–24.

62 Coburn RF, Forster RE, Cane PB. Considerations of the physiological variables that determine the blood carboxyhemoglobin concentration in man. *J Clin Invest* 1965; **44**: 1899–910.

63 Petersen JE, Stewart RD. Predicting carboxyhemoglobin levels from carbon monoxide exposures. *J Appl Physiol* 1975; **39**: 633–8.

64 Chiodi H, Dill DB, Conzalazio F *et al*. Respiratory and circulatory responses to acute carbon monoxide poisoning. *Am J Physiol* 1941; **134**: 683–93.

65 Pirnay F, Dujardin J, Deroanne R *et al*. Muscular exercise during intoxication by carbon monoxide. *J Appl Physiol* 1971; **31**: 573–5.

66 Vogel JA, Gleser MA, Wheeler RC *et al*. Carbon monoxide and physical work capacity. *Arch Environ Health* 1972; **24**: 198–203.

67 Vogel JA, Gleser MA. Effect of carbon monoxide on oxygen transport during exercise. *J Appl Physiol* 1972; **32**: 235–9.

68 Ekblom B, Huot R. Response to submaximal and maximal exercise at different levels of carboxyhemoglobin. *Acta Physiol Scand* 1972; **86**: 473–4.

69 Raven PB, Drinkwater BL, Ruhling RO *et al*. Effect of carbon monoxide and peroxyacetylnitrate on man's maximal aerobic capacity. *J Appl Physiol* 1974; **36**: 288–93.

70 Drinkwater BL, Raven PB, Horvath SM *et al*. Air pollution, exercise and heat stress. *Arch Environ Health* 1974; **28**: 177–82.

71 Raven PB, Drinkwater BL, Horvath SM *et al*. Age, smoking habits, heat stress and their interactive effects with carbon monoxide and peroxyacteylnitrate on man's aerobic power. *Int J Biometeorol* 1974; **18**: 222–32.

72 Horvath SM, Raven PB, Dahms TE *et al*. Maximal aerobic capacity at different levels of carboxyhemoglobin. *J Appl Physiol* 1975; **38**: 300–3.

73 Nielson B. Thermoregulation during work in carbon monoxide poisoning. *Acta Physiol Scand* 1971; **82**: 98–106.

74 Chevalier RB, Bowers JA, Bondurant S *et al*. Circulatory and ventilatory effects in smokers and nonsmokers. *J Appl Physiol* 1963; **18**: 357–60.

75 Gliner JA, Raven PB, Horvath SM *et al*. Man's physiologic response to long-term work during thermal and pollutant stress. *J Appl Physiol* 1975; **39**: 628–32.

76 Aronow WS, Harris CN, Isbell MS *et al*. Effect of freeway travel on angina pectoris. *Ann Intern Med* 1972; **77**: 669–76.

77 Aronow WS, Isbell MW. Carbon monoxide effect on exercise-induced angina pectoris. *Ann Intern Med* 1973; **79**: 392–5.

78 Anderson EW, Andelman RJ, Strauch JM *et al*. Effect of low-level carbon monoxide exposure on onset and duration of angina pectoris: a study of ten patients with ischemic heart disease. *Ann Intern Med* 1973; **79**: 46–50.

79 Aronow WS, Cassidy J. Effect of carbon monoxide on maximal treadmill exercise: a study in normal persons. *Ann Intern Med* 1975; **83**: 496–9.

80 Ayres SM, Grannelli S Jr, Mueller H. Effects of low concentrations of carbon monoxide: myocardial and systemic response to carboxyhemoglobin. *Ann N Y Acad Sci* 1970; **17**: 268–93.

81 Debias DA, Baneyu CM, Burkhead NC *et al*. Carbon monoxide inhalation effects following myocardial infarction in monkeys. *Arch Environ Health* 1973; **27**: 161–7.

82 Folinsbee LJ, Horvath SM, Raven PB *et al*. Influence of exercise and heat stress on pulmonary function during ozone exposure. *J Appl Physiol* 1977; **43**: 409–13.

83 Raven PB, Gliner JA, Sutton JC. Dynamic lung function changes following long-term work in polluted environments. *Environ Res* 1976; **12**: 18–25.

245

Prolonged exercise and the immune system

DR BENTE K PEDERSEN

DEPARTMENT OF INFECTIOUS DISEASES, RIGSHOSPITALET (UNIVERSITY HOSPITAL),
COPENHAGEN, DENMARK

It has been known for more than a century that muscular exercise influences the immune system and resistance towards infections. Charrin and Roger published the first report on exercise and immunology in 1890, and noted an increased risk of infections in fatigued rats[1]. The first publication on exercise-induced leucocytosis was written by Schulz in 1893[2] and one decade later, in 1902, Larrabee described 'violent leukocytosis' experienced by runners after the Boston marathon[3]. Only sporadic reports on exercise and immunology were available in the years that followed, but during the past 15 years there has been growing interest in understanding to which degree and by which mechanisms exercise influences the immune system[4,5].

Today, much research is stimulated by the acceptance of exercise as a tool to study the immune system. Exercise can be employed as a model for temporary immuno-suppression, which occurs after severe physical stress. The exercise-stress model can be easily manipulated and allows for the study of interactions between the nervous, the endocrine and the immune systems. This chapter will focus on the immune changes that occur in response to prolonged acute and chronic exercise, the mechanisms underlying these changes, and their clinical consequences.

Acute exercise

Effects on leucocyte subpopulation

Several consistent patterns involving leucocyte subpopulations in the blood have been observed in response to acute exercise. For instance, neutrophil concentrations increase during and after exercise, while lymphocyte concentrations increase during exercise and fall below pre-exercise levels after long-duration physical work (Figure 1)[5]. Exercise-induced changes seen in subsets of blood mononuclear cells (BMNC) have also been described in several reports[4,6]. The increase in lymphocyte concentrations may be due to the recruitment of its subpopulations (eg CD4+ T cells, CD8+ T cells, CD19+ B cells, CD16+ natural killer (NK) cells and CD56+ NK cells) to the blood. CD4+ and CD8+ T cells contain both CD45RO+ memory and CD45RA+ virgin or naive cells which are identified by the absence of 45RO and the presence of CD62L. Data show that recruitment is mainly of CD45RO+ lymphocytes[7]. Recent studies reveal that concentrations of CD45RO+, CD45RO- and CD62L- increase

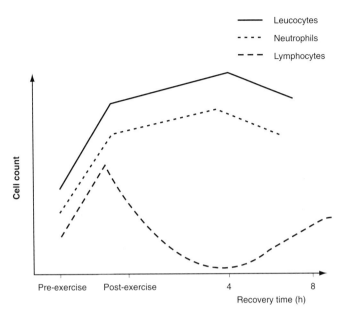

Figure 1

Relative leucocyte, neutrophil and lymphocyte counts before and after two-and-a-half hours of treadmill running

during exercise, suggesting that memory, but not naive, lymphocytes are rapidly mobilized to the blood in response to physical exercise[7].

Lymphocyte turnover in cells recruited during exercise was recently investigated at the Copenhagen Muscle Research Center, Denmark, by analysing the length of the telomeric terminal restriction fragment. Telomeres are the extreme ends of chromosomes that consist of repeats of a TTAGGG sequence. After each cycle of cell division, the telomeric sequence was found to be missing because of the inability of deoxyribonucleic acid (DNA) polymerase to fully replicate the 5' end of the chromosome[7]. Telomere length has been used as a marker for replication history and for the proliferation potential of cells. CD8+ T cell cultures, which have reached replicate senescence after multiple rounds of cell division, lack expression of the CD28 co-stimulatory molecule and have short telomere lengths. In response to exercise, lymphocytes lacking the CD28 molecule were mobilized to the circulation, and telomere lengths in CD4+ and CD8+ lymphocytes were significantly shorter than cells isolated at rest[7]. The characterization of lymphocytes mobilized to the blood is summarized in Table 1.

Most lymphocyte subpopulations increase in number during physical exercise; however, the percentage of CD4+ cells declines mainly because NK cells increase more than other lymphocyte subpopulations; this contributes to the exercise-induced alterations in in vitro immune assays in which a fixed number of BMNC is studied. Human studies

Table 1 *Characteristics of lymphocytes mobilized to blood during exercise*

- Activated cells
- Memory cells
- Cells lacking CD28
- Low proliferative capacity
- Short telomere length

reveal that lymphocyte responses to T cell mitogens, phytohaemagglutinin and concanavalin A, decline during and for up to several hours after exercise[4,8]; this is also consistently found in animal studies[4,8]. This may partly be due to the increase in NK cells in circulation and the reduction of CD4+ cells in in vitro assays. When cellular immune function is assessed by in vitro measurements, the NK and lymphokine activated killer (LAK) cell activities, as well as the proliferative responses and the in vitro production of immunoglobulins (Igs), decline. In vivo measurements have shown that the delayed type hypersensitivity reaction to recall antigens introduced into the skin is impaired following strenuous exercise, whereas the antibody responses following vaccination have been reported not to be influenced by exercise[9].

Origin of leucocytes

The movement of neutrophils from marginal pools located intravascularly and from extravascular storage pools contributes to exercise-related neutrocytosis. With respect to lymphocytosis during exercise, the role of margination is less clear. Research indicates that lymphocytes are recruited to the circulation from peripheral tissue compartments during exercise, including the spleen, lymph nodes and gastrointestinal (GI) tract. The spleen may contribute to lymphocytosis as it is a major storage pool for lymphocytes. Splenectomized subjects demonstrate a low lymphocyte count when injected with adrenaline; subjects without a spleen show a smaller increase in lymphocyte numbers during exercise[10,11].

As the cells that move to the blood have short telomere lengths, it does not seem likely that these cells are mobilized from the bone marrow or from thymus. The number of cells entering the circulation is determined by the intensity of the stimulus. Prolonged and/or very high intensity exercise causes a reduction in the total concentration of lymphocytes. The mechanisms for this probably include the lack of mature cells that can be recruited, as well as the redistribution of lymphocytes from the circulation to organs.

Fate of the lymphocytes

Strenuous exercise is characterized by increased oxygen consumption and a disturbance in intracellular pro-oxidant and antioxidant homeostasis. Increased oxygen consumption leads to greater generation of reactive oxygen species (ROS) through the mitochondrial electron transport chain. Xanthine oxidase reaction, due to adenosine triphosphate degradation and activated neutrophils, may also play an important role in the formation of ROS during the recovery period after exercise. At rest and during mild oxidative stress, the antioxidant defence system maintains homeostasis but this may fail during extensive oxygen stress[12]. ROS have a strong tendency to interact with other molecules and to damage various cellular components. Azenabor and Hoffman-Goetz demonstrated that oxidative damage in mice lymphoid tissues occurred after running and could contribute to lymphocyte damage or apoptosis (programmed cell death) after acute exercise[13]. It is well documented that ROS are mediators of apoptosis. Other physiological stimuli such as exposure to glucocorticoids and pro-inflammatory cytokines also trigger induction of apoptosis. The available data concerning apoptosis in response to exercise are still controversial, but it is clear that many mechanisms able to induce apoptosis are present during and after a heavy run. One issue still to be addressed is whether or not apoptosis plays a role in the different cellular changes, or whether or not the antioxidant defence system can prevent the apoptotic cascade that is initiated.

Several studies have shown that exhaustive exercise increases superoxide dismutase in different tissues. The fat-soluble antioxidant vitamin E does not seem to be significantly affected by one acute bout of exercise. Similarly, the water-soluble antioxidant vitamin C is not depleted following an acute bout of exercise in humans; however, Azenabor and Hoffman-Goetz revealed significantly reduced plasma levels of vitamin C in mice 24 hours after a run to exhaustion[13].

Local production of antibodies

The secretory immune system of mucosal tissues, such as the upper respiratory tract, is considered by many clinical immunologists to be the first barrier to its colonization by pathogenic microorganisms. Lower concentrations of salivary IgA have been reported in cross-country skiers after a race[14]. This finding was confirmed by a 70% decrease in salivary IgA, which persisted for several hours after completion of intense, long-duration ergometer cycling[15]. Reduced salivary IgA was also found after intense swimming, running and incremental treadmill running to exhaustion. Submaximal exercise had no effect on this Ig[15,16].

Nilssen *et al* showed that intestinal IgA- and IgM-producing cells were not reduced in marathon runners after completing the race[17]. They hypothesized that a stress-induced hormonal influence on the homing of primed B cells to the mucosa, or an immune response to elevated influx of stimulatory luminal antigens, could course the different observations. Many marathon runners suffer GI tract side-effects after a long run.

Cytokines

Strenuous exercise induces increased levels of cytokines in the blood, especially interleukin (IL)-6 (Figure 2)[4], which has been shown to increase 100-fold after running a marathon. Although initial research suggested that IL-1 levels increased in response

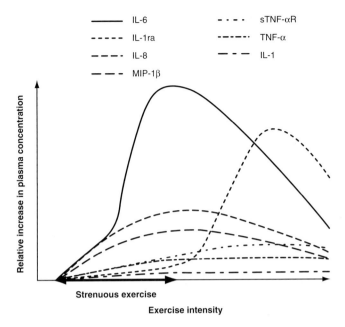

Figure 2

Effect of strenuous exercise on plasma levels of IL-1, IL-1ra, IL-6, IL-8, macrophage inflammatory protein (MIP)-1β, tumour necrosis factor (TNF)-α and soluble TNF α-receptor (sTNF-αR)

to exercise, recent studies using more specific assays have shown no increase or only a small increase in the concentrations of IL-1. The rise in IL-6 is followed by an increase in the concentration of IL-1ra, a naturally occurring inhibitor of IL-1[18-21]. Thus, the level of IL-6 peaks immediately after cessation of exercise, whereas IL-1ra does not increase until after the exercise and peaks approximately two hours post-exercise.

One source of IL-6 has recently been identified. Ostrowski *et al* detected IL-6-messenger ribonucleic acid (mRNA) in skeletal muscle biopsies obtained from runners after a marathon[21], which indicates that IL-6 is locally produced in response to strenuous exercise or exercise-induced muscle damage. IL-1ra-mRNA was not present in skeletal muscle but was expressed by BMNC obtained after, but not before, the race. This suggests that locally produced IL-6 induces a systemic anti-inflammatory response. The latter finding of IL-6 mRNA has also been confirmed in an animal model (Jonsdottir, unpublished data). The biological role of locally produced IL-6 needs to be defined. Ongoing research at the Copenhagen Muscle Research Center, Denmark, indicates the possibility that IL-6 induces signal transduction in the working muscle and, thus, acts as a growth factor. Table 2 summarizes the characteristics of IL-6.

In addition to IL-6, concentrations of tumour necrosis factor (TNF)-α have been shown to increase two to threefold after strenuous exercise[19]. Also, recent data from

Table 2 *Characteristics of IL-6 during prolonged exercise*

IL-6:
- is produced early
- is related to duration and intensity of exercise
- is related to heart rate
- increases exponentially
- is locally produced in the muscle
- induces signal transduction in the muscle

the Copenhagen Muscle Research Center, Denmark, have indicated that circulating levels of soluble TNF receptors (sTNF-R) 1 and 2 and the chemokines IL-8 and macrophage inflammatory protein (MIP)-1 are increased in response to strenuous exercise. Thus, exercise induces a strong anti-inflammatory response.

Neuroendocrinological mechanisms for immune change

The mechanisms underlying exercise-associated immune changes are multifactorial and include neuroendocrinological factors such as adrenaline, noradrenaline, growth hormone, cortisol and β-endorphin[4,22,23]. The concentrations of these hormones increase during exercise and return to pre-exercise values shortly afterwards, but appear to affect lymphocytes and neutrophils in the recovery period of exercise. Studies in which hormone receptors were blocked by drugs or when hormone production was inhibited by epidural blockade in relation to physical stress contribute to our understanding of the mechanisms of action. These studies suggest that adrenaline and, to a lower degree, noradrenaline are responsible for acute exercise effects on lymphocyte dynamics, including the effects of exercise on NK cell activity and T cell function. Increases in growth hormone and catecholamines mediate the acute effects on neutrophils, whereas cortisol exerts its effects within a time lag of at least two hours and, thus, may contribute to maintain the lymphocytopenia and neutrocytosis only after long-term exercise[24,25]. The role of β-endorphins is less clear, but they are not thought to play an important role in the immediate recruitment of NK cells to the blood. They are, however, likely to mediate some of the chronic exercise effects on the immune system.

Chronic exercise

The influence of chronic exercise on the immune system has been investigated in both animal and human models, the latter including both longitudinal and cross-sectional studies. Cross-sectional studies have shown increased natural immunity in elite cyclists, runners and highly conditioned elderly subjects, while other studies have found no difference in natural immunity between trained and untrained subjects. Longitudinal studies found no effect of eight weeks of training on NK cell activity in neither elderly subjects nor patients with rheumatoid arthritis. Other studies found enhanced resting levels of NK cell activity following 16 weeks of training in elderly women and after 15 weeks of moderate training in previously inactive mildly obese women.

In contrast to the human studies which show variable influence of training, several animal studies, using training protocols of varying length and intensity and different animal species, support the findings of increased resting levels of natural cytotoxicity after voluntary exercise[4].

The observations on NK cell activity and training are controversial. It is possible that the increased NK cell activity reported in some groups of athletes is not directly related to training but may, in fact, be due to other factors such as the diet. This was demonstrated in a recent study where NK cell activity was enhanced following seven weeks of training on a carbohydrate-rich diet, but not after training on a fat-rich diet[26].

Clinical consequences

Although moderate exercise seems to enhance the immune system, it is a common perception among elite athletes and their coaches that heavy exercise lowers resistance to infection. Thus, an important question is whether or not the exercise-induced changes in lymphocyte concentrations in the circulating pool, the proportional distribution of lymphocyte subpopulations and the function of these cells are of clinical significance, especially with respect to resistance to infectious disease and malignancy. Athletes do not seem to be immunocompromised by a clinical definition. Upper respiratory tract infections (URTI) are the only illnesses to which they appear to be more susceptible.

Anecdotal evidence suggests that, while regular training promotes resistance to URTI, severe exertion, especially when coupled with mental stress, places athletes at increased risk of URTI. The epidemiological studies on exercise and URTI are mostly based on self-reported symptoms rather than clinical verification. Using these studies, Nieman has proposed a 'J'-shaped relationship between exercise and URTI[27] (Figure 3). The link between exercise-associated immune changes and sensitivity to infections may be explained by the so-called 'open window' of altered immunity. Based on the open window hypothesis and the fact that high-performance athletes often train more than once a day, chronic immunosuppression may occur if the immune system has not fully recovered before the next training session. However, whether athletes showing the most extreme immunosuppression after heavy exertion are those that contract an infection within the following one to two weeks remains to be demonstrated.

According to the immune surveillance theory, it is to be expected that moderate exercise protects against malignancy while exhaustive exercise is linked with increased

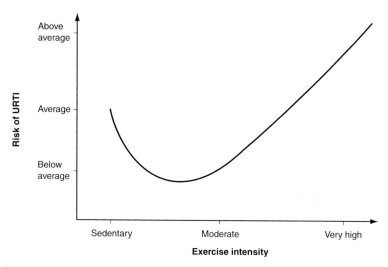

Figure 3

Relative risk of URTI in correlation to duration and intensity of exercise, proposed by Nieman[27]

cancer risk. Accumulating results to date support the idea that exercise protects against colon cancer and breast cancer[4], but there is little or no published evidence that strenuous exercise is associated with increased risk of cancer.

Role of dietary intervention

Altered protein metabolism, such as declined glutamine concentrations in plasma as a result of muscular activity, has been suggested to influence lymphocyte function[28], and reduced plasma glucose is thought to increase stress-hormone levels and, thus, immune function[29]. Free oxygen radicals and prostaglandins (PG) released by the increased number of neutrophils and monocytes may also influence the function of lymphocytes. Thus, nutritional supplementation with glutamine, carbohydrate, PG-inhibitors or antioxidants may, in principle, influence exercise-associated immune function.

Glutamine hypothesis

The demands on muscle and organs for glutamine under intense physical exercise may force the lymphoid system into a glutamine debt, which will temporarily affect its function. Factors that directly or indirectly influence glutamine synthesis or release could, therefore, influence the function of lymphocytes and monocytes[30].

Following intense long-term exercise and other physical stress disorders, the glutamine concentration in plasma declines. Glutamine in vitro enhances lymphocyte proliferation and LAK cell activity, but has no effect on NK cell activity. It also stimulates IL-2 and IFN production in vitro without influencing the production of IL-1,

IL-6 or TNF-α. When added to in vitro assays, glutamine was shown to be unable to abolish the post-exercise decline in proliferative responses and did not normalize the low lymphocyte proliferation in human immunodeficiency virus (HIV) seropositive patients.

Castell *et al* found that glutamine supplementation decreased the incidence of URTI after a marathon[31]. In contrast, MacKinnon *et al* found no difference in plasma-glutamine levels in swimmers who did or did not develop URTI following intensive swimming training[32]. Two recent placebo-controlled glutamine intervention studies revealed that glutamine abolished the post-exercise decline in plasma glutamine without influencing post-exercise impairment of NK and LAK cell function, or mitogen-induced proliferative responses[33,34]. These studies did not support the hypothesis that post-exercise decline in immune function is caused by a decrease in the plasma glutamine concentration. This is consistent with the fact that reduced immune function in vitro is seen only if glutamine concentrations in assays are <10% of the physiological concentrations.

Carbohydrate hypothesis

Earlier research had established that a reduction in blood glucose levels is associated with hypothalamic-pituitary-adrenal activation, increased release of adrenocortico-trophic hormone and cortisol, increased plasma growth hormone, decreased insulin, and a variable effect on blood adrenaline level[24]. Given the link between stress hormones and immune responses to prolonged and intensive exercise[23], carbohydrate ingestion should maintain plasma glucose concentrations, attenuate increases in stress hormones and, thus, diminish changes in immunity.

This hypothesis has been tested in several studies using double-blind, placebo-controlled randomized designs. Carbohydrate beverage ingestion before, during (about 1 l/h) and after two-and-a-half hours of exercise was associated with: higher plasma glucose levels, an attenuated cortisol and growth hormone response, fewer perturbations in blood immune cell counts, lower granulocyte and monocyte phago-cytosis and oxidative burst activity, and increases in IL-6 and IL-1ra. Overall, the hormonal and immune responses to carbohydrate compared with placebo ingestion were diminished. Some immune variables (eg granulocyte and monocyte function) were slightly affected by carbohydrate ingestion, while others (eg plasma cytokine concentrations and blood cell counts) were strongly influenced[29].

Further investigation is needed to determine the clinical significance of carbohydrate-induced effects on the endocrine and immune systems. Current data indicate that athletes ingesting carbohydrate beverages before, during and after prolonged and intensive exercise should experience reduced physiological stress. Research to estab-lish whether or not carbohydrate ingestion will improve protection against viruses in athletes during intense training or following competitive endurance events is war-ranted. Also, it remains to be established whether or not the diminished IL-6 response is due to a reduced signal for IL-6 production or if carbohydrate exerts its effect directly on IL-6 production. Furthermore, the effect of carbohydrate supplementation on initial and prolonged muscle damage needs to be determined. It would also be interesting to investigate whether or not carbohydrate supplementation alters the acute phase response to clinical stress disorders such as sepsis and trauma, as it is known that some immune changes in these conditions are similar to those elicited by exercise.

n-3 PUFA hypothesis

Polyunsaturated fatty acids (PUFA) can be divided into two main classes: n-6 and n-3 families[35]. The precursor of both families is linoleic acid. Linoleic acid is converted to arachidonic acid, the precursor of PG and leukotrienes (LT) which have potent proinflammatory and immunoregulatory properties. If the n-6:n-3 ratio decreases by administration of a diet rich in n-3 fatty acids, the PGE_2-mediated immunosuppression may be abolished. Acute exercise induces high levels of PGE_2. Although conflicting results have been obtained for the effect of PG inhibitors on post-exercise immune impairment, some believe the theory that n-3 PUFA supplementation may alter exercise-induced immune changes by a mechanism involving PG or alteration of the fluidity and the structure of the cell membranes.

The possible interaction between intense acute exercise, immune function and PUFA was examined in inbred female C57BI/6 mice[36]. The animals received either a natural ingredient diet or a diet supplemented with various oils such as beef tallow, safflower, fish oil or linseed oil for an eight-week period. The group receiving linseed oil (which contained >50% 18:3 (n-3) α-linoleic acid) showed a marked immunomodulatory effect of 18:3 (n-3) α-linoleic acid on exhaustive exercise-related immunosuppression compared to the effects of other selected PUFA; linseed oil abolished post-exercise immunosuppression of IgM plaque forming cell response.

Antioxidant hypothesis

Antioxidants may neutralize the ROS that are produced by neutrophilic leucocytes during phagocytosis. This was demonstrated by Peters *et al*[37] who evaluated the effect of vitamin C on the incidence of URTI during the two-week period after the Comrades Ultramarathon[37]. The incidence was 68% in the placebo group, significantly higher than in the vitamin C supplementation group where only 33% reported URTI when taking 600 mg vitamin C daily supplementation for three weeks before the race. In another study, Peters *et al* found that vitamin A supplementation had an insignificant effect on the incidence of URTI in marathon runners[38].

Only one study has evaluated the effect of vitamin C on lymphocyte function and stress hormone levels after exercise[39]. It showed that supplementation with vitamin C did not influence leucocyte subsets, NK cell activity, lymphocyte proliferative responses, granulocyte phagocytosis, catecholamines or cortisol. Nielsen *et al* recently found that *N*-acetylcysteine (6 g daily for three days) had no effect on exercise-induced suppression of lymphocyte proliferation or NK cell activity[40].

Conclusions

In response to prolonged exercise, lymphocytes are mobilized to the blood; these cells are activated and have a reduced proliferative capacity. There is evidence to suggest that the cells are mobilized from peripheral compartments such as the spleen. During the post-exercise period, the lymphocyte count decreases below resting value. Recent studies indicate that exercise-induced apoptosis may play a mechanistic role.

Prolonged exercise also induces a cascade of pro- and anti-inflammatory cytokines. In particular, high levels of IL-6 are found in plasma which increase exponentially and are related to both duration and intensity of exercise. IL-6 is produced locally in skeletal muscle and may mediate some of the exercise effects on the muscle. The clinical consequence of exercise-induced immune changes is increased risk of obtaining an infection. Interventional studies have shown that carbohydrate supplementation abolishes some of the exercise effects on leucocytes and cytokines. However, the clinical significance remains to be identified.

References

1 Charrin, Roger. A l'etude experimentale du surmenage; son influence sur l'infection. *Arch de Physiol Norm Path* 1890; **2**: 273–83.

2 Schulz. Diagnostische bedeutung der leucocytose. *Dtsch Arch Kli Med* 1893; **51**: 234–81.

3 Larrabee RC. Leucocytosis after violent exercise. *J Med Res* 1902; **7**: 76–82.

4 Pedersen BK, Hoffman-Goetz L. Exercise and the immune system: regulation, integration and adaption. *Physiol Rev* 2000; **80**: 1055–81.

5 Brines R, Hoffman-Goetz L, Pedersen BK. Can you exercise to make your immune system fitter? *Immunol Today* 1996; **17**: 252–4.

6 Fitzgerald L. Exercise and the immune system. *Immunol Today* 1988; **9**: 337–9.

7 Bruunsgaard H, Jensen MS, Schjerling P *et al*. Exercise induces recruitment of lymphocytes with an activated phenotype and short telomeres in young and elderly humans. *Life Sci* 1999; **65**: 2623–33.

8 Nielsen HB, Pedersen BK. Lymphocyte proliferation in response to exercise. *Eur J Appl Physiol* 1997; **75**: 375–9.

9 Mackinnon LT, Hooper S. Mucosal (secretory) immune system responses to exercise of varying intensity and during overtraining. *Int J Sports Med* 1994; **15**(suppl 3): S179–83.

10 Steel CM, French EB, Aitchison WR. Studies on adrenaline-induced leucocytosis in normal man. I. The role of the spleen and of the thoracic duct. *Br J Haematol* 1971; **21**: 413–21.

11 Nielsen HB, Secher NH, Kristensen JH *et al*. Splenectomy impairs lymphocytosis during maximal exercise. *Am J Physiol* 1997; **272**: R1847–52.

12 Ji LL. Antioxidants and oxidative stress in exercise. *Proc Soc Exp Biol Med* 1999; **222**: 283–92.

13 Azenabor AA, Hoffman-Goetz L. Intrathymic and intrasplenic oxidative stress mediates thymocyte and splenocyte damage in acutely exercised mice. *J Appl Physiol* 1999; **86**: 1823–7.

14 Tomasi TB, Trudeau FB, Czerwinski D, Erredge S. Immune parameters in athletes before and after strenuous exercise. *J Clin Immunol* 1982; **2**: 173–8.

15 Mackinnon LT, Chick TW, van As A, Tomasi TB. The effect of exercise on secretory and natural immunity. *Adv Exp Med Biol* 1987; **216A**: 869–76.

16 McDowell SL, Hughes RA, Hughes RJ *et al*. The effect of exhaustive exercise on salivary immunoglobulin A. *J Sports Med Phys Fitness* 1992; **32**: 412–5.

17 Nilssen DE, Oktedalen O, Lygren I *et al*. Intestinal IgA- and IgM-producing cells are not decreased in marathon runners. *Int J Sports Med* 1998; **19**: 425–31.

18 Bruunsgaard H, Galbo H, Halkjaer-Kristensen J *et al*. Exercise-induced increase in serum interleukin-6 in humans is related to muscle damage. *J Physiol* 1997; **499**: 833–41.

19 Ostrowski K, Rohde T, Asp S *et al*. Pro- and anti-inflammatory cytokine balance in strenuous exercise in humans. *J Physiol* 1999; **515**: 287–91.

20 Ostrowski K, Hermann C, Bangash A *et al*. A trauma-like elevation of plasma cytokines in humans in response to treadmill running. *J Physiol* 1998; **513**: 889–94.

21 Ostrowski K, Rohde T, Zacho M *et al*. Evidence that interleukin-6 is produced in human skeletal muscle during prolonged running. *J Physiol* 1998; **508**: 949–53.

22 Pedersen BK, Nieman DC. Exercise immunology: integration and regulation. *Immunol Today* 1998; **19**: 204–6.

23 Hoffman-Goetz L, Pedersen BK. Exercise and the immune system: a model of the stress response? *Immunol Today* 1994; **15**: 382–7.

24 Pedersen BK, Bruunsgaard H, Klokker M *et al*. Exercise-induced immunomodulation — possible roles of neuroendocrine and metabolic factors. *Int J Sports Med* 1997; **18**(suppl 1): S2–7.

25 Shinkai S, Watanabe S, Asai H, Shek PN. Cortisol response to exercise and post-exercise suppression of blood lymphocyte subset counts. *Int J Sports Med* 1996; **17**: 597–603.

26 Pedersen BK, Helge JW, Richter EA *et al*. Training and natural immunity — effects of diets rich on fat or carbohydrate. *Eur J Appl Physiol* 2000; **82**: 98–102.

27 Nieman DC. Exercise, upper respiratory tract infection, and the immune system. *Med Sci Sports Exerc* 1994; **26**: 128–39.

28 Newsholme EA, Parry-Billings M. Properties of glutamine release from muscle and its importance for the immune system. *JPEN J Parenter Enteral Nutr* 1990; **14**(suppl 4): 63S–7S.

29 Nieman DC, Pedersen BK. Exercise and immune function. Recent developments. *Sports Med* 1999; **27**: 73–80.

30 Newsholme EA. Biochemical mechanisms to explain immunosuppression in well-trained and overtrained athletes. *Int J Sports Med* 1994; **15**(suppl 3): S142–7.

31 Castell LM, Poortmans JR, Newsholme EA. Does glutamine have a role in reducing infections in athletes? *Eur J Appl Physiol* 1996; **73**: 488–90.

32 Mackinnon LT, Hooper SL. Plasma glutamine and upper respiratory tract infection during intensified training in swimmers. *Med Sci Sports Exerc* 1996; **28**: 285–90.

33 Rohde T, MacLean DA, Pedersen BK. Effect of glutamine supplementation on changes in the immune system induced by repeated exercise. *Med Sci Sports Exerc* 1998; **30**: 856–62.

34 Rohde T, Asp S, MacLean DA, Pedersen BK. Competitive sustained exercise in humans, lymphokine activated killer cell activity, and glutamine — an intervention study. *Eur J Appl Physiol* 1998; **78**: 448–53.

35 Calder PC. Fat chance of immunomodulation. *Immunology Today* 1998; **19**: 244–7.

36 Benquet C, Krzystyniak K, Savard R *et al*. Modulation of exercise-induced immunosuppression by dietary polyunsaturated fatty acids in mice. *J Toxicol Environ Health* 1994; **43**: 225–37.

37 Peters EM, Goetzsche JM, Grobbelaar B, Noakes TD. Vitamin C supplementation reduces the incidence of postrace symptoms of upper-respiratory-tract infection in ultramarathon runners. *Am J Clin Nutr* 1993; **57**: 170–4.

38 Peters EM, Cambell A, Pawley L. Vitamin A fails to increase resistance to upper respiratory in distance runners. *S Afr J Sports Med* 1992; 3–7.

39 Nieman DC, Henson DA, Butterworth DE *et al*. Vitamin C supplementation does not alter the immune response to 2.5 hours of running. *Int J Sport Nutr* 1997; **7**: 173–84.

40 Nielsen HB, Secher NH, Kappel M, Pedersen BK. N-Acetylcysteine does not affect the lymphocyte proliferation and natural killer cell activity responses to exercise. *Am J Physiol* 1998; **275**: R1227–31.

257

DISCUSSION

Professor Peter Raven: With the pollution cascade of interleukin 6 and the cytokines, do you think the acute immunosuppression may put the person at greater risk?

Dr Bente Pedersen: Yes, this is most likely. We know from other studies that if you have two stressors, eg exercise and hypoxia, the effect on the immune system is additive.

Attendee: Are there any studies which show that those athletes who are immunosuppressed are likely to have the most infections?

Dr Bente Pedersen: This is a very important question, but until now there have not been any studies trying to link the degree of immunosuppression, the severity of symptoms and upper respiratory tract infections. We are, of course, largely talking about self-reported symptoms. Dr Tunstall Pedoe's story (in his *Marathon myths and marathon medicine* chapter) about the lung transplant patient who developed septicaemia and died after running a marathon actually supports the idea that we are not just talking about symptoms but infections with some clinical significance.

Dr Dan Tunstall Pedoe: Can we be sure that the reported upper respiratory tract infections after a marathon really are viral infections? I have heard the suggestion that this may not always be the case and the symptoms may be produced by other mechanisms.

Dr Bente Pedersen: I agree. Exercise induces a very dramatic inflammatory response and it is possible that high levels of interleukin 6 and other cytokines will induce feelings of inflammation. Maybe we ought to talk about symptoms of inflammation and not infections. However, animal experiments very convincingly show that hard exercise induces immunosuppression and increases the risk of infections.

Attendee: We have heard about extreme prolonged exercise. What is the effect of repeated bouts of exercise?

Dr Bente Pedersen: The cross-sectional data and the longitudinal data showed either no effect or an improvement of the natural immunity. If you start on a higher level then you may tolerate a decrease. There are some new interesting data from Ola Ronssen showing that, with repeated bouts of severe exercise with short recovery periods, as short as three hours, the second bout of exercise provokes an extreme amount of stress hormones and extreme changes in the cellular immune system. If you perform extreme exercise, then you should allow your immune system time for recovery.

Attendee: What is the role of the central nervous system in relation to the immune system?

Dr Bente Pedersen: The neuroendocrine and immune systems are tightly interrelated. The redistribution of cells seen during exercise is mediated by catecholamines, and both cortisol and β-endorphins play mechanistic roles.

Attendee: Is there any one measurement that can be used to indicate exercise-induced immune suppression?

Dr Bente Pedersen: Yes, the lymphocyte count relates very well to immune function such that if the lymphocyte count is reduced and remains low, then there is functional immune impairment.

Attendee: When would you make that measurement?

Dr Bente Pedersen: If you have a certain exercise protocol where you exercise for about two hours, it might be advisable to check the lymphocyte count after two, four, six and eight hours, to see when the individual returns to baseline and then advise him or her not to start a new session until baseline is reached.

Professor Peter Raven: One anecdote was Nadia Comanec, the Olympic gymnast in the world championships held in 1984 in Fortworth, US. She was hospitalized just after getting a blister and could not respond to the sort of septic shock that she was experiencing. This raises the question of the relationship between calorie deficiency, overtraining and immune suppression. On a related topic can AIDS patients use exercise in some way to protect themselves by generating more CD4 lymphocytes?

Dr Bente Pedersen: There have been seven longitudinal studies on exercise training in patients with human immunodeficiency virus. They have all shown negative results and, thus, do not demonstrate enhancement of CD4 count. On the other hand, they do not find any harmful effects.

Professor Eric Newsholme: There is evidence that ingestion of branched-chain amino acids can reduce mental fatigue. There is also some evidence that ingestion of glutamine, after hard endurance training or competition, can reduce the incidence of upper respiratory tract infections over the next few weeks[1,2].

Reference

1 Castell LM, Newsholme EA. Glutamine and the effect of exhaustive exercise upon the immune response. *Can J Physiol Pharmacol* 1998; **76**: 524–32.

2 Blomstrand E, Hassmen P, Ekblom B. Newsholme EA. Administration of branched-chain amino acids during sustained exercise-effects on performance and on plasma concentration of some amino acids. *Eur J Appl Physiol Occup Physiol* 1991; 63: 83–8.

Cardiovascular health benefits of aerobic exercise

PROFESSOR ADRIANNE HARDMAN

DEPARTMENT OF PHYSICAL EDUCATION, SPORTS SCIENCE AND RECREATION MANAGEMENT,
LOUGHBOROUGH UNIVERSITY, LEICESTERSHIRE, UK

Aerobic exercise has been shown to have significant effects on cardiovascular diseases. Results of studies showing the effect of occupational work have been confirmed through research into levels of leisure time physical activity. Potential mechanisms have been explored but still remain unclear.

One objective of research in this area is the input into public health. The challenging process of defining desirable and optimal levels and patterns of exercise has already begun, but more extensive work is needed. This chapter will focus on how the evidence on exercise and cardiovascular disease has been extended and strengthened during the past 25 years. Proposed mechanisms for these effects will also be outlined.

Evidence for the association between physical activity, CHD risk and all-cause mortality

Much research has been carried out on the relationship between physical activity and the risk of coronary heart disease (CHD)[1,2]. Powell *et al* examined 43 studies published before 1986, mainly of North American and European working age men, for their measures of physical activity and CHD and to determine the epidemiological methods[1]. An inverse association was consistently observed, especially in the better-designed studies: the association was strong, with a median relative risk of 1.9. Thus, the least active individuals had nearly twice the risk of CHD as the most active. The association was also appropriately sequenced (measures of activity pre-dated the onset of CHD) and graded. The better-designed studies tended to show a more substantial benefit from physical activity than those less well-designed. Meta-analysis of the same and subsequent studies confirmed these findings[2].

Observations from a prospective study in US alumni graduates[3] and from a study of English civil servants[4] contributed significantly to this body of evidence. In the US, Paffenbarger and colleagues studied cohorts of men entering Harvard and Pennsylvania Universities between 1916 and 1950 for their activity in student days and in middle-age. A 12–6-year follow-up revealed that the risk of death was about one-quarter to one-third lower in men who expended >2,000 kcal (8.4 MJ)/week in physical activity (eg playing sports, gardening, walking and stair-climbing) than in classmates whose exercise energy expenditure was less. Thus, high levels of exercise energy expenditure were shown to be a determinant of risk[5]. Cardiovascular and respiratory diseases showed the strongest disease-specific association.

Prospective study over nine years of English civil servants found that men reporting 'vigorous' exercise on initial survey subsequently experienced a lower CHD risk than sedentary men[4]. In contrast with the Harvard alumni findings, total energy expended in exercise was not associated with the lower risk. This inconsistency may be explained by the fact that, as the civil servants were a 'healthy worker' cohort, more vigorous exercise was needed to produce the necessary overload than in a general population sample such as the Harvard alumni[6]. Moreover, 'vigorous' exercise was defined as that likely to involve peaks of energy expenditure of 7.5 kcal/min (31 kJ/min) which, in the context of exercise as a whole, may be better described as 'moderately vigorous'[6].

Thus, by the beginning of the 1990s, there was substantial evidence that physical inactivity was a strong risk factor for CHD and death in men. Evidence on women and older men was scant, and there was insufficient information on the dose–response aspects of the relationships on which to build secure public health recommendations.

Physical fitness and CHD

One important development was the measurement of physical fitness. Fitness was assumed to reflect mainly the outcome from physical activity (a behaviour) and there is evidence that it may be a stronger predictor for reduced risk of CHD than physical activity, possibly due to greater measurement deficiencies in the latter. This may be particularly true for women, for whom the questionnaires traditionally employed to measure physical activity may be inappropriate.

Low physical fitness, measured by a variety of laboratory methods, has been reported to be associated with a high risk of myocardial infarction, cardiovascular mortality

Table 1 *Maximal oxygen uptake values (METs)* *for low and high fitness** for adult men and women*

Age category	Men (Low–high fitness)	Women (Low–high fitness)
30–39 years	10.1–13.4	7.1–11.1
40–49 years	9.1–12.5	6.6–9.7
50–59 years	8.4–11.7	6.0–8.9
≥60 years	7.0–10.5	5.4–8.0

* 1 MET (metabolic equivalent) is resting metabolic rate in oxygen consumption units and equals 3.5 ml oxygen/kg/min

** Low fitness=bottom 20% within each age category; high fitness=top 20% within each age category

and all-cause mortality in men[7–10]. Attempts to estimate desirable fitness levels, expressed as maximal oxygen uptake values, can be made on the basis of available evidence. Data from the Aerobics Center Longitudinal Study show that a level of fitness that can reduce the risk of CHD in middle-aged men is about 10 metabolic equivalents (METs) (35 ml/kg/min) (Table 1)[9]. In this study, maximal oxygen uptake was predicted from treadmill times, and the fitness categories were based on Blair *et al*'s study on 10,224 men and 3,120 women. Independent data from Finnish men are consistent with these values — men with a maximal oxygen uptake >34 ml/kg/min had 50% less risk of myocardial infarction than the least fit men[9,10].

Observations in different population groups

There is still inadequate evidence for the effects of physical activity on groups other than middle-aged Caucasian men, but new information is gradually emerging. For women, the most comprehensive prospective data are from the US Nurses Health Study (*n*=72,488). As previously reported for men, there was a strong, graded inverse association between total exercise energy expenditure and CHD — even after multivariate analysis. Both brisk walking (⩾3 hours/week) and vigorous exercise (>6 METs) were associated with a 30–40% reduction in CHD risk[11]. Among a random sample of Swedish women (*n*=1,405), both occupational physical activity and leisure time activity were associated with a lower mortality risk relative to inactivity (relative risks 0.28 and 0.56 respectively)[12]. Data on fitness (as opposed to physical activity) for women are limited to that from Blair *et al*[9,13] and, because the number of subjects was much smaller than for men, analyses performed have been more restricted. Nevertheless, it is clear that mortality rates are lower among women with moderate levels of fitness than in those with low fitness, both in the presence and absence of smoking, high plasma cholesterol concentrations and hypertension[13].

One of the weaknesses of earlier literature was a dearth of information on older men; however, some data are now available. For example, among the subgroup of older British civil servants, those who reported that their usual walking speed was fast (>4 mph or 6.4 km/h) experienced less than half the CHD incidence of less active men[4]. The older Harvard alumni who reported walking more than nine miles/week had a 21% lower risk of death over the follow-up period than those who walked <3 miles (4.8 km)/week[5]. In the British Regional Heart Study, men >60 years who walked 40–60 min/day to and from work showed a decreased risk of heart attack[14]. Also, the Honolulu Heart Program, which reported data for 2,678 men aged between 71 and 93 years, revealed after a two to four-year follow-up that those who walked <0.25 miles/day had twice the risk of CHD as those who walked >1.5 miles/day[15].

Strength of risk of inactivity/low fitness in relation to other risk factors

Earlier studies concluded that cardiovascular disease risk due to inactivity was of the same order of magnitude as that associated with traditional risk factors such as smoking, hypertension and hypercholesterolaemia[1,2]. These conclusions were, however, based on estimates derived from different population samples. Relative risks of all-cause mortality were computed for Harvard alumni for four risk factors after 12–6 years follow-up: the average independent relative risks for a sedentary lifestyle (defined as expending <2,000 kcal (8.4 MJ)/week in playing sports, gardening, climbing stairs and walking), hypertension, cigarette smoking and early parental death were 1.31, 1.73, 1.76 and 1.15, respectively ($p<0.02$)[5]. This suggests that physical inactivity is a strong and significant risk factor of death but may be less powerful than hypertension and smoking.

The results of recent data on physical fitness from attendees at the Cooper Institute for Aerobics Research have been analysed[13]. Relative risks for cardiovascular mortality were 1.70, 1.57, 1.34, 1.65 and 1.18 for low fitness (20% least fit vs 40% most fit), smoking (current or recent), hypertension (systolic >140 mmHg), hypercholesterolaemia (>6.2 mmol/l) and parental death from CHD (all statistically significant and adjusted for these and other risk factors measured) respectively. Thus, low fitness, which probably includes a stronger constitutional factor than activity levels, was an even stronger predictor of cardiovascular mortality than traditional risk factors. More detailed analyses of all-cause mortality data revealed the protective effect of fitness among smokers and non-smokers, and those with and without hypertension and hypercholesterolaemia.

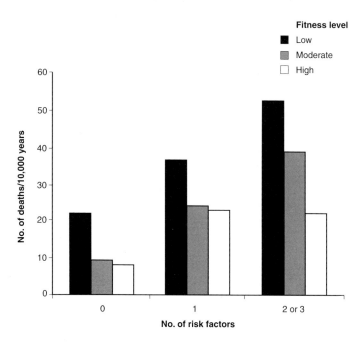

Figure 1

Risk of all-cause mortality according to level of fitness and number of traditional risk factors exhibited in men from the Aerobics Institute Longitudinal Study[13]

These comparisons could not be made for women because of the smaller numbers, but men and women exhibiting high levels of fitness and two or three other cardio-vascular risk factors had lower death rates than those exhibiting low fitness levels with no other risk factors. This suggests that moderate fitness protects against the influence of some other risk factors (Figure 1)[13]. Recent reports on the interactions of fitness and obesity, another risk factor, emphasize this point. Lean men with a low fitness level experience higher cardiovascular and all-cause mortality than men with body mass index >30 kg/m² with a high fitness level[16]. Thus, physical inactivity and low fitness are strong predictors of cardiovascular and all-cause mortality, which appear to confer protection against the influence of other predictors.

Effects of changes in lifestyle and fitness/activity

A fundamental problem with survey data is selection bias; this limits the conclusions that can be drawn from findings based on point observations of physical activity or fitness levels. Changes in lifestyle and fitness may provide more convincing evidence for the argument that adequate exercise reduces the risk of death from CHD and all-causes. Several reports are available. For example, the Harvard Alumni study relates changes in physical activity over a 11–5-year period to mortality risk — men who were initially sedentary but subsequently participated in moderately vigorous sports had a 41% lower risk of CHD death than men who remained sedentary[17]. Such activity was as important in risk reduction as smoking cessation (Figure 2). Similar

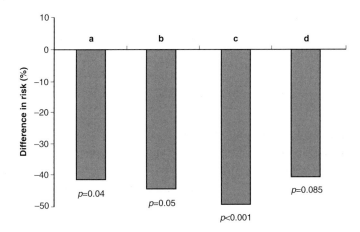

Figure 2

Difference in risk of death from CHD in men who changed their lifestyle between 1962 or 1966 and 1977. Men who: (a) took up moderately vigorous exercise, compared with those who remained inactive; (b) stopped smoking, compared with those who continued; (c) avoided becoming hypertensive, compared with those who became hypertensive; (d) remained lean, compared with those whose body mass index increased to at least 26 kg/m²[17]

benefits were observed among older men in the British Regional Heart Study, who took up at least light physical activity having been inactive at first observation. Their all-cause, cardiovascular and non-cardiovascular mortality rates were lower than for men who were inactive at both observation points[18].

Swedish women who reduced leisure activity over a six-year interval were shown to have a twofold higher risk of all-cause mortality than those who maintained their activity[12]. Findings for changes in fitness are similar to those for physical activity. Middle-aged unfit men who improved their fitness between two observation points separated by a period of years had a significantly lower risk of cardiovascular mortality and all-cause mortality than men who remained unfit[19,20].

Dose-response issues

Data are now available to describe the relationships of the frequency, intensity and duration of activity, allowing the study of dose-response issues which have recently become a main focus area for research. It is clear that a gradient exists between physical activity (or fitness) levels and the risk of CHD[21]. There is evidence that the relationship may be curvilinear, where CHD risk decreases steeply at the lower end of the continuum but reaches an asymptote in the mid-range. For example, the difference in all-cause death rates among participants in the Aerobics Center Longitudinal Study was greatest between the least fit groups of men and women and those with the next higher level[9]. Among Harvard alumni, an inverse relationship was observed between all-cause mortality and increment of physical activity. The risk of death in men expending 3,500 kcal (14.7 MJ)/week in activity was less than half that associated with the lowest level of activity (<500 kcal (2.1 MJ)/week), and those in categories <2,000 kcal (8.4 MJ) had a 38% greater risk than those in higher activity groups[5].

The role of exercise intensity in determining CHD risk still remains uncertain. Several key studies have shown substantial reductions in risk with accumulation of physical activity, most of which was at moderate intensity[21,22]. However, the work of Morris[4] and, more recently, Lee[23] (data for total mortality as opposed to CHD mortality) argues that more vigorous physical activity may provide unique benefits. For example, a dose response was observed in British male civil servants for frequency of activity >7.5 kcal/min (31.4 kJ/min vigorous exercise) but not for exercise of lower intensity[4]. Further investigation is needed before this important issue can be clarified.

Data on stroke

Data on the relationship of physical activity with stroke is less extensive than that for CHD or other cardiovascular diseases, and information on fitness is not available. Data from the British Regional Heart Study, therefore, make a substantial contribution to this area[24]. Physical activity (an index combining elements of intensity and frequency) was inversely related to the risk of stroke, independent of CHD risk factors, heavy drinking and pre-existing heart disease or stroke. Moderately active men had 60% and vigorously active men only 30% of the incidence of stroke among inactive men. Findings from the US Nation Health and Nutrition Examination Survey I (NHANES 1) Epidemiologic Follow-up Study also reveal that reduced physical activity is related to a higher risk of stroke, and extend this finding to white women and black persons[25]. The dose-response aspects of the relationship of physical activity with the risk of stroke have been described in men. There was a significant linear trend for decreased risk for energy expenditures up to 3,000 kcal (12.6 MJ)/week, but not beyond — walking was associated with significantly lower risk, independently of other activity[26].

Influence of physical inactivity on specific cardiovascular risk factors

Physical activity influences several major risk factors for cardiovascular disease, including insulin resistance, high blood pressure, dyslipidaemia and overweight. Although much research has been carried out, only recent information that extends our understanding or opens up a potentially fruitful area of research is discussed.

Diabetes

Physical inactivity has been shown to increase the risk of developing type 2 diabetes in men and women (including postmenopausal women); a few studies in men demonstrate that this is also true for low fitness. Participation in vigorous exercise was associated with a lower risk of developing the disease during follow-up among US nurses and doctors[27,28]. For men, the risk decreased with increasing frequency of such exercise. Among male alumni from the University of Pennsylvania, each 500 kcal (2.1 MJ)/week increment in energy expenditure was associated with a 6% reduction in risk[29]. When classified according to maximal oxygen uptake, men with levels >31.0 ml/kg/min exhibited only 26% of the risk of less fit men[30]. In these studies, the effect of physical activity persisted when adjusted for likely confounders. The protection provided by exercise was strongest in those at high risk, ie those who were overweight, had hypertension or had parental history of diabetes.

Insulin resistance is, of course, the primary pathology in type 2 diabetes. It has been known since the 1970s that men who exercise regularly have better insulin sensitivity than sedentary controls. Recent studies have increased our understanding of the mechanisms involved, how rapidly these benefits are lost or gained, and the dose-response relationships. Both vigorous and non-vigorous exercise have been positively associated with insulin sensitivity, as measured by an intravenous glucose tolerance test[31]. The high level of insulin sensitivity seen in regular exercisers is lost after three to four days without exercise, however, so only frequent exercise will maintain this. Laboratory studies suggest that an exercise session only increases insulin sensitivity in trained muscle so that, although this is a genuine effect of training, it is short-lived. One mechanism is an increase in the expression of GLUT-4, the glucose transporter found in muscle. The concentration of GLUT-4 has been shown to increase with training[32] and to decrease when training is interrupted[33].

Hypertension

Several large prospective studies have reported an inverse relationship between blood pressure and either physical activity or fitness. Among Harvard alumni, men who did not engage in vigorous sports were at 35% greater risk of subsequently developing hypertension than those who did[34]. In a recent study, increased physical activity and at least weekly participation in vigorous exercise were associated with a reduced risk of developing hypertension in men but not in women[35].

Endurance exercise causes moderate reductions in resting arterial blood pressure in normotensive and hypertensive individuals. The average reduction in better-designed studies is 6–7 mmHg for both systolic and diastolic pressures[36], which are independent of weight loss suggesting that weight loss achieved through exercise may have a more important effect. Ambulatory monitoring shows that blood pressure post-exercise remains lower for at least 12 hours[37], which is in line with the overall picture that daily exercise is more effective than three times per week. These effects appear to be independent of exercise intensity; moderate exercise is at least as effective in reducing blood pressure as more vigorous exercise.

Lipoprotein metabolism

Early studies showed particularly elevated concentrations of high density lipoprotein (HDL) cholesterol in runners[38], but recent reports indicate that more moderate exercise may be sufficient to increase the levels, at least in some groups. For example, among older adults, regular walking as a means of exercise has been associated with a low ratio of total to HDL cholesterol[39]. Walking for exercise has also been reported to increase HDL cholesterol in women[40]. However, increased exercise seems likely to confer more benefit, which is the case for HDL cholesterol and other lipoprotein lipid risk factors. Data describing the relations between such factors and training regimens in male (n>8,200) and female (n>1,800) distance runners in the US Runners' Health Study demonstrate that vigorous exercise which is greatly in excess of current guidelines is associated with a further decline in CHD risk. Running distance was six times more important as a determinant of HDL cholesterol than running speed in both men and women, suggesting that total energy expended may be an important factor. Based on these cross-sectional data, every additional kilometre run per week (up to 64–79 km) was associated with an average of 0.003 to 0.004 mmol/l higher HDL cholesterol (for women and men, respectively)[41,42]. Higher distance runners were less likely to have clinically low concentrations of HDL cholesterol or high concentrations of low density lipoprotein (LDL) cholesterol (Figure 3).

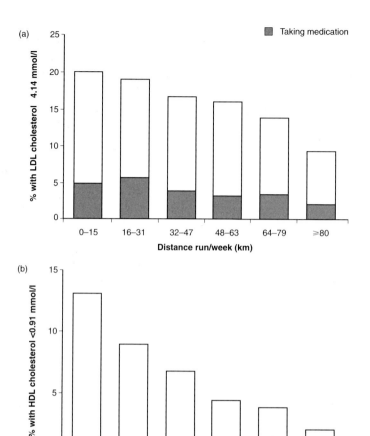

Figure 3

Proportion of 8,283 male runners with (a) LDL cholesterol ≥4.14 mmol/l and taking lipid-lowering medication and (b) low HDL cholesterol (<0.91 mmol/l)

Adapted from[40].

Results from longitudinal studies are much less consistent, probably due to biological and analytical variation as well as the difficulty of performing studies over many months. One way to overcome this is to challenge the system which mainly determines HDL cholesterol concentration, and examine the effects of exercise on the response to this challenge. A fundamental determinant of HDL cholesterol concentration is triglyceride clearance. Repeated episodes of high postprandial lipaemia, mainly reflecting poor triglyceride clearance, lead to low HDL cholesterol and to other atherogenic disturbances to lipoprotein metabolism. For these reasons, and because case-control studies report higher lipaemia in patients, exaggerated postprandial lipaemia is now recognized as an independent risk marker for coronary artery disease. Exercise has profound effects on postprandial lipaemia, a single session resulting in a 20–30% decrease in the subsequent lipaemic response to a fatty meal[43]. Although the mechanisms responsible are not clear — and may differ for moderate compared with more vigorous exercise — there is evidence on the relative efficacy of different intensities and patterns of exercise. Longer duration, low intensity exercise reduces lipaemia by the same extent as a shorter period of moderate exercise expending the same energy[44]. Intermittent exercise has similar effects as one longer session of equivalent duration, and even three 10-minute brisk walks during a day have been shown to decrease day-long plasma triglyceride concentrations[45].

As exaggerated postprandial lipaemia may contribute to the development of a preponderance of small, dense LDL (which are particularly atherogenic), these effects on the handling of dietary fat may account for findings that regular exercisers exhibit lower concentrations of these particles than sedentary controls. Changes to the chemical composition of LDL (more cholesterol enriched, protein-poor) have also been reported in the same individuals after a period of training[46] and, in a different study, training decreased the proportion of circulating oxidized LDL[47]. Exercise, therefore, appears to influence lipoprotein metabolism in multiple ways which may decrease the progression of atherogenic stimulus, the chronic phase of cardiovascular disease.

Obesity

Obesity is epidemic in the US, and the prevalence has increased significantly in the UK and its substantial co-morbidities make this a serious public health concern. Strategies for prevention of weight gain must include physical activity. Recent prospective studies support a strong role for exercise in the maintenance of desirable body weight, with findings that low leisure time physical activity is inversely related to weight gain. For example, Finnish men and women who reported no regular activity at the end of the follow-up were 2.5 times more likely to experience a clinically significant weight gain (defined as >5 kg, alongside a body mass index of >26 kg/m at follow-up)[48].

Balancing physical activity and risks

A period of strenuous exertion, among other external stimuli, can trigger myocardial infarction. Solid evidence for this can now be added to anecdotal and descriptive evidence; in about 5% of patients, such exertion immediately precedes the onset of symptoms. Epidemiological studies (case-control and case-crossover) have quantified the transient increase in risk associated with exertion and the magnitude of this depends on habitual exercise levels. Among people who regularly engage in vigorous exercise, the risk associated with such exercise is between 1.3 to 2.4 times greater than at all other times[49,50]. By contrast, in sedentary people risk is increased by between seven and 100 times during vigorous exercise. The balance of risks (ie during and not during vigorous exercise) determines the overall risk and this, as shown by numerous prospective studies and from a study in which both risks were quantified in the same population[51], is much lower in habitual exercisers. Thus, the challenge for exercise promotion initiatives is to find ways to enable sedentary people to progress their exercise habit gradually so that they achieve the long-term cardioprotective effect with minimal increase in the transient risk.

Possible mechanisms

Despite many years of research, the precise mechanisms by which exercise reduces the risk of cardiovascular disease remain unclear. The influences on traditional risk factors, such as hypertension, diabetes, dyslipidaemia and obesity, may decrease the progression of atherosclerosis. However, a consistent feature of the epidemiological evidence is that only current and continuing exercise is protective. For example, among Harvard alumni, men who were active in their youth but became sedentary in middle-age exhibited a risk similar to that of men who had never been active[5]. This points to effects on the acute phases of the disease.

Atherosclerosis is now thought to be a chronic inflammatory condition converted to an acute event by induction of plaque rupture. Although exercise may influence plaque development by decreasing concentration-dependent lipid transport into the artery wall and/or by decreasing oxidation of trapped lipoproteins, it may also influence thrombosis, myocardial ischaemia or arrhythmia. There is growing epidemiological evidence for lower levels of fibrinogen and factor VII activity in men who engage vigorous exercise, and scientific evidence that acute exercise increases fibrinolytic activity[52]. Based on a short-term intervention in patients with coronary artery disease, exercise may also improve endothelium-dependent vasodilatation of coronary vessels[53]. This could help maintain the crucial link between myocardial demand and coronary blood flow, decreasing the likelihood of myocardial ischaemia. Speculatively, endothelium-independent dilatation may also develop with long-term endurance training, further increasing dilating capacity in coronary arteries[54].

Exercise recommendations

Evidence that the effects of exercise on postprandial lipaemia, insulin sensitivity and blood pressure persist only for a short time when the exercise stimulus is withdrawn, coupled with the recognition that exercise may influence the acute phases of cardiovascular disease, underpin increased emphasis in current exercise recommendations on the frequency of regular exercise. Thus, as in the US, guidelines in the UK are for at least 30 minutes of dynamic endurance activity at a moderate level or higher on most, preferably all, days of the week. There are clear indications that more intense exercise probably confers greater benefits but, because this also increases risks, these guidelines constitute sensible advice for the many presently sedentary individuals.

References

1 Powell KE, Thompson PD, Casperson CJ, Kendrick JS. Physical activity and the incidence of coronary heart disease. *Ann Rev Public Health* 1987; **8**: 253–87.

2 Berlin JA, Colditz GA. A meta-analysis of physical activity in the prevention of coronary heart disease. *Am J Epidemiol* 1990; **132**: 612–28.

3 Paffenbarger RS, Wing AL, Hyde RT. Physical activity as an index of heart attack risk in college alumni. *Am J Epidemiol* 1978; **108**: 161–75.

4 Morris JN, Clayton DG, Everitt MG *et al*. Exercise in leisure time: coronary attack and death rates. *Br Heart J* 1990; **63**: 325–34.

5 Paffenbarger RS, Hyde RT, Wing AL, Hsieh C-C. Physical activity, all-cause mortality, and longevity of college alumni. *N Engl J Med* 1986; **314**: 605–13.

6 Morris JN. Exercise in the prevention of coronary heart disease: today's best buy in public health. *Med Sci Sports Exerc* 1994; **26**: 807–14.

7 Lakka TA, Venäläinen JM, Raurama R *et al*. Relation of leisure-time physical activity and cardiorespiratory fitness to the risk of acute myocardial infarction in men. *N Engl J Med* 1994; **330**: 1549–54.

8 Ekelund L-G, Haskell WL, Johnson MS *et al*. Physical fitness as a predictor of cardiovascular mortality in asymptomatic North American men. *N Engl J Med* 1988; **319**: 1379–84.

9 Blair SN, Kohl HW, Paffenbarger RS *et al*. Physical fitness and all-cause mortality: a prospective study of healthy men and women. *JAMA* 1989; **262**: 2395–401.

10 Sandvik L, Erikssen J, Thaulow E *et al*. Physical fitness as a predictor of mortality among healthy, middle-aged Norwegian men. *N Engl J Med* 1993; **328**: 533–7.

11 Manson J, Hu FB, Rich-Edwards JW *et al*. A prospective study of walking as compared with vigorous exercise in the prevention of coronary heart disease in women. *N Engl J Med* 1999; **341**: 650–8.

12 Lissner L, Bengtsson C, Björkelund C, Wedel H. Physical activity levels and changes in relation to longevity. *Am J Epidemiol* 1996; **143**: 54–62.

13 Blair SN, Kampert JB, Kohl HW *et al*. Influences of cardiorespiratory fitness and other precursors on cardiovascular disease and all-cause mortality in men and women. *JAMA* 1996; **276**: 205–10.

14 Hakim AA, Curb JD, Petrovitch H *et al*. Effects of walking on coronary heart disease in elderly men. The Honolulu Heart Program. *Circulation* 1999; **100**: 9–13.

15 Wei M, Kampert JB, Barlow CE *et al*. Relationship between low cardiorespiratory fitness and mortality in normal-weight, overweight, and obese men. *JAMA* 1999; **282**: 1547–53.

16 Paffenbarger RS, Hyde RT, Wing AL *et al*. The association of changes in physical activity level and other lifestyle characteristics with mortality among men. *N Engl J Med* 1993; **328**: 538–45.

17 Wannamethee SG, Shaper AG, Walker M. Changes in physical activity, mortality, and incidence of coronary heart disease in older men. *Lancet* 1998; **351**: 1603–8.

18 Blair SN, Kohl HW, Barlow CE *et al*. Changes in physical fitness and all-cause mortality. A prospective study of healthy and unhealthy men. *JAMA* 1995; **273**: 1093–8.

19 Erikssen G, Liestøl K, Bjørnholt J *et al*. Changes in physical fitness and changes in mortality. *Lancet* 1998; **352**: 759–62.

20 Haskell WL. Health consequences of physical activity: understanding and challenges regarding dose-response. *Med Sci Sports Exerc* 1994; **26**: 649–60.

21 Blair SN, Connelly JC. How much physical activity should we do? The case for moderate amounts and intensities of physical activity. *Res Q Exerc Sport* 1996; **67**: 193–205.

22 Lee I-M, Hsieh C-C, Paffenbarger RS. Exercise intensity and longevity in men. The Harvard alumni health study. *N Engl J Med* 1995; **273**: 1179–84.

23 Shaper AG, Wannamethee G. Physical activity and ischaemic heart disease in middle-aged British men. *Br Heart J* 1991; **66**: 384–94.

24 Wannamethee G, Shaper AG. Physical activity and stroke in British middle-aged men. *BMJ* 1992; **304**: 597–601.

271

25 Gillum RF, Mussolino ME, Ingram DD. Physical activity and stroke incidence in women and men. The NHANES 1 Epidemiologic Follow-up Study. *Am J Epidemiol* 1996; **143**: 860–9.

26 Lee I-M, Paffenbarger RS. Physical activity and stroke incidence. The Harvard Alumni Health Study. *Stroke* 1998; **29**: 2049–54.

27 Manson JE, Rimm EB, Stampfer MJ *et al*. Physical activity and incidence of non-insulin-dependent diabetes mellitus in women. *Lancet* 1991; **338**: 774–8.

28 Manson JE, Nathan DM, Krolewski AS *et al*. A prospective study of exercise and incidence of diabetes among US male physicians. *JAMA* 1992; **268**: 63–7.

29 Helmrich SP, Ragland DR, Leung RW, Paffenbarger RS. Physical activity and reduced occurrence of non-insulin-dependent diabetes mellitus. *N Engl J Med* 1991; **325**: 147–52.

30 Lynch J, Helmrich SP, Lakka TA *et al*. Moderately intense physical activities and high levels of cardiorespiratory fitness reduce the risk of non-insulin-dependent diabetes mellitus in middle-aged men. *Arch Int Med* 1996; **156**: 1307–14.

31 Mayer-Davis EJ, D'Agostino R, Karter AJ *et al*. Intensity and amount of physical activity in relation to insulin sensitivity. The Insulin Resistance Atherosclerosis Study. *JAMA* 1998; **279**: 669–74.

32 Houmard JA, Shinebarger MH, Dolan PL *et al*. Exercise training increases GLUT-4 protein concentration in previously sedentary middle-aged men. *Am J Physiol* 1993; **264**: E896–901.

33 Vukovich MD, Arciero PJ, Kohrt WM *et al*. Changes in insulin action and GLUT-4 with 6 days of inactivity in endurance runners. *J Appl Physiol* 1996; **80**: 240–4.

34 Paffenbarger RS, Wing AL, Hyde RT, Jung DL. Physical activity and incidence of hypertension in college alumni. *Am J Epidemiol* 1983; **117**: 247–57.

35 Haapanen N, Miilunpalo S, Vuori I *et al*. Association of leisure time physical activity with the risk of coronary heart disease, hypertension and diabetes in middle-aged men and women. *Int J Epidemiol* 1997; **26**: 739–47.

36 Arroll B, Beaglehole R. Does physical activity lower blood pressure: a critical review of the clinical trials. *J Clin Epidemiol* 1992; **45**: 439–47.

37 Pescatello LS, Fargo AE, Leach CN, Scherzer HH. Short-term effect of dynamic exercise on arterial blood pressure. *Circulation* 1991; **83**: 1557–61.

38 Wood PD, Haskell WL, Stern MP *et al*. Plasma lipoprotein distributions in male and female runners. *Ann N Y Acad Sci* 1977; **301**: 748–63.

39 Tucker LA, Friedman GM. Walking and serum cholesterol in adults. *Am J Public Health* 1990; **80**: 1111–3.

40 Duncan JJ, Gordon NF, Scott CB. Women walking for health and fitness. How much is enough? *JAMA* 1991; **266**: 3295–9.

41 Williams PT. High density lipoprotein cholesterol and other risk factors for coronary heart disease in female runners. *N Engl J Med* 1996; **334**: 1298–303.

42 Williams PT. Relationship of distance run per week to coronary heart disease risk factors in 8,283 male runners. *Arch Int Med* 1997; **157**: 191–8.

43 Hardman AE, Herd SL. Exercise and postprandial lipid metabolism. *Proc Nutr Soc* 1998; **57**: 63–72.

44 Tsetsonis NV, Hardman AE. reduction in postprandial lipemia after walking: influence of exercise intensity. *Med Sci Sports Exerc* 1996; **28**: 1235–42.

45 Murphy MH, Nevill AM, Hardman AE. Different patterns of brisk walking are equally effective in decreasing postprandial lipaemia. *Int J Obesity* 2000; **24**: 1303–9.

46 Houmard JA, Bruno NJ, Bruner RK *et al*. Effects of exercise training on the chemical composition of plasma LDL. *Arterioscler Thromb* 1994; **14**: 325–30.

47 Vasankari TJ, Kujala UM, Vasankari TM, Ahotupa M. Reduced oxidized LDL levels after a 10-month exercise program. *Med Sci Sports Exerc* 1998; **30**: 1496–501.

48 Haapanen N, Miilunpalo S, Pasanen M *et al*. Association between leisure time physical activity and 10-year body mass change among working-aged men and women. *Int J Obesity* 1997; **21**: 288–96.

49 Mittleman MA, Maclure M, Tofler GH *et al*. Triggering of acute myocardial infarction by heavy physical exertion. Protection against triggering by regular exertion. *N Engl J Med* 1993; **329**: 1677–83.

50 Willich SN, Lewis M, Löwel H *et al*. Physical exertion as a trigger of acute myocardial infarction. *N Engl J Med* 1993; **329**: 1684–90.

51 Siscovick DS, Weiss NS, Fletcher RH, Lasky T. The incidence of primary cardiac arrest during vigorous exercise. *N Engl J Med* 1984; **311**: 874–7.

52 Meade TW. Exercise and haemostatic function. *J Cardiovasc Risk* 1995; **2**: 323–9.

53 Hambrecht R, Wolf A, Gielen S *et al*. Effect of exercise on coronary endothelial function in patients with coronary artery disease. *N Engl J Med* 2000; **342**: 454–60.

54 Haskell WL, Sims C, Myll J *et al*. Coronary artery size and dilating capacity in ultradistance runners. *Circulation* 1993; **87**: 1076–82.

DISCUSSION

Attendee: Does exercise improve insulin sensitivity in type 2 diabetic patients, as well as in healthy people?

Professor Adrianne Hardman: Yes. Exercise training improves fasting plasma insulin concentrations and insulin action in type 2 diabetics. In healthy people, this may be largely due to the acute effects of recent exercise sessions.

Attendee: I have a predisposition to laziness but wish to obtain maximum benefit from exercise. How can I achieve this?

Professor Adrianne Hardman: This is another way of asking, 'How little exercise can I get away with?'. Because it is now known that the acute effects of each exercise session are important and that many benefits die quickly once training stops, I would emphasize that exercise should be frequent as well as regular. The recommendations from the US Centers for Disease Control and Prevention are for at least 30 minutes of activity at a moderate level or above, on most (preferably all) days of the week. Brisk walking is a good recommendation for the population at large, because it carries little risk. It is cheap, attainable by most (including the elderly) and is an excellent basis for the transition to more vigorous exercise.

Non-cardiovascular benefits of exercise

DR ALAN MARYON-DAVIS

SENIOR LECTURER IN PUBLIC HEALTH MEDICINE,
DEPARTMENT OF PUBLIC HEALTH SCIENCES, KING'S COLLEGE LONDON, LONDON, UK

The 1977 New York Academy of Sciences book on the marathon covered many aspects of the race, but did not include in detail the non-cardiovascular benefits of exercise due to a paucity of studies at that time on which to frame a review. The focus for considering the health consequences of physical activity in the late 1970s was dominated by the cardiovascular agenda, and in particular the great studies linking physical activity and coronary heart disease (CHD) (discussed in Professor Hardman's chapter).

However, during the 1980s, interest extended into non-cardiovascular health outcomes. By the late 1980s and early 1990s, evidence was accumulating of associations between physical activity and reductions in a number of non-cardiovascular diseases, mainly diabetes[1], colon cancer[2] and depression[3]. The US Surgeon General's 1996 report, *Physical activity and health*[4], devoted 30 pages to non-cardiovascular health effects compared to only 26 for cardiovascular disease. This chapter will focus on the role of exercise in obesity control, cancer prevention and musculoskeletal health.

Exercise and obesity control

Size of the problem

Obesity, defined as a body mass index (BMI) >30, is associated with a number of threats to health and wellbeing[5]. It is a known risk factor for CHD, both independently and partly through its association with hypertension, non-insulin-dependent diabetes and hypercholesterolaemia. It is also a well-established risk factor for breast cancer in postmenopausal women, bowel cancer in men, complications in pregnancy and childbirth, gallstones and sleep apnoea. Obesity has also been linked to social exclusion, depression, substance abuse, risk of accidents, and a wide range of other disorders including back pain and degenerative joint disease. In addition, it has been shown to have a negative effect on self-esteem, the level of functioning and perceived health[6].

The prevalence of overweight (BMI 25.0–29.9) and obesity has recently increased in much of the developed world, including the UK. For example, between 1980 and 1996, the prevalence of overweight adults in England increased from 39% to 62% in men and from 32% to 53% in women, and the percentage of clinically obese from 6% to 17% in men and from 8% to 20% in women[7]. Similar trends have been found in children and adolescents[8]. These increases have taken place against a background of reduced average energy intake and are thought to be mainly due to decreased physical activity levels[9]. The 1992 Allied Dunbar National Fitness Survey revealed exceptionally low levels of physical activity in much of the adult population[10]. A wide variety of genetic, psychological, social and cultural factors are also involved.

The health, social and economic costs of overweight/obesity are substantial. Costs for diagnosis and treatment of overweight/obesity and its co-morbidities have been estimated at 2–8% of total healthcare expenditure in a range of developed countries[11].

Physical activity, diet and obesity

In theory, people gain weight if their caloric intake is greater than their caloric expenditure; conversely, weight is lost if their expenditure exceeds their intake.

In practice, however, changes in metabolic rate and body composition may produce varying effects. For example, as weight is lost, energy expenditure declines due to a combination of reduced resting metabolic rate, reduced thermic effect of food, and reduced caloric cost of physical activity[12]. These and other complexities make it difficult to interpret studies investigating the physiological effects of physical activity on energy balance. Energy expenditure is clearly increased during a bout of exercise, but whether or not regular physical activity increases resting metabolic rate, the thermic effect of food, and the energy cost of exercise is not yet firmly established[13].

At a clinical level, several studies have shown that adding an exercise regimen to a calorie-restricted diet promotes the loss of body fat, but tends to be accompanied by a less than expected weight loss[14,15]. This may partly be explained by the observation that exercise maintains lean mass during caloric restriction and, because lean tissue is more dense than fat, offsets weight loss. Recent reviews and meta-analyses have concluded that the rate of weight loss with exercise is positively related, in a dose-response manner, to the frequency, intensity and duration of the activity. Perhaps more importantly from a public health point of view, the addition of increased physical activity to a calorie-restricted diet appears to be more effective for long-term weight loss maintenance than dieting alone[16,17].

Independent of its effect on weight and total fat mass, physical activity may also favourably affect fat distribution. Several large cross-sectional studies report an inverse association between physical activity and central body fat distribution[18], the latter being a risk factor for type 2 diabetes and CHD.

Cross-sectional studies carried out to examine the role of physical activity in the prevention of obesity reveal that patients with higher levels of self-reported physical activity or fitness had lower weight, BMI or skin-fold measures. However, it is difficult to disentangle the effects of obesity on the take-up of exercise. Prospective studies, some of which were initiated as child cohorts, have shown less consistent results, with some finding a significant inverse relationship between physical activity and later development of obesity, and others finding no association. In general, a preventive effect was more consistently observed among women than men. The range of results probably reflects the difficulties of controlling for confounding variables in such long-term cohort studies[4].

Exercise and cancer prevention

Colon cancer

The most studied link between exercise and cancer, and the most consistent inverse relationship found, has been that with colon cancer. To date, about two-thirds of these 40 studies have shown a statistically significant 'protective' effect[4,19]; several indicate a clear dose-response gradient. The methods used and populations studied have been diverse. For example, some have been case-control studies while others cohort studies. The populations have comprised all ages drawn from many cultures and ethnic groups. Some studies have used occupational physical activity as their key variable, others leisure time or total activity. In a few, incidence has been used as the endpoint, and in others mortality. Apart from adjusting for age and BMI, few of the studies have attempted to compensate for other potential confounders such as dietary habits, social class or family history of colon cancer. However, the consistency of findings across such a diversity of populations suggests that the association is a real one[4].

Results of studies that included leisure time as well as occupational activities broadly suggest that 'sedentary' people have up to double the risk of developing colon cancer than 'active' people of either sex. For example, one of the larger and better-designed studies was carried out on 47,723 US male health professionals aged between 40 and 75 years[20]. Their leisure time activity was coded to eight categories, and the endpoint was colon cancer incidence (n=201). After adjusting for age, BMI, family history, endoscopic history, diet, smoking and aspirin use, results showed that the most active quintile had a relative risk of 0.53 compared with the least active quintile (p=0.03).

Regular physical activity has been shown to decrease the food residue transit time in the large bowel, thereby reducing epithelial exposure to carcinogenic waste products[21]. A proposed mechanism for this is a change in the synthesis of local prostaglandin, where strenuous exercise stimulates prostaglandin F_2 production which increases intestinal motility[22].

Rectal cancer

A number of studies have looked for a link between physical activity and rectal cancer, including some of those also investigating colon cancer. Results have been conflicting, and there does not seem to be a consistent relationship between occupational, leisure time or total physical activity and rectal cancer[4].

Breast cancer

Of the hormone-dependent cancers in women, breast cancer is the most common and, in terms of possible links with exercise, has been the most studied. As with colon cancer, a variety of methods have been used and populations studied; also in common with colon cancer, age and BMI are obvious confounders. However, the link with breast cancer is further complicated by many reproductive factors — ie age at menarche, use of contraceptives, age at first pregnancy, number of pregnancies and age at menopause — and some researchers have been more fastidious than others in controlling for these. Thus, results have generally been inconsistent. However, two recently published large case-control studies have examined the associations between vigorous physical activity in youth and subsequent breast cancer; the studies were carefully adjusted for reproductive confounders and the results support the suggestion that increased activity in teens and the early 20s reduces the likelihood of developing breast cancer in middle age[23,24].

Mittendorf et al studied 6,888 cases of breast cancer and 9,539 matched controls in the US; they focused on the strenuous activity of women between 14 and 22 years[24]. Adjustments were made for age, parity, age at first birth, family history, BMI, previous breast disease, age at menopause, menopausal status and alcohol use. The results showed that women who were active on a daily basis had a relative risk of 0.5 compared with women who were not active.

A large cohort study, which involved 25,624 pre- and postmenopausal Norwegian women who were followed up for a mean of 13.7 years, revealed that greater leisure time activity was associated with a reduced risk of breast cancer[25]. After adjusting for age, BMI, height, parity and county of residence, the relative risk was 0.63 (95% CI 0.42–0.95) among women who exercised regularly compared with sedentary women (p=0.04). The reduction was greater in pre- than postmenopausal women, and the lowest relative risk was seen in lean women (BMI <22.8) who exercised at least four hours a week. Risk was also lowered at higher levels of activity at work. The investigators concluded that physical activity during leisure and at work is associated with a reduced risk of breast cancer. However, no adjustment was made for social class and it is known that both leisure time activity and breast cancer are higher in non-manual groups. Also, no information on use of the contraceptive pill was collected.

Among the proposed mechanisms for a putative link between vigorous exercise in early life and reduced incidence of subsequent breast cancer are the well-documented observations that:

- vigorous exercise may suppress the release of pituitary gonadotrophins and, thus, reduce the influence of the menstrual cycle on susceptibility to breast cancer
- reduced body fat accompanying an active life leads to lower levels of circulating oestradiol, another known risk factor for breast cancer.

Adjusting for factors such as age at menarche and BMI to determine the independent effect of exercise, these secondary effects may be lost.

Other hormone-dependent cancers in women

Only a few studies have been carried out to examine the effects of exercise on ovarian, endometrial or cervical cancer, and the resulting data have been either too limited or inconsistent to firmly establish any relationships[4,19].

Prostate cancer

About 50% of the published papers support a relationship between regular exercise and lower risk of prostate cancer. Oliviera et al recently studied a cohort of 12,975 men aged 20–80 years at entry and who were followed for up to 20 years at the Cooper Clinic, Dallas, US[26]. Subjects were treadmill-tested at baseline. Self-complete questionnaires were posted at intervals of several years, which sought information about the development of a range of disorders including cancer of the prostate gland. After adjusting for age, BMI and smoking habits, the results showed that higher cardiorespiratory fitness levels at baseline were inversely associated with the incidence of prostate cancer. A significant dose-related reduction in relative risk was found in men under 60 years, from 1.1 in the least active quartile to 0.26 in the most active; similar findings were observed for physical activity.

The beneficial effects of cardiorespiratory fitness and physical activity may be explained by the fact that habitual physical activity reduces the levels of free circulating endogenous testosterone which is a putative risk factor for prostate cancer[27].

Testicular cancer

The case-control UK Testicular Cancer Study revealed that men who pursued ≥15 h/week of leisure time physical activity were 50% less likely to develop testicular cancer as sedentary men[28]. A significant trend was also observed in the relative risk across six categories of time spent exercising. However, other studies have revealed conflicting results[29,30] and, as there are insufficient consistent data available, meaningful conclusions about the association between physical activity and testicular cancer cannot be drawn.

Exercise and musculoskeletal benefits

The immediate effects of exercise on muscles, joints and bones are well documented. Exercise increases: the size, strength and endurance of muscles; the thickness and strength of tendons and ligaments; and the mineral density and strength of bones. These changes are functional adaptations to the demands exerted on the different tissues. For example, where the demand is to use a force against firm resistance (isometric exercise, eg weight-training), the response is increased musculoskeletal strength. Where the demand is for continuous rhythmic movement against little resistance for long periods (isokinetic exercise, eg distance running), the response is increased muscular endurance. Most forms of physical activity involve a combination of these demands. However, the changes can only be maintained as long as the demands continue. Improvements in strength and endurance are lost within four to six weeks of returning to pre-training exercise levels.

The main beneficial effects of physical activity on musculoskeletal health include improved mobility and avoidance of injury. Specifically, exercise can help prevent osteoporotic fractures, especially in postmenopausal women who are especially susceptible to these fractures, and can provide greater freedom of movement, physical capability and independence for older people.

Prevention of osteoporosis

Osteoporosis is characterized by reduced bone mass and structural weakness leading to increased fragility and susceptibility to fractures. It is primarily a disorder of old age, as bone mass and strength progressively decline in both sexes. However, the problem is exacerbated in older women mainly because women: have a lower peak bone mass than men, rapidly lose bone mineral after the menopause due to lower oestrogen levels, and tend to live longer than men[31]. Fractures can occur with minimal trauma, eg vertebral compression fractures on coughing or bending, and wrist, humerus and hip fractures on slipping and falling. Hip fractures are associated with more deaths, disability and healthcare costs than all other osteoporotic fractures combined.

Physical activity may positively affect susceptibility to osteoporosis by increasing peak bone mass in early life and by reducing bone mineral loss in later life. Bone adapts to the mechanical stresses and strains exerted on it. The loading that occurs in exercise, particularly through weight-bearing activities, can contribute to bone mass and can strengthen bone structure by a process of remodelling, provided appropriate nutritional and hormonal co-factors are present. Conversely, inactivity or lack of mechanical loading has been clearly shown to result in decreased bone mass. For example, a young adult at bed rest for one week loses about 1% of spinal density, which would be regained after about four months of mobilization[32].

The evidence that exercise increases peak bone mass in young adults is provided by cross-sectional and prospective studies. Cross-sectional studies suggest that highest bone mineral densities are achieved in strength-trained individuals, particularly men, when compared with age- and sex-matched endurance-trained or sedentary controls, although these differences may partly be explained by selection bias[33]. Prospective studies examining physical activity and subsequent bone mineral density have been mainly conducted on women because of their susceptibility to osteoporotic fractures in later life. Most studies suggest a positive association between premenopausal exercise levels and postmenopausal bone mineral density; however, the results are not yet sufficiently consistent to allow firm conclusions. This variability may be due to the range of activity types, exercise protocols, durations of training, and somatotypes of subjects in the different studies[33].

Several trials have now been conducted on postmenopausal women, which suggest that appropriately tailored exercise can also maintain or improve bone mineral density in later life[34]. Although most attention has been focused on postmenopausal women, it is important to recognize that osteoporosis can also affect younger women and men but to a lesser degree. Strategies for prevention of bone mineral loss must begin in childhood and continue throughout life.

Advantages to older people

The World Health Organization definition of health includes social, as well as physical and mental, wellbeing. Quality of life, independence and social integration are increasingly being recognized and assessed as important elements of older people's health[35]. It is also becoming clear that physical, mental and social health are interdependent. For example, social health is often a consequence of physical and mental health — if you lack mobility or motivation, it is more difficult to maintain social links. Physical activity, by promoting functional ability and positive mental outlook, can improve social wellbeing.

Current levels of functional ability in the UK reveal a considerable challenge. For instance, a recent analysis of data from the Allied Dunbar National Fitness Survey and the Health Education Authority's National Survey of Activity and Health has found that[36]:

- 9% of men aged 64–74 and 40% of women cannot maintain a 3 mph walking pace
- 7% of men aged 70–74 and 25% of women cannot get out of a chair without using their arms.

Prevention of falls

A key benefit of improved functional ability among older people is in the prevention of falls[37]. Few studies have examined the effectiveness of exercise in preventing falls. One notable example is the meta-analysis of pooled results of the Frailty and Injuries Cooperative Studies of Intervention Techniques (FICSIT) trials, which showed the risk of falling to be reduced by: 10% by targeted exercise, 25% by balance training, and by 37% by regular tai chi[38]. In the UK, a recent randomized controlled trial of home-based strength and balance training in women aged ≥80 years demonstrated large reductions in fall incidence and injury on first fall compared with control[39].

Thus, there is evidence to suggest that exercise, such as balance training, is effective in improving postural stability and in reducing the risk of falls in older people[40]. A recent review has highlighted the importance of the functional gains and health benefits derived from fairly low amounts of exercise in this age group, and that 'the greatest benefits are seen when one goes from doing nothing to doing something'[41].

Looking to the future

Since the late 1970s, our understanding of the potential health benefits of physical activity at all stages of life has improved, but there are still large lacunae of ignorance. More research needs to be directed at the potential benefits, both short- and long-term, of increased exercise in childhood. The advantages for adolescent girls and young women need particular attention, especially with regard to certain minority ethnic groups such as those from south Asia who are less likely to take up or maintain exercise. The potential benefits of exercise in pregnancy also need further examination.

In all age groups, the dose-response effect of frequency, intensity, type and duration of exercise should be investigated in more depth. Although the ACSM Guidelines are well suited to general public education messages about healthy living, patients and the general public should know precisely which activities, how intensively, how often, and for how long they must exercise to make the advantages specifically tailored to their particular needs.

Perhaps the greatest challenge is in communicating to people the real health benefits of exercise, and encouraging them to keep active. As the global population becomes increasingly aged, the important need for people to maintain physical activity becomes ever more apparent. The 21st century, however, promises a life of even more advanced convenience and labour-saving comfort. We urgently need to research the barriers to keeping active if we are to reduce the public health burden of inactivity.

References

1 Manson JE, Nathan DM, Krolewski AS *et al*. A prospective study of exercise and incidence of diabetes among US male physicians. *JAMA* 1992; **268**: 63–7.

2 Garabrant DH, Peter JM, Mack TM, Bernstein L. Job activity and colon cancer risk. *Am J Epidemiol* 1984; **119**: 1005–14.

3 Martinsen EW. Benefits of exercise for the treatment of depression. *Sports Med* 1990; **9**: 380–9.

4 US Surgeon General. *Physical activity and health: a report of the Surgeon General*. Pittsburg: US Department of Health and Human Services, 1996.

5 British Nutrition Foundation Task Force. *Obesity*. Oxford: Blackwell Science, 1999.

6 Fontaine KR, Bartlett SJ. Estimating health-related quality of life in obese individuals. *Dis Man Health Outcomes* 1998; **3**: 61–70.

7 Prescott-Clarke P, Primatesta P. *Health survey for England 1997*. London: The Stationery Office, 1999.

8 Hughes J, Li L, Chinn S, Rona RJ. Trends in growth in England and Scotland, 1972–1994. *Arch Dis Chil* 1997; **76**: 182–9.

9 Prentice AM, Jebb SA. Obesity in Britain: gluttony or sloth? *BMJ* 1995; **311**: 437–9.

10 Allied Dunbar National Fitness Survey. *Main findings*. London: Health Education Authority and Sports Council, 1992.

11 Seidell JC. The burden of obesity and its sequelae. *Dis Man Health Outcomes* 1999; **5**: 13–21.

12 Melchionda N, Parenti M, Pasquali R *et al*. Economy of energy expenditure and body composition after weight loss. Meta-analysis of experiments from 1900 to 1990. In: Belfiore F, Jeanrenaud B, Papalia D, eds. *Obesity: basic concepts and clinical aspects, front diabetes, Vol 11*. Basel: Karger, 1992: 134–50.

13 Hill JO, Drougas HJ, Peters JC. Physical activity, fitness and moderate obesity. In: Bouchard C, Shephard RJ, Stephens T, eds. *Physical activity, fitness and health. International Proceedings and Consensus Statement*. Champaign, Illinois: Human Kinetics, 1994: 684–95.

14 Sweeney ME, Hill JO, Heller PA *et al*. Severe vs moderate energy restriction with and without exercise in the treatment of obesity: efficiency of weight loss. *Am J Clin Nutr* 1993; **57**: 127–34.

15 Miller Wc, Koceja DM, Hamilton EJ. A meta-analysis of the past 25 years of weight loss research using diet, exercise or diet plus exercise intervention. *Int J Obes Relat Metab Disord* 1997; **21**: 941–7.

16 Stefanick ML. Exercise and weight control. *Exerc Sport Sci Rev* 1993; **21**: 363–96.

17 Ballor DL, Keesey RE. A meta-analysis of the factors affecting exercise-induced changes in body mass, fat mass, and fat-free mass in males and females. *Int J Obes* 1991; **15**: 717–26.

18 Slattery ML, McDonald A, Bild DE *et al*. Associations of body fat and its distribution with dietary intake, physical activity, alcohol, and smoking in blacks and whites. *Am J Clin Nutr* 1992; **55**: 943–50.

19 McTiernan A, Ulrich C, Slate S, Potter J. Physical activity and cancer etiology: associations and mechanisms. *Cancer Causes Control* 1998; **9**: 487–509.

20 Giovannucci E, Ascherio A, Rimm EB *et al*. Physical activity, obesity and risk for colon cancer and adenoma in men. *Ann Internal Med* 1995; **122**: 327–34.

21 Cordain L, Latin RW, Behnke JJ. The effects of an aerobic running program on bowel transit time. *J Sports Med Phys Fitness* 1986; **26**: 101–4.

22 Shephard RJ, Verde TJ, Thomas SG, Shek P. Physical activity and the immune system. *Can J Sport Sci* 1991; **16**: 163–85.

23 Bernstein L, Henderson BE, Hanisch R *et al*. Physical exercise and reduced risk of breast cancer in young women. *J Nat Cancer Inst* 1994; **86**: 1403–8.

24 Mittendorf R, Longnecker MP, Newcomb PA *et al*. Strenuous physical activity in young adulthood and risk of breast cancer (United States). *Cancer Causes Control* 1995; **6**: 347–53.

25 Thune I, Brenn T, Lund E, Gaard M. Physical activity and the risk of breast cancer. *N Eng J Med* 1997; **336**: 1269–75.

26 Oliviera SA, Kohl HW, Trichopoulos D, Blair SN. The association between cardiorespiratory fitness and prostate cancer. *Med Sci Sports Exerc* 1996; **28**: 97–104.

27 Lee IM, Paffenbarger RS Jr, Hsieh CC. Physical activity and risk of prostatic cancer among college alumni. *Am J Epidemiol* 1992; **135**: 169–79.

28 United Kingdom Testicular Cancer Study Group. Aetiology of testicular cancer: association with congenital abnormalities, age at puberty, infertility, and exercise. *BMJ* 1994; **308**: 1393–9.

29 Thune I, Lund E. Physical activity and the risk of prostate and testicular cancer: a cohort study of 53,000 Norwegian men. *Cancer Causes Control* 1994; **5**: 549–56.

30 Srivastava A, Kreiger N. Relation of physical activity to risk of testicular cancer. *Am J Epidemiol* 2000; **151**: 78–87.

31 Hunter DJ, Sambrook PN. Bone loss: epidemiology of bone loss. *Arthritis Res* 2000; **2**: 441–5.

32 Krolner B, Toft B. Vertebral bone loss: an unheeded side effect of therapeutic bed rest. *Clin Sci* 1983; **64**: 537–40.

33 Blair SN, Horton E, Leon AS *et al*. Physical activity, nutrition, and chronic disease. *Med Sci Sports Exerc* 1996; **28**: 335–49.

34 Nelson M, Fiatarone M, Morganti C *et al*. Effects of high-intensity strength training on multiple risk factors for osteoporotic fractures — a randomised controlled trial. *JAMA* 1994; **272**: 1909–14.

35 Ginn J, Archer S, Cooper H. *Researching older people's health needs and health promotion issues.* London: Health Education Authority, 1998.

36 Skelton DA, Young A, Walker A, Hoinville E. *Physical activity in later life: further analysis of the Allied-Dunbar National Fitness Survey and the Health Education Authority's National Survey of Activity and Health.* London: Health Education Authority, 1999.

37 Nuffield Institute for Health. *Preventing falls and subsequent injury in older people. Effective Health Care Bulletin series.* York: Centre for Reviews and Dissemination, 1996.

38 Province MA, Hadley EC, Hornbrook MC *et al.* The effects of exercise on falls in elderly patients. A pre-planned meta-analysis of the FICSIT trials. *JAMA* 1995; **273**: 1341–7.

39 Campbell AJ, Robertson MC, Gardner MM *et al.* Randomised controlled trial of a general practice programme of home-based exercise to prevent falls in elderly women. *BMJ* 1997; **315**: 1065–9.

40 American College of Sports Medicine. Position stand on exercise and physical activity for older adults. *Med Sci Sports Exerc* 1998; **30**: 992–1008.

41 Galloway MT, Jokl P. Aging successfully: the importance of physical activity in maintaining health and function. *J Am Acad Orthop Surg* 2000; **8**: 37–44.

Ups and downs of training and performance — the underperformance syndrome

DR RICHARD BUDGETT

DIRECTOR OF MEDICAL SERVICES, BRITISH OLYMPIC MEDICAL CENTRE, LONDON, UK

Unexplained underperformance in athletes is a common problem, occurring in about 10–20% of elite endurance squads including marathon runners[1]. In the absence of any other medical cause, this is sometimes called: the overtraining syndrome, burnout, staleness, sports fatigue syndrome or chronic fatigue in athletes[1–3]. The condition is often secondary to the stress of training but the exact aetiology and pathophysiology is not known[4]. Many factors may lead to failure to recover from training or competition.

There has been some confusion in the literature on the definition and diagnostic criteria of underperformance[5]. The term 'overtraining syndrome' implies a cause that limits investigation of this problem in athletes. Much confusion exists as to whether or not athletes suffering from frequent respiratory infections, a depressed mood state, fatigue or underperformance are all, in fact, overtrained[6]. To help researchers and clinicians investigate this problem, a broader definition was created at a round table discussion in St Catherine's College, Oxford, on 19 April 1999[7]. However, several distinct subgroups may exist, some of which may overlap. It is, therefore, important that those conducting research and producing case reports define exactly which group(s) they are investigating or whether or not they have included all athletes with persistent unexplained underperformance.

This chapter will define unexplained underperformance syndrome (UPS), and will focus on its pathophysiology, prevention strategies and management.

Definition of UPS

UPS can be defined as a persistent unexplained performance deficit that is recognized and agreed by coach and athlete, even after two weeks of relative rest[7]. This contrasts with the definition of chronic fatigue syndrome, where symptoms must last at least six months[8].

The following symptoms have been reported in UPS[4,6,7,9]:

- fatigue and an unexpected sense of effort during training
- history of heavy training and competition
- frequent minor infections
- unexplained or unusually heavy, stiff and/or sore muscles
- mood disturbance
- change in expected sleep quality
- loss of energy
- loss of competitive drive
- loss of libido
- loss of appetite.

If underperformance may be explained in terms of a major disease, then UPS cannot be diagnosed. For this reason, all marathon runners diagnosed with UPS should have a thorough history and physical examination. In most cases, the coach and athlete will be best able to measure performance and compare it to that of previous weeks, months or years. The performance deficit may be agreed by the sports scientist or sports physician if appropriate ergometer or field tests have been carried out. It may be most appropriate to compare performance to the same stage of previous marathon cycles.

Although relative rest cannot be defined exactly, it should involve a significant reduction in training and an increase in recovery time.

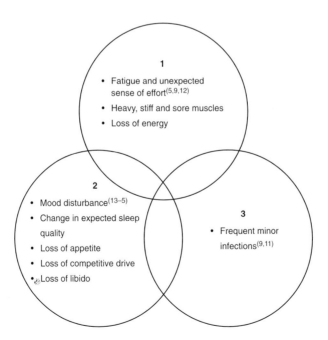

Figure 1
Pattern of symptoms in UPS

Marathon runners present with fatigue and underperformance with secondary changes in mood specific to the sport and individual[10]. Those suffering from frequent minor infections, particularly upper respiratory tract infections (URTI), may form a separate overlapping subgroup (Figure 1)[11]. As a result of these overlapping groups and the confusion of definitions, the British Olympic Medical Centre, London, UK, definition of unexplained underperformance is broad and all-inclusive — it does not include over-reaching (discussed below) or so-called short-term overtraining from which runners recover with two weeks of relative rest[1].

Normal response to training

Marathon runners must train hard. Although, the initial hard training causes underperformance, supercompensation takes place and an improvement in performance is seen if recovery is allowed[16]. Training for the marathon is designed in a cyclical way (periodization), allowing time for recovery with progressive overload. During the hard training/overload period, transient signs and symptoms and changes in diagnostic tests may occur — this is called over-reaching[5].

In the state of over-reaching, changes take place in the Profile of Mood State (POMS) questionnaire which shows reduced vigour and increased tension, depression, anger, fatigue and confusion (see Professor Morgan's chapter)[15]. Muscle glycogen stores are depleted and resting heart rate increases. The testosterone:cortisol ratio is reduced as a result of lower testosterone and high cortisol levels. Microscopic damage to muscle also leads to increased creatine kinase levels if there is eccentric exercise[17]. All these changes are physiological and normal if recovery occurs within two weeks. Over-reaching is an important part of training for improved performance[6].

Abnormal response to training

There is a risk of developing UPS if training is prolonged, heavy and monotonous (where, in this context, monotonous means lacking in variation or periodization and not necessarily boring). Nevertheless, most athletes recover fully after two weeks of adequate rest no matter how hard the training. The cyclical nature of most training programmes allows this recovery and full benefit from hard exercise (Figure 2)[16]. Eventually, fatigue becomes so severe that recovery does not occur despite the two-week rest. A diagnosis of UPS can be made at this stage.

Signs

Reported signs of UPS are often caused by associated illness and are inconsistent and generally unhelpful in making the diagnosis. Cervical lymphadenopathy is very common. There may be an increased postural drop in blood pressure and postural rise in heart rate, probably related to the underlying pathophysiology[18]. Physiological testing

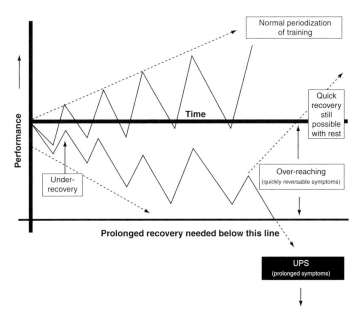

Figure 2

Overtraining or under-recovery, leading to unexplained underperformance syndrome (UPS)

may show a reduced maximal oxygen uptake and maximal power output; an increased submaximal oxygen consumption and pulse rate may also been observed, with the pulse rate slowly returning to normal after exercise. In a standard step test, the pace is increased until lactate levels rise sharply which is the 'onset of blood lactate accumulation' (OBLA). If this occurs at a higher workload, performance is considered to have improved. If there is insufficient glucose (as in glycogen depletion) then there will be a reduced production of lactate. In athletes with UPS, the OBLA is sometimes at a higher workload than in previous tests (called the lactate paradox) and glycogen depletion has been excluded, which suggests a problem in mobilizing or using glucose.

Prevention and early detection

Overtraining for one marathon runner may be insufficient training for another. Runners tolerate different levels of training, competition and stress at different times, depending on their level of health and fitness. The training load must, therefore, be individualized and reduced or increased according to the runner's response. Other stresses, ie examinations, should also be taken into account[10].

In practice, it is difficult to distinguish between over-reaching and UPS. Researchers have attempted to follow blood parameters such as haemoglobin, haematocrit and creatine kinase, but these only measure the stress of training and do not predict who will be unable to recover. Mood state profiling on a regular basis, however, can provide useful guidance[19]. Many runners monitor their own heart rate. Although this is nonspecific, it provides objective evidence that something is wrong[20]. Other prevention strategies are a good diet, full hydration and rest between training sessions. It is more difficult for athletes with full-time jobs and other commitments to recover quickly after training. Many sports scientists and coaches are advising alternate day hard and light training within the normal cyclical programme[12].

The intensity and spacing of training are the two most important factors in optimizing performance and minimizing UPS risk. Morton used a complex mathematical model to optimize periodization of athletic training, and suggested intensive training on alternate days over a 150-day period season with a build up over the first half and taper over the second half. This was more effective than moderate training throughout the whole year[16].

Many athletes use supplements but these do not seem to offer any protection from chronic fatigue. Trace elements and minerals such as magnesium have been investigated but there is no proven link to UPS or chronic fatigue syndrome[5].

Pathophysiology

Training and psychology

Studies have shown a reduction in the lactate:rating of perceived exertion ratio with heavy training[21] — thus for a set lactate level, the perceived exertion is higher. This may represent central fatigue, but could be due to glycogen depletion causing lower lactate levels or the lactate paradox.

The POMS questionnaire was completed by a group of collegiate swimmers in the US[19], which revealed that training was increased whenever the mood state improved and was reduced whenever the POMS deteriorated. The incidence of burnout, which was previously about 10% per year, reduced to zero[22]. Similar studies have not been carried out in marathon runners.

Hormonal changes

The role of hormones in UPS is still not fully understood. The levels of stress hormones, such as adrenaline and cortisol, have been shown to increase more in underperforming athletes than in controls. Salivary cortisol levels (reflecting free cortisol levels) in a group of swimmers were significantly higher in stale, underperforming athletes and this correlated with the depressed mood state[23].

A low testosterone:cortisol ratio has been suggested as a marker of UPS, reflecting a change in the balance of anabolism to catabolism. This ratio falls in response to overreaching, so only a very low ratio is useful. In some athletes, no significant change is seen despite the symptoms of UPS[23].

A reduced response to insulin-induced hypoglycaemia was demonstrated by Baron and Noakes, which suggests hypothalamic dysfunction[24].

Noradrenaline levels have been shown to be higher in fatigued underperforming swimmers than in controls, particularly during tapering, but levels were generally proportional to the training stress. There was no change in cortisol levels[25]. Plasma catecholamine levels and stress ratings (by questionnaire) were useful predictors of staleness, and a well-being rating questionnaire during tapering predicted performance[26]. The rise in noradrenaline levels and the fall in basal nocturnal plasma dopamine and adrenaline have been proposed as a method of monitoring training because these levels correlate with symptoms. There may be a reduction in the sensitivity of β-adrenergic receptors due to overstimulation, which could lead to undermobilization of glucose in exercise and may explain the lactate paradox[27].

Amino acids and central fatigue

The neurotransmitter 5-hydroxytryptamine (5-HT), or serotonin, is widespread in the brain and its effect includes fatigue, sleep and control of hormone levels. It is postulated that changes in the levels of 5-HT and the sensitivity of its receptors in the brain lead to some of the symptoms of UPS.

Prolonged hard training has been shown to cause a fall in branched-chain amino acids and glutamine levels, both acutely and chronically, in runners with UPS. Branched-chain amino acids compete with tryptophan to cross the blood–brain barrier, thus a fall in levels of branched-chain amino acids will result in more tryptophan entering the brain where it is immediately converted into 5-HT. Crossing the blood–brain barrier is the rate limiting step[28,29]. Higher levels of 5-HT could lead to a down regulation of 5-HT receptors and this may account for many of the symptoms seen in UPS. Runners with UPS seem to have difficulty in maximally recruiting all muscle fibres when tested in the laboratory and this may be due to a sensitivity which may be related to changes in the 5-HT receptors[30].

Immunosuppression and glutamine

There is evidence that moderate regular exercise helps reduce the level of infection in normal individuals. However, intense heavy exercise increases the incidence of infections[11]. URTI have been shown to occur more frequently with higher training mileage and after a marathon[31]. Several factors may contribute to this apparent immunosuppression, such as raised cortisol levels, reduced salivary immunoglobulin levels and low glutamine levels. Glutamine is an essential amino acid that rapidly divides cells such as lymphocytes. Low levels of glutamine have been found in chronically fatigued and underperforming athletes, including marathon runners, and levels are known to be lower after hard training[32]. Thus, in addition to a possible role in central fatigue, glutamine may have a role in immunosuppression.

Glutamine intervention studies have provided evidence that the incidence of infection in endurance athletes after prolonged exercise is lower than those taking glutamine compared to placebo, and that recovery from a period of intense training (over-reaching) is quicker[33].

Management

Athletes suffering from UPS are different from chronic fatigue sufferers — they present much earlier, tend to recover more quickly and have an opportunity to change major stresses in their lives (training and competition). However, management of the UPS patient is very similar to that of the chronic fatigue patient and requires an holistic approach. Rest and regeneration are central to recovery[1].

Studies at the British Olympic Medical Centre, London, UK, have shown that both performance and mood state improve following five weeks of physical rest[15]. Low level exercise has also been shown to speed recovery from the chronic fatigue syndrome[34,35].

As most athletes will usually not comply if instructed to rest, they should be given positive advice and told to exercise aerobically at a pulse rate of 120–40 beats/min for five to 10 minutes each day, ideally in divided sessions, and slowly build this up over six to 12 weeks. The exercise programme should be individually designed and will depend on the clinical picture and rate of improvement. The cycle of partial recovery followed by hard training and recurrent breakdown needs to be stopped. It is often necessary to avoid the athlete's own sport using cross-training because of the tendency to increase the exercise intensity too quickly. A positive approach is essential, with an emphasis on slowly building up volume instead of intensity to about one hour/day. Once this volume is tolerated, more intense work can be incorporated above the onset of blood lactate accumulation (OBLA)[21].

Very short (<10 s) sprints/power sessions with at least three to five minutes of rest are safe and allow some hard training to be done[36].

There are no trials of regeneration strategies (including rest, relaxation, counselling and psychotherapy) which were widely used in the old Eastern Block countries[30]. Massage and hydrotherapy are used and nutrition is looked at carefully. Large quantities of vitamins and supplements are administered but no evidence exists to suggest they are effective. Stresses outside sport are reduced as much as possible.

Depression may need to be treated with antidepressants but normally drugs are of no value, although any concurrent illness must be treated. There is one report of the (prohibited) use of anabolic steroids to treat UPS[37].

Marathon runners who have been underperforming for many months are often surprised at the good performance they can produce after 12 weeks of extremely light exercise. At this point, care must be taken not to increase the training intensity too rapidly and to allow full recovery after difficult parts of the training cycle. The British Olympic Medical Centre, London, UK, recommends that athletes recover completely at least once a week.

Conclusions

UPS is a condition of undeperformance with persistent fatigue and an increased vulnerability to infection, leading to recurrent infections in some runners. It is a common syndrome in marathon runners. Central, peripheral, hormonal and immunological factors may all contribute to the failure to recovery from exercise.

Optimizing training and careful monitoring of athletes may help prevent UPS. Symptoms have been seen to resolve between six and 12 weeks with regeneration strategies and a structured exercise programme.

Acknowledgements

Adapted with permission from: Budgett R. Fatigue and underperformance in athletes: the overtraining syndrome. *Brit J Sports Med* 1998; **32**: 107–10.

References

1 Budgett R. The overtraining syndrome. *BMJ* 1994; **309**: 4465–8.

2 Fry RW, Morton AR, Keast D. Overtraining syndrome and the chronic fatigue syndrome. *N Zeal J Sports Med* 1991; **19**: 48–52.

3 Lehmann M, Foster C, Keull J. Overtraining in endurance athletes: a brief review. *Med Sci Sports Exerc* 1993; **25**: 854–62.

4 Lehmann M, Foster C, Gastmann U *et al*. Definition, types, symptoms, findings, underlying mechanisms, and frequency of overtraining and overtraining syndrome. In: Lehmann M, Foster C, Gastmann U *et al*, eds. *Overload, performance incompetence, and regeneration in sport*. New York: Plenum, 1999: 1–6.

5 Budgett R. The overtraining syndrome. *Br J Sports Med* 1990; **24**: 231–6.

6 Budgett R. Fatigue and underperformance in athletes: the overtraining syndrome. *BMJ* 1998; **32**: 107–10.

7 Budgett R, Newsholme E, Lehmann M *et al*. Redefining the overtraining syndrome as the unexplained underperformance syndrome. *Br J Sports Med* 2000; **34**: 67–8.

8 Royal Colleges. *Chronic fatigue syndrome: report of a joint working group of the Royal Colleges of Physicians, Psychiatrists and General Practitioners*. London: Royal College of Physicians, 1996.

9 Smith C, Kirby P, Noakes TD. The worn-out athlete: a clinical approach to chronic fatigue in athletes. *J Sports Sci* 1997; **15**: 341–51.

10 Budgett R. The overtraining syndrome. *Coaching Focus* 1995; **28**: 4–6.

11 Nieman D. Exercise infection and immunity. *Int J Sports Med* 1994; **15**: S131.

12 Fry RW, Morton AR, Keast D. Periodisation and the prevention of overtraining. *Can J Sports Sci* 1992; **17**: 241–8.

13 Morgan WP, Costill DC, Flynn MG *et al*. Mood disturbance following increased training in swimmers. *Med Sci Sports Exerc* 1988; **20**: 408–14.

14 Dyment P. Frustrated by chronic fatigue? *Physician Sports Med* 1993; **21**: 47–54.

15 Koutedakis Y, Budgett R, Faulmann L. Rest in underperforming elite competitors. *Br J Sports Med* 1990; **24**: 248–52.

16 Morton RH. Modelling training and overtraining. *J Sports Sci* 1997; **15**: 335–40.

17 Costill DL, Flynn MG, Kirway JP *et al*. Effects of repeated days of intensified training on muscle glycogen and swimming performance. *Med Sci Sports Exerc* 1988; **20**: 249–54.

18 Kindermann W. Das Ubertraining-Ausdruck einer vegetativen Fehlsteurung. *Deutsche Zeitschrift fur Sportsmedizin* 1986; **37**: 138–45.

19 Morgan WP, Brown DR, Fascm Raglin JS *et al*. Psychological monitoring of overtraining and staleness. *Br J Sports Med 1987*; **21**: 107–14.

20 Dressendorfer RH, Wade CE, Scaff JH. Increased morning heart rate in runners: a valid sign of overtraining? *Physician Sports Med* 1985; **13**: 77–86.

21 Synder AC. A physiological/psychological indicator of overreaching during intensive training. *Int J Sports Med* 1993; **14**: 29–32.

22 O'Connor PJ, Carson Smith J. Using mood responses to overtraining to optimize endurance performance and prevent staleness. *Flemish J Sports Med Sports Sci* 1999; **80**: 14–9.

23 Flynn MG, Pizza FX, Boone JB *et al*. Indices of training stress during competitive running and swimming seasons. *Int J Sports Med* 1994; **15**: 21–6.

24 Barron JL, Noakes TD, Levy W *et al*. Hypothalamic dysfunction in overtrained athletes. *J Clin Endocrinol Metab* 1985; **60**: 803–6.

25 Hooper SL, Mackinnon LT, Gordon RD, Bachmann AW. Markers for monitoring overtraining and recovery. *Med Sci Sports Exerc* 1995; **27**: 106–12.

26 Hooper SL, Mackinnon LT. Monitoring overtraining in athletes. *Sports Med* 1995; **20**: 231–7.

27 Lehmann M, Dickhuth HH, Gendrisch E *et al*. Training-overtraining. A prospective experimental study with experienced middle and long distance runners. *Int J Sports Med* 1991; **12**: 444–52.

28 Blomstrand E, Hassmen P, Newsholme EA. Administration of branched-chain amino acids during sustained exercise. *Eur J Appl Physiol* 1991; **63**: 83.

29 Blomstrand E, Perrett D, Parry-Billings M, Newsholme EA. Effect of sustained exercise on plasma amino acid concentrations and on 5-hydroxtryptamine metabolism in six different brain regions in the rat. *Acta Physiol Scand* 1989; **136**: 473.

30 Koutedakis Y, Frishknecht R, Vrbová G *et al*. Maximal voluntary quadriceps strength patterns in Olympic overtrained athletes. *Med Sci Sports Exer* 1995; **27**: 566–72.

31 Nieman D, Johanssen LM, Lee JW, Arabatzis K. Infections episodes before and after the Los Angeles Marathon. *J Sports Med Phys Fitness* 1990; **30**: 289–96.

32 Parry-Billings M, Budgett R, Kouttedakis Y *et al*. Plasma amino acid concentrations in the overtraining syndrome: possible effects on the immune system. *Med Sci Sports Exerc* 1992; **24**: 1353–8.

33 Castell LM, Poortmans J, Newsholme EA. Does glutamine have a role in reducing infection during intensified training in swimmers. *Med Sci Sports Exerc* 1996; **28**: 285–90.

34 Fultcher KY, White PD. Randomised controlled trial of graded exercise in patients with chronic fatigue syndrome. *BMJ* 1997; **314**: 1647–52.

35 Wearden AJ, Morris RK, Mullis R *et al*. A randomised, double blind, placebo controlled treatment trial of fluoxetine and a graded exercise programme for chronic fatigue syndrome. *Br J Psychiatry* 1998; **172**: 485–90.

36 Fry AC, Kraemer WJ. Does short-term near-maximal intensity machine resistance training induce overtraining? *J Strength Cond Res* 1994; **8**: 188–91.

37 Kereszty A. Overtraining. In: Larson L, ed. *Encyclopedia of sports science and medicine*. New York: MacMillan, 1971: 218–22.

Psychological factors associated with distance running and the marathon

PROFESSOR WILLIAM MORGAN

DIRECTOR, EXERCISE PSYCHOLOGY LABORATORY, DEPARTMENT OF KINESIOLOGY,
UNIVERSITY OF WISCONSIN-MADISON, MADISON, WISCONSIN, USA

It is only the arbitrary vantage point we adopt that allows us to speak in terms of 'mind' and 'body' as independent or unitary constructs. There is now an extensive literature from the fields of psychology, neuroscience and psychosomatic medicine demonstrating that mind and body should be viewed as one. I will, therefore, focus on the 'mind' of the marathon runner in this chapter with the understanding that mind–body oneness is a given.

A number of reviews have been published dealing with the psychology of endurance performance since the appearance of a report in the 1977 New York Academy of Sciences publication[1]. The first review was prepared by Dishman and Landy[2], and was followed by updates on the general subject[3–5] — these updates contain summaries of research related to the principles and findings outlined in the original report, and included discussions of additional endurance events in sports such as cycling, middle-distance running and swimming. This chapter will discuss mainly the marathon.

There is much research evidence supporting the view that performance in endurance events is influenced to a substantial degree by factors of a psychological nature[1–5], and numerous anecdotal observations can also be cited. Perhaps the most dramatic example was the record-setting performance of Roger Bannister in the mile run on 6 May 1954. His world record of three minutes and 59.4 seconds (3:59.4) on that day was significant for many reasons. For example, other runners had come close to breaking the four-minute barrier and there was a continuing question as to whether or not the barrier was physical or mental. Gunder Hägg and Arne Anderson of Sweden had run 4:01.4 and 4:01.6 respectively but were unable to go under four minutes in the mile. Hägg was an exceptional runner in his time — he held world records in the one-, two- and three-mile, as well as 1,500 m, 3,000 m and 5,000 m at the same point in time. The famous Swedish sport psychologist, Dr Lars-Eric Unestahl, has speculated that Hägg and other runners had convinced themselves that no man would ever run faster than four minutes in the mile[6]. It is Unestahl's view that a 'psychological barrier' prevented runners from running faster than four minutes in the mile.

The views expressed by Unestahl have been held by others[2–5], and it is clear that a different mindset characterized Bannister and his running mates[7,8]. They were confident that the mile could be run in less than four minutes, and the question became one of where and when the attempt should be made. Bannister later wrote: 'Though physiology may indicate respiratory and circulatory limits to muscular effort, psychological and other factors beyond the ken of physiology set the razor's edge of defeat or victory and determine how close an athlete approaches the absolute limits of performance'[7].

Bannister has also prepared a detailed account of the assault on the four-minute barrier and this instructive volume is recommended reading for those interested in maximal physical performance[8]. Bannister not only broke the four-minute mile barrier but, once he removed it, others were able to quickly follow. His performance opened the doorway for other sub, four-minute milers, and it forced us to start thinking about maximal physical performance in a fundamentally different way. Athletes, coaches, trainers and specialists in sports medicine began to think in different terms regarding goal-setting and physical limitations as a direct consequence of Bannister's phenomenal performance in 1954.

Earlier reports

The psychological characteristics of a selected sample of male marathon runners were described by Morgan and Costill nearly three decades ago[9]. These runners completed a battery of psychological questionnaires designed to measure introversion–extroversion, neuroticism–stability, anxiety and depression. While many authors in the popular press, as well as the quasi scientific literature, had previously speculated about the unique nature of the marathon runner's psyche, runners in this study were found to score well within the published norms for each of the variables evaluated with the exception of anxiety. The mean anxiety score was much lower than the published norm — this may have been due to many years of running, although selection or sampling may also have been a factor. It was reported in this investigation that none of the psychological variables were correlated with performance in the marathon, but the absence of a significant relationship may have been due to the small sample size in concert with the homogenous nature of the group.

It has been recognized by personality theorists for many years that individual differences in personality structure must be taken into consideration when advancing generalizations about the influence of personality on behaviour. In their seminal volume titled *Theories of personality*, Hall and Lindzey conceptualized the nature of this issue in terms of idiographic and nomothetic phenomena[10]. Emphasis is placed on the unique nature of the individual when using idiographic models in research or practice, whereas principles of behaviour derived from the study of groups are emphasized when nomothetic models are employed. This is an important principle that must be considered in any discussion involving the contribution of psychological factors to performance in the marathon.

An example from the study by Morgan and Costill illustrates the importance of making a distinction between idiographic and nomothetic observations[9]. While the marathon runners in their study scored slightly below the population average on extroversion–introversion (ie more introverted), the top runner in this sample, and the winner of the Boston marathon the following year, scored significantly higher than the population average on extroversion. This could be important since it has been reported that: pain tolerance is higher in extroverts; extroverts consistently rate an absolute exercise intensity to be less effortful; and, when given an opportunity to select an exercise intensity (ie preferred exertion), extroverts have been reported to adopt a higher intensity than introverts[11].

The psychological characteristics of elite middle- and long-distance runners were compared with those of elite marathon runners by Morgan and Pollock[1] — the subgroups were found to be remarkably similar. Furthermore, the psychological profile for this group of elite runners was similar to that observed earlier in the study by Morgan and Costill[9]. These runners possessed what has been termed the 'iceberg' profile (Figure 1). This stereotypical profile has been observed in subsequent research involving independent samples of both men and women marathon runners classified in the elite category[12,13]. These runners tend to score below the population average on mood states such as tension, depression, anger, fatigue and confusion as measured by the Profile of Mood States (POMS)[14], and score above the population average on vigour. It should be emphasized that this profile represents a nomothetic characterization and there are elite marathon runners who do not possess this profile. Also, the profile is subject to change, and this usually occurs during periods of overtraining where individual and group profiles are often observed to flatten or invert. Thus, the 'iceberg' profile is commonly observed in elite distance runners under baseline conditions, but it is not typically observed during periods of overtraining.

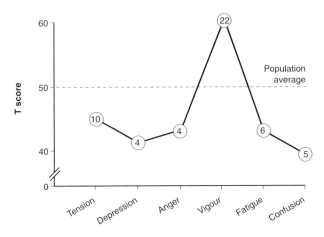

Figure 1

Summary of the Profile of Mood States (POMS) data from selected samples of elite men and women marathon runners

Adapted from[1,12,13,53].

Perhaps the most important observation made in this earlier study was the finding that the elite runners employed a predominant cognitive strategy that was labelled association, compared with non-elite marathon runners who relied on a cognitive strategy known as dissociation[1,3]. Thus, instead of ignoring distressful sensations by dissociating sensory input, the elite runners reported that they paid close attention to multiple signals of a somatic nature (eg muscle pain, cramps, parathesias, respiration, effort sense). It was common for these runners to make a conscious decision to slow the pace if they began to experience respiratory distress. One of the top marathon runners in this group reported that: 'If I am having trouble getting enough air, I know I have to slow the pace'[3]. These runners paid attention to the 'clock', but pace was moderated by how they felt at any given point in a race. There is a compelling theoretical rationale, along with empirical research evidence, in support of relying on 'effort sense' to dictate the pace in a competitive run[11,15]. While these runners agreed that it was preferable to stay in contact with selected opponents during a given competition, they also preferred to 'read their own bodies' and 'run their own race'. Many of the runners constantly reminded themselves to 'stay loose', 'relax', 'don't get tight', 'remember to drink', and so on. It was also remarkable that these runners did not regard 'pain zones' and 'the wall' as being as important as did the non-elite runners[1,3]. These elite runners tended to minimize the importance of 'pain zones' and 'the wall', and one elite runner reported that: 'If I am having trouble during a marathon, I know that everyone else is in trouble as well. If others do not slow the pace when I do, they will probably crash at some point down the line. I don't worry about what the other runners are doing in a race. I pay attention to my body... I read the signs... I sort of have the equivalent of a shopping list that I keep going over... I seem to dehydrate very easily, and I know that I have to drink a lot during a marathon so I am constantly reminding myself to drink... I pick up the pace, and I slow my pace based on how I feel'[3].

There is considerable evidence that the most efficient running pattern is one involving a steady pace (pay-as-you-go) as opposed to one in which the runner accelerates and decelerates (buy-now-pay-later) throughout the race[3,14,16]. Nevertheless, there are a number of anecdotal reports[3,16-20], as well as experimental research evidence, demonstrating that a dissociative cognitive strategy can actually result in the enhancement of endurance performance. There are also anthropological reports that Tibetan monks (Mahetangs) trained in 'swiftness of foot' were able to run long distances (eg 300 miles) in a remarkable time[21,22]. These reports have been challenged by Scott[23] who has reported that: 'A final comment about the "monk runners" of Tibet: they do not really run as fast as has been reported because the distance was miscalculated. You can only run 100 miles in 16 hours at altitude; 300 miles in 30 hours is absolutely impossible'[20].

At any rate, it has been shown that application of the cognitive strategy allegedly employed by these Tibetan monks can produce a significant increase in endurance performance under controlled laboratory conditions[20]. Furthermore, since the performance enhancement noted in this experimental research was not associated with observable physiological changes (ie cardiovascular, lactate and catecholamine levels remained the same), it would appear that the participants were able to tolerate the distress associated with prolonged efforts by using the dissociative strategy. It is also known that perception of effort can be systematically increased and decreased with hypnotic suggestion[11,16,24], and changes in effort sense are often associated with changes in heart rate and ventilatory minute volume. Furthermore, the hypnotic perturbation of effort sense during steady state exercise has recently been shown to alter regional cerebral blood flow (rCBF) in selected brain regions[25].

The original research describing the predominant cognitive strategies employed by elite and non-elite distance runners[1] has generated considerable research, but the only follow-up studies designed to directly replicate and extend the original findings have been carried out by Morgan and colleagues[12,13]. The direct replications involved the same research protocol (discussed below). While the related studies have generally confirmed the basic premise originally advanced, it is not possible to make direct comparisons between these studies owing to different methods, research designs and types of athletes. The qualitative methodology involved taped interviews that included both structured and unstructured components. The quantitative data collection was based on physiological, perceptual and psychometric variables, and these data were analysed with conventional statistical procedures. The subsequent research has not relied on the use of qualitative and quantitative designs; most of this related research cannot be compared with the earlier work[1] due to methodological differences.

Related research

Some of the related research has dealt with recreational athletes and college students involved in sports other than distance running. These studies have included sports and exercises such as swimming[26], rowing[27] and race walking[28]. Despite the fact that different populations have been sampled, the findings have been consistent with the original observations for the most part. However, this more recent research has been restricted to individuals classified as non-elite in terms of athleticism[29–39]. While some of the related research has actually dealt with marathon runners, none of these investigations involved the study of elite performers. For example, one investigation involved the study of ultramarathon runners[39], but the participants were not elite performers. Also, the cognitive taxonomy employed in this study differed from that used in the original work.

A number of investigators have attempted to reconceptualize and make operational the nature of the associative–dissociative construct. This restructuring has consisted of efforts to add a dimension of directionality (ie internal vs external)[31,39–41], while others have introduced the added dimension of task specificity (ie task related vs

297

unrelated)[32]. The effort to develop a more precise measure of the psychological construct in question may be premature, as well as unnecessary. In some respects the situation might be likened to efforts designed to create an interval scale measure of physical activity. That is, investigators can usually identify sedentary and active individuals, but efforts to precisely quantify the degree of physical activity have been associated with psychometric problems involving objectivity, reliability and validity. In other words, it might be relatively simple to identify the predominant cognitive style employed by a runner (eg associative vs dissociative) during training and competition, but quite another matter to create an instrument that possesses the interval scale properties and assumptions required when employing conventional statistical models. In one sense, the various questionnaires and scaling procedures that have been advanced for use in assessing association and dissociation should probably be viewed as experimental scales that lack construct validity.

The research carried out following the original report by Morgan and Pollock[1] has been characterized by a number of methodological problems; one of the most significant has been the restructuring and interpretation of the association–dissociation construct. In a paper by Couture et al, for example, participants in the association group were given the following instructions: 'While you are swimming, I want you to try to think of the word air every time you inhale. Try to think of nothing else but the word air'[26]. In the earlier research by Morgan et al, a similar set of instructions was employed, but it was conceptualized as a dissociative cognitive strategy[20]. Furthermore, it is problematic to contrast the effect of cognitive strategies employed by young beginning swimmers with those of older adults tested on a treadmill — the absence of external validity in such a comparison restricts the ability of generalization. It appears that confirmation or refutation of the original findings presented by Morgan and Pollock[1] and Morgan et al[20] has suffered to a large degree by the operationalism of association and dissociation, along with major differences in exercise mode and performance status (ie elite vs non-elite). There has also been a general tendency for investigators to ignore the impact of the original research findings with the passage of time. Stevenson and Biddle[31] have stated, for example, that 'The assertion of Morgan that non-elite athletes tend to dissociate in races is not supported'. An alternative explanation has been offered by Raglin and Wilson[5] who pointed out that: 'Description of these cognitive strategies and their impact have been widely reported in running magazines, and this may account for the widespread adoption of association as a racing strategy by many recreational runners'.

The explanation by Raglin and Wilson[5] is probably closer to the truth as more than two decades have passed since the original reports appeared in the scientific[1] and lay literature[42]. One would hope that athletes and coaches would adopt research findings as they become available, and this appears to have taken place in the case of the predominant cognitive strategies employed by marathon runners[5]. The suggestion that the original findings by Morgan and Pollock[1] have not been confirmed in more recent research[31] fails to account for the passage of time. Further support for this view comes from the later research by Morgan *et al* carried out with elite and non-elite women marathon runners[13]. These sub-groups were found to be similar on each of the variables included in this study and, in particular, the elite and non-elite runners did not differ in the cognitive strategies employed during training or competition.

Following a review of the early work describing dissociation as the cognitive strategy employed by non-elite marathon runners during competition, and association as the predominant strategy used by elite runners, Stevinson and Biddle[31] stated that: 'No support for either of these positions exists from other studies'. These authors proceed to support this unusual position by citing the reports of Summers *et al*[34], Okwumabua *et al*[36,37] and Masters *et al*[29], none of whom included elite marathon runners in their research. Stevinson and Biddle also discuss the methodological issues characteristic of studies by Schomer[32], Clingman and Hilliard[28], Pennebaker and Lightner[43], Padgett and Hill[42], Goode and Roth[40], and Acevedo *et al*[39] dealing with this subject, but none of these investigators employed elite runners in their research either. Some did not even study runners! Furthermore, the study by Stevinson and Biddle was restricted to a questionnaire survey of non-elite runners[31], and the authors omitted reference to any research dealing with the cognitive strategies of elite and non-elite marathon runners published after the original report by Morgan and Pollock in 1977. Later research by Morgan *et al*[12,13] appeared in 1986 and 1987, more than a decade before the report by Stevinson and Biddle in 1998[31]. The report by these investigators dealt with the cognitive orientations in non-elite marathon runners with special emphasis on the phenomenon known as 'hitting the wall', but all runners (*n*=66) in their study completed the marathon. Hence, by definition, none of the runners in their study 'hit the wall', presumably due to their use of association, the preferred cognitive strategy previously identified.

The failure of Stevinson and Biddle[31] to confirm the earlier research by Morgan and colleagues[1,3,12,13,16,18,20,42] is probably due to the widespread adoption of the associative cognitive strategy by recreational runners during competition as proposed by Raglin and Wilson[5]. The report by Stevinson and Biddle[31] is characterized by a number of serious methodological and design flaws. A commentary by Scully[44] follows the report by Stevinson and Biddle[31], and this uncritical evaluation accepts the author's views as being factual. Unfortunately, Scully goes on to state that the report has '… obvious clinical relevance in providing evidence to support practical recommendations for marathon runners…' An alternative view would be that:

- the study was based on several misconceptions
- the literature on which the study was based was selective in the sense that irrelevant reports were reviewed and relevant research was ignored
- the sample of recreational marathon runners included in the study was restricted to volunteers who completed a questionnaire following the completion of a marathon (ie, drop-outs were not included in the analysis)

- this descriptive study suffers from the problem of volunteerism
- there is an absence of external validity.

This study clearly lacks the basis for the application and clinical relevance suggested by Scully[44]. Stevinson and Biddle do not offer an explanation for the decision to exclude runners who failed to complete the marathon under investigation[31]. The inclusion of both finishers and drop-outs would have been instructive, and this would have enabled them to evaluate the cognitive strategies employed by marathon runners differing in performance.

Thus, to summarize, the published literature involving the cognitive strategies employed by distance runners and marathon runners is fairly consistent on a number of points. First, it is apparent that dissociation of sensory input based on distress, fatigue and general discomfort not only reduces the sensation of distress, but can also result in the enhancement of endurance performance[20]. However, it is also recognized that use of such a strategy as a means of coping with distress can result in various problems ranging from blisters, strains and sprains, to bone fractures, hyperthermia, hypothermia and myocardial infarction[42]. It would, therefore, seem prudent to rely on an associative cognitive strategy during periods of intense and prolonged physical activity of the type encountered in running a marathon. This was found to be the predominant strategy employed by elite distance runners first studied by Morgan and Pollock[1], and this has been replicated in samples of elite men and women marathon runners studied later[12,13]. This does not mean that elite runners do not employ dissociation at times. Although this is especially true during training runs, elite runners also employ dissociation during competition when association is not needed[12,13]. In addition, there are anecdotal reports of elite marathon runners relying on the judicious use of dissociation to effectively negotiate a critical component of a race[19].

The original research by Morgan and Pollock revealed that elite runners tended to employ association while non-elite runners relied primarily on dissociation. These characteristic cognitive patterns have changed as a function of time, and it has been suggested by Raglin and Wilson that recreational runners have adopted the use of associative strategies as the original research was assimilated by non-elite runners[5]. There can be little question about the impact of packaging and disseminating scientific research in lay publications, and the original work[1,20] was published for the lay public in *Psychology Today* under the title 'Mind of the marathoner'[42]. It is concluded that marathon runners can effectively employ associative and dissociative cognitive strategies during training and competition. The extent to which one strategy becomes predominant at any given point in time should be governed by both internal (ie the runner's bodily responses) and external (eg temperature, course, opponents) factors. Put simply, one might enjoy running in the pleasurable state that accompanies dissociation, but he or she would be well advised to shift into an associative mode when circumstances dictate. This is precisely the type of selective attention employed by elite marathon runners[1,12,13].

Health benefits of running

The importance of the general health benefits that accompany long-distance running are quite apparent to workers in the exercise and sport sciences. However, it has only been in recent years that the mental health benefits of distance running and other physical activities have become widely recognized[45]. There is now considerable evidence that regular physical activity is associated with affective beneficence in general[46], and reduced depression and anxiety in both patient groups and normal individuals is now well documented[45,47]. Despite the observation that regular exercise results in acknowledged health benefits, to include the widely documented improved sense of wellbeing, about half of the sedentary individuals who adopt exercise programmes become recidivists within a short period of time[48,49]. Nevertheless, there is a sector of the general population that continues to exercise on a regular basis throughout their life. In a longitudinal study of ageing marathon runners, for example, it was noted at 20–5 years of follow-up that >90% of these individuals continued to run on a regular basis[50]. The adherence rate for this sample was remarkable, and the individual who no longer took part in long-distance running because of a medical problem continued to work in the garden, walk and perform other physical activities into the seventh decade of life. These ageing marathon runners were characterized by the stereotypical 'iceberg' profile illustrated in Figure 1 when first evaluated in the late 1960s and early 1970s, and were found to be remarkably similar when evaluated 20–5 years later. It is probable that the positive mood states (eg low anxiety and depression) noted in this sample were due in part to the active life styles maintained by these individuals. Of course, one cannot rule out the possibility that the individuals were unique in a number of ways from the outset of the study[50].

Exercise abuse and deprivation

Given the powerful effect of vigorous exercise as an antidepressant and anxiolytic agent, it is reasonable to assume that exercise abuse might occur in some individuals. The beneficial effects resulting from regular exercise could lead to such a positive feeling that some individuals might engage in excessive levels of exercise in order to insure ever increasing levels of positive affect. Conversely, it is also possible that negative mood effects might occur when regular exercisers are prevented from exercising for a period of time (ie exercise deprivation).

The runner's high

There has been considerable discussion in the lay literature regarding the phenomenon that has been termed the 'runner's high'. Many authors of popular articles have suggested that exercise produces a euphoric-like state as a consequence of endorphin production in the central nervous system. However, these views are largely speculative as far as the human is concerned[46]. Research carried out with humans has been of an indirect nature in the sense that β-endorphin levels in the circulating plasma (not brain) have been studied[15]. Although increases in β-endorphin/β-lipotropin immunoreactivity have been shown to further elevate in the plasma following vigorous exercise on the treadmill, this cannot be viewed as evidence that alterations in brain levels have occurred[15]. Hoffmann has stated that '... because the blood-brain barrier is rather impermeable to circulating peptides, peripheral concentrations of β-endorphin would not be expected to modify CNS [central nervous system] opioid activity'[51]. Another approach that has been employed with humans has consisted of administering opiate antagonists such as naltrexone and naloxone to humans before and/or during exercise in an effort to block the production of β-endorphins in the central nervous system. When naltrexone and placebo have been administered to runners in a double-blind manner before exercise, it has been reported that tension decreases (ie mood improvement occurs) in both conditions[52]. Research of this nature has tended to discount the hypothesis that the improved sense of wellbeing following exercise is mediated by brain levels of endorphin. On the other hand, Hoffmann has argued that such findings may simply reflect the use of small doses of opioid antagonists in this research[51]. The failure to find consistent support for the hypothesis that exercise results in the activation of endogenous opioids in humans may be due to methodological problems as pointed out by Hoffmann[51]. Also, Hoffmann's research relying on a rat model suggests that prolonged aerobic exercise not only results in the activation of endogenous opioids, but it is also associated with behavioural changes. Hoffmann has termed this the 'endorphin calm'[51].

It appears that most individuals enjoy a general sense of wellbeing following exercise, and there is objective evidence that transitory shifts in mood state (eg anxiety, depression) occur in the post-exercise period[45-7]. Should this sense of exhilaration be termed an 'exercise high'? One of the original papers that led to the proposal that a 'runner's high' exists was written by Mandell, who wrote[53]:

> 'Thirty minutes out, and something lifts. Legs and arms become light and rhythmic... The fatigue goes away and feelings of power begin. I think I'll run twenty-five miles today. I'll double the size of the research grant request. I'll have that talk with the dean... Then, sometime into the second hour comes the spooky time. Colors are bright and beautiful, water sparkles, clouds breathe, and my body, swimming, detaches from the earth. A loving contentment invades the basement of my mind, and thoughts bubble up without trails. I find the place I need to live if I'm going to live. The running literature says that if you run six miles a day for two months, you are addicted forever. I understand. A cosmic view and peace are located between six and ten miles of running... After the run I can't use my mind. It's empty. Then a filling begins. By afternoon I'm back into life with long and smooth energy, a quiet feeling of strength, the kind wisdom afforded those without fear, those detached yet full. The most delicious part is the night's sleep. Long an illusive, fickle dealer with me, Father Sandman now stands ready whenever I want. Maybe the greatest power of the second cycle is the capacity to decide when to fall asleep.'

This provocative thought piece was written at a theoretical level, and it drew on the neurochemical literature involving the recognized influence of various drugs on the central nervous system. Parallels between various drugs and physical exercise are illustrated in this paper. While the mechanisms proposed by Mandell must continue to be viewed as yet-to-be-confirmed hypotheses in some cases, the proposals possess biological plausibility. The suggested role of serotonin by Mandell has more recently been confirmed by Chauloff[54], and other monoamines such as norepinephrine have also been shown to have a significant central effect following exercise[55]. It might be inappropriate to think of β-endorphin activation as the principal mechanism of action since neurotransmitters such as dopamine, norepinephrine and serotonin are known to influence mood, and these monoamines can be altered in a dramatic way by exercise and various drugs[53-5].

The research dealing with the influence of exercise on brain levels of peptides and neurotransmitters[51,54,55] has been based on the use of animal models (mice and rats), and there is sometimes a reluctance to accept this research when attempting to understand the human condition. However, a rat model of psychopathology has been advanced for use in exercise science[56], and its biological plausibility has been demonstrated in that rat brain levels of monoamines have been shown to be associated with behavioural assessments of emotional stability[57].

Exercise addiction

Since there is evidence that vigorous exercise can lead to changes in brain levels of β-endorphin, dopamine, norepinephrine and serotonin, and as these peptides and neurotransmitters are known to influence mood states, it is understandable that exercise might become a habit. It is also conceivable that habitual exercise could lead to a form of dependence or addiction. The concept of an 'exercise addiction' was introduced by Morgan in 1979[58] and was based largely on a qualitative analysis of selected exercisers who reported an inability to function without daily exercise. Some of the runners went so far as to label this their daily 'fix'! These individuals appeared to be 'addicted' to exercise since they regarded it as being more important than jobs or careers, significant others and personal health — when given the choice of running or losing their job, running received a higher priority; when given the choice of running versus interacting with a spouse, children or friends, running was regarded as being more important; and when given the option of running versus resting at the recommendation of his or her physician, the runner would elect to run through the pain. This latter point is similar to Mandell's comment that 'I find the place I need to live if I'm going to live'. The paper describing 'exercise addiction' was actually titled 'Negative addiction in runners' in order to alert the sports medicine community to this syndrome and counter the 'positive addiction' movement that was developing as part of the 'inward' movement ('me' generation) that characterized the hedonistic 70s.

The report of a phenomenon known as exercise addiction[58] was met with a number of responses from the exercise establishment. One of the most common was that the runners described in this paper were not addicted but were motivated, committed, dependent or compulsive. It is not possible to review all of these counter arguments here, but it is interesting to note that most of this literature has been ignored in a recent paper discussing 'exercise abuse'[59]. It is important that we remain undivided by terms, labels and diagnostic categories such that the phenomenon or syndrome of concern does not receive the attention it warrants — both in terms of research and practice. After all, what is the difference if a runner is addicted, dependent, motivated, obligatory, committed or merely 'abusing' exercise if he or she: elects to exercise even though his/her physician recommends rest in order for a body part to heal; skips an important staff meeting or conference to not miss a daily run; is confronted by a running widow/widower with the ultimatum that 'its running or me' sides with the more attractive running option (ie 'fix'). If the runner is confronted with an external force resulting in exercise deprivation for 24–72 hours, finds him- or herself becoming anxious, aggressive, hostile, irritable, confused, depressed, unable to focus, concentrate or sleep, and experiences rapid and irregular heart beat, hypertension, ticks in the facial/neck areas, along with a generalized tension in the skeletal musculature, how should one label these symptoms? Does it make a difference if we classify the individual as an 'obligatory' runner, an 'addicted' runner or merely one who is suffering from 'exercise abuse'? It is known, for example, that the behaviour of mice addicted to exercise and then deprived of it is the same as those first addicted to morphine and then deprived of the drug[46]. Both groups experience 'wet dog' shakes along with other behavioural changes that are viewed as withdrawal symptoms. While the epidemiology of exercise addiction and dependence has never been addressed in an adequate manner, it is fair to say that both conditions exist to some degree among a small number of individuals who exercise evangelicals would prefer to classify with other labels.

Overtraining

Despite the extensive literature supporting the psychological beneficence of both acute and chronic physical activity, it is also recognized that overtraining can actually produce the opposite effect. It is now apparent that an optimal amount of exercise is needed in order to achieve the desired outcomes, and exercise in excess of this level can produce dysphoric mood[59–63]. Furthermore, there is evidence that >50% of all elite men and women marathon runners have overtrained at some point in their careers to the degree that staleness has resulted[12,13]. The staleness syndrome is associated with mood disturbance, insomnia, hypertension, muscle soreness, chronic fatigue, loss of appetite, reduced libido, and elevation in resting levels of creatine kinase and cortisol[61–5]. The mood disturbance that follows an overtraining stimulus is not only predictable in a law-like manner, but changes in variables such as anxiety and depression are associated with exercise volume in a dose–response manner[61]. The relationship between overtraining and mood disturbance can be viewed as causal for the following reasons:

- the observation has been replicated across laboratories in a consistent manner
- there is a temporal sequence associated with this phenomenon such that increased training is followed by increased mood disturbance, and decreased training is followed by improvement in mood
- there is a dose–response relationship between training volume and the development of disturbances in mood
- the causal nature of this relationship possesses biological plausibility[63,64].

Exercise deprivation

Another important phenomenon associated with the complex relationship known to exist between exercise and mood state involves the problem of exercise deprivation. It is likely that the positive mood state reported in the longitudinal study of ageing marathon runners is due in part to the physically active lifestyles pursued by these individuals[50]. Furthermore, the research suggesting that habitual exercisers at times exhibit compulsive behaviour[60] that can initiate exercise addiction[58] or exercise abuse[59], along with research suggesting that vigorous exercise can cause changes in brain levels of opioid peptides and monoamines[51,54,55], leads to the prediction that exercise deprivation could become problematic for such individuals.

The seminal work of Little involving the problem of exercise deprivation in habitual exercisers is instructive in this regard[66]. The patients described by Little were all men and had experienced a sudden emotional breakdown at about the age of 40 years[66,67]. These individuals were preoccupied with physical fitness, and the emotional disturbances experienced by these fitness fanatics were preceded by some type of threat to their physical well-being that reduced or prevented continued physical activity. Little reported that the emotional disturbance observed in these individuals was characterized by anxiety and neurotic depressive symptoms. Little proposed a diagnostic category he dubbed the 'athlete's neurosis' to describe this condition. While a minority of these patients recovered quickly, he reported that a '… majority proceeded to an intractable chronic neurotic state extremely resistant to psychological and physical therapies'. Earlier research by Carmen, Zerman and Blaine demonstrated that athletes were less likely to use a college psychiatric service than non-athletes, and these authors reported a '… seeming reluctance of athletes to come to a service that requires that they articulate their feelings'[68]. These authors also suggested that many athletes rely on physical activity as a means of expressing feelings and aggressions rather than '… talking things out'. Hence, athletes would lose a principal coping strategy if confronted with an injury that would prevent them from using physical activity in this manner.

The research by Little and Carmen *et al* has implications for our understanding of exercise dependence and the problems that can arise when a physically active individual is prevented from exercising. Although it might be possible to test this hypothesis experimentally, it could be problematic if the individuals one hopes to study are dependent on, or addicted to, exercise. It would probably be difficult to enlist such individuals as volunteers for experiments of the type needed in order to study the problem. In one of the earliest attempts to study this problem, Baekeland tried without success to recruit habitual exercisers to take part in a study of exercise deprivation[69]. It was not possible to enlist the participation of 'hard-core' exercisers who engaged in daily physical activity, and this led Baekeland to study individuals who exercised less frequently. Even though the individuals studied probably did not have an exercise dependence, voluntary exercise deprivation was associated with anxiety and disturbances in sleep. There has also been related research demonstrating that exercise deprivation is associated with an increase in somatic symptoms along with increased anxiety, depression, anger and confusion[70–2]. Furthermore, there is survey research by Robbins and Joseph involving 'deprivation sensations' in a group of 345 runners[73]. The symptoms most often reported by runners who missed a run or series of runs included restlessness, irritability and general fatigue.

Much of the research in the area of exercise deprivation has suffered from a number of methodological problems. One of the most serious problems has been the study of individuals deprived of regular exercise because of an injury. This is problematic since Little has reported that habitual exercisers can experience a 'deprivation crisis' following injuries[66,67]. Also, investigators have employed psychological instruments that lack validity, inappropriate statistical analyses have been common, and there has been a failure to make operational or quantify physical activity patterns. In addition, some investigators have studied individuals who were exercising as few as three days/week, and these individuals would obviously not experience distress with a day or so of exercise deprivation since their regular pattern of exercise would be unchanged.

In a more recent investigation by Mondin *et al*, a group of 10 habitual exercisers was studied who worked out at least once daily on six to seven days of each week[74]. These individuals volunteered to take part in a study dealing with the influence of exercise deprivation on mood state. They were characterized by the 'iceberg' profile but experienced a significant increase in mood disturbance (eg increased anxiety and depression) within 48 hours of the voluntary cessation of regular exercise. The group's mood improved on the fourth day of exercise deprivation and, while this may have represented a form of adaptation, it is more likely that it reflected the anticipation of the study's completion. Indeed, the transitory mood disturbance disappeared with the resumption of regular exercise in these individuals.

Conclusions

The predominant cognitive strategy employed by the elite distance runners described by Morgan and Pollock was of an associative nature, whereas the non-elite runners in this work relied primarily on a dissociative cognitive strategy. There is evidence that non-elite marathon runners today are just as likely to employ association[12,31], and

Raglin and Wilson[5] have attributed this to recreational runners adopting the cognitive strategies reported earlier for elite runners. Nevertheless, there is evidence that a dissociative strategy can actually lead to enhanced performance under controlled laboratory conditions[20], and, furthermore, there are anecdotal reports from the anthropological literature[21,22], as well as the contemporary sport literature[3,19], indicating that dissociation can at times be an effective strategy[3,23]. The psychological profile of the elite marathon runner, as well as the middle- and long-distance runner, is characterized by positive mental health[75]. The stereotypical profile reported for these runners has been found to persist at 20–5 years of follow-up[50].

There is considerable evidence that both elite marathon runners and recreational runners enjoy considerable health benefits that are attributed to the adoption of a lifestyle that incorporates regular physical activity[45–8]. These individuals, for example, typically score one or more standard deviations below the mean for sedentary persons on standardized measures of anxiety, depression, and other mood states[12,13,50]. However, overtraining can lead to increased anxiety and depression[61–4], and the mood disturbance associated with excessive exercise appears to follow a dose–response pattern. There is also evidence that some individuals can become compulsive exercisers[60], and this can result in what has been termed exercise addiction[58] or exercise abuse[59]. In other words, regular physical activity has both a bright and a dark side. There is also evidence that physically active individuals often experience dysphoric mood when deprived of their regular exercise[66,67,69–74]. This observation lends further support to the view that compulsive exercisers can experience a form of dependence or addiction, and there is considerable psychoendocrine research suggesting that opioid peptides and monoamines may be implicated in both the 'feeling good' sensation that accompanies exercise, as well as the dysphoria associated with both exercise deprivation and overtraining.

References

1 Morgan WP, Pollock ML. Psychologic characterization of the elite distance runner. In: Milvy P, ed. *Ann N Y Acad Sci* 1977; **301**: 382–403.

2 Dishman RK, Landy FJ. Psychological factors and prolonged exercise. In: Lamb DR, Murray R, eds. *Perspectives in exercise science and sports medicine. Volume 1: prolonged* exercise. Indianapolis: Benchmark Press, 1988: 140–167.

3 Morgan WP. Mind games: the psychology of sport. In: Lamb DR, Murray R, eds. *Perspectives in exercise science and sports medicine: optimizing sport performance. Volume 10.* Carmel: Cooper Publishing, 1997: 1–62.

4 O'Connor PJ. Psychological aspects of endurance performance. In: Shephard RJ, Åstrand PO, eds. *Endurance in sport.* Oxford: Blackwell Scientific, 1992: 139–45.

5 Raglin JS, Wilson GS. Psychology in endurance performance. In: Shephard RJ, Åstrand PO, eds. *Endurance in sport.* Oxford: Blackwell Scientific, 2000: 211–9.

6 Unestahl LE. *Use of hypnosis in sport psychology.* Indianapolis: Society of Clinical and Experimental Hypnosis Workshop, 1982.

7 Bannister RG. Muscular effort. *Br Med Bull* 1956; **12**: 222–5.

8 Bannister RG. *The four-minute mile.* New York: Dodd, Mead & Co, 1981.

9 Morgan WP, Costill DL. Psychological characteristics of the marathon runner. *J Sports Med Phy Fitness* 1972; **12**: 42–6.

10 Hall CS, Lindzey G. *Theories of personality*. New York: John Wiley, 1957.

11 Morgan WP. Psychological components of effort sense. *Med Sci Sports Exerc* 1994; **26**: 1071–7.

12 Morgan WP, O'Connor PJ, Ellickson KA, Bradley PW. Personality structure, mood states and performance in elite male distance runners. *Int J Sport Psych* 1986; **19**: 247–63.

13 Morgan WP, O'Connor PJ, Sparling BP, Pate RR. Psychological characterization of the elite female distance runner. *Int J Sports Med* 1987; **8**: 124–31.

14 McNair M, Lorr M, Droppleman F. *Profile of mood states*. San Diego: Educational and Industrial Testing Service, 1992.

15 Farrell PA, Gates WK, Maksud MG, Morgan WP. Increases in plasma beta-endorphin/beta-lipotropin immunoreactivity after treadmill running in humans. *J Appl Physiol* 1982; 1245–9.

16 Morgan WP. Psychophysiology of self-awareness during vigorous physical activity. *Res Q Exerc Sport* 1981; **52**: 385–427.

17 Newsholme LE, Leech T, Duester G. *Keep on running: the science of training and performance*. West Sussex, England: John Wiley & Sons, 1994.

18 Morgan WP. Mind over matter. In: Straub WF, Williams JM, eds. *Cognitive sport psychology*. New York: Sport Sciences Associates, 1984: 315–22.

19 Olsen E. Dixon's the one. *Runner* 1984; **1**: 30–6.

20 Morgan WP, Horstman DH, Cymerman A, Stokes J. Facilitation of physical performance by means of a cognitive strategy. *Cognit Ther Res* 1983; **7**: 252–64.

21 David-Neel A. *Magic and mystery in Tibet*. London: Souvenir Press, 1967.

22 Watson W. *Super nature*. New York: Anchor Press/Doubleday, 1973.

23 Scott W. The psychology of sport. Discussion. In: Lamb DR, Murray R, eds. *Perspectives in exercise science and sports medicine: optimizing sport performance. Volume 10*. Carmel, IN: Cooper Publishing, 1997: 60–1.

24 Morgan WP. Hypnosis and sport psychology. In: Rhue J, Lynn SJ, Kirsch I, eds. *Handbook of clinical hypnosis*. Washington, DC: American Psychological Association, 1993: 649–70.

25 Williamson JW, McColl R, Mathews D *et al*. Hypnotic manipulation of effort sense during dynamic exercise: cardiovascular responses and brain activation. *J Appl Physiol* 2001, **90**: in press.

26 Couture RT, Jerome W, Tihanyi J. Can associative and dissociative strategies affect the swimming performance of recreational swimmers. *Sport Psychologist* 1999; **13**: 334–43.

27 Scott LM, Scott D, Bedic SP, Dowd J. The effect of associative and dissociative strategies on rowing ergometer performance. *Sport Psychologist* 1999; **13**: 57–68.

28 Clingman JM, Hilliard VD. Race walkers quicken their step by tuning in, not stepping out. *Sport Psychologist* 1990; **4**: 25–32.

29 Masters KS, Lambert MJ. The relations between cognitive coping strategies: reasons for running, injury, and performance of marathon runners. *J Sport Exerc Psych* 1989; **11**: 161–70.

30 Silva JM III, Appelbaum MI. Association–dissociation patterns of United States Olympic trial contestants. *Cognitive Ther Res* 1989; **13**: 185–92.

31 Stevinson CD, Biddle SJH. Cognitive orientations in marathon running and 'hitting the wall'. *Br J Sports Med* 1998; **32**: 229–35.

32 Schomer HH. Mental strategy and the perception of effort of marathon runners. *Int J Sport Psychol* 1986; **17**: 41–59.

33 Tammen VV. Elite middle and long distance runners associative/dissociative coping. *J Appl Sport Psychol* 1996; **8**: 1–8.

34 Summers JJ, Sargent GI, Levey AJ, Murray KD. Middle-aged, non-elite marathon runners: a profile. *Percep Mot Skills* 1982; **54**: 963–9.

35 Wrisberg CA, Pein RL. Past running experience as a mediator of the attentional focus of male and female recreational runners. *Percep Mot Skills* 1990; **70**: 427–32.

36 Okwumabua TM, Meyers A, Santille L. A demographic and cognitive profile of master runners. *J Sport Behavior* 1987; **10**: 212–20.

37 Okwumabua TM, Meyers A, Schlesser R, Cooke R. Cognitive strategies and running performance: an exploratory study. *Cog Ther Res* 1983; **7**: 363–9.

38 Ungerleider S, Golding JM, Porter K, Foster J. An exploratory examination of cognitive strategies used by masters track and field athletes. *Sport Psychologist* 1989; **3**: 245–53.

39 Acevedo EO, Dzewaltowski DA, Gill DL *et al.* Cognitive orientations of ultramarathoners. *Sport Psychologist* 1992; **6**: 242–52.

40 Goode KT, Roth DL. Factor analysis of cognitions during running: association with mood change. *J Sport Exerc Psychol* 1993; **15**: 375–89.

41 Padgett VR, Hill AK. Maximizing athletic performance in endurance events: a comparison of cognitive strategies. *J Appl Soc Psychol* 1989; **19**: 331–40.

42 Morgan WP. The mind of the marathoner. *Psych Today* 1978; **11**: 38–40.

43 Pennebaker JW, Lightner JW. Competition of internal and external information in an exercise setting. *J Pers Soc Psychol* 1980; **39**: 165–74.

44 Scully D. Commentary. *Br J Sports Med* 1998; **32**; 234.

45 Morgan WP. *Physical activity and mental health*. Washington: Taylor and Francis, 1997.

46 Morgan WP. Affective beneficence of vigorous physical activity. *Med Sci Sports Exerc* 1985; **17**: 94–100.

47 Morgan WP. Psychological outcomes of physical activity. In: Maughan RJ, ed. *Basic science for sports medicine*. Oxford: Butterworth-Heinemann, 1999: 237–59.

48 Morgan WP. Involvement in vigorous physical activity with special reference to adherence. In: Gedvilas LI, Kneer MW, eds. *Proceedings of the National College Physical Education Association*. Chicago: University of Illinois-Chicago Publications Service, 1977: 235–46.

49 Dishman RK, ed. Exercise adherence: its impact on public health. Champaign: Human Kinetics Publishers, 1988.

50 Morgan WP, Costill DL. Selected psychological characteristics and health behaviors of aging marathon runners: a longitudinal study. *Int J Sports Med* 1996; **17**: 305–12.

51 Hoffmann P. The endorphin hypothesis. In: Morgan WP, ed. Physical activity and mental health. Washington: Taylor and Francis, 1997: 163–77.

52 Farrell PA, Gustafson AB, Morgan WP, Pert CB. The effect of prolonged exercise on circulating enkephalins, catecholamines, and psychological mood alterations. *Med Sci Sports Exerc* 1987; **19**: 347–53.

53 Mandell AJ The *second* second wind. *Psychiat Annals* 1979; **9**: 57–69.

54 Chauloff F. The serotonin hypothesis. In: Morgan WP, ed. *Physical activity and mental health*. Washington: Taylor and Francis, 1997: 179–98.

55 Dishman RK. The norepinephrine hypothesis. In: Morgan WP, ed. Physical activity and mental health. Washington: Taylor and Francis, 1997: 199–212.

56 Morgan WP, Olson EB, Pedersen NP. A rat model of psychopathology for use in exercise science. *Med Sci Sports Exerc* 1982; **14**: 91–100.

57 Olson EB, Morgan WP. Rat brain monoamine levels related to behavioral assessment. *Life Sci* 1982; **30**: 2095–100.

58 Morgan WP. Negative addiction in runners. *Phys Sportsmed* 1979; **7**: 57–70.

59 Davis C. Exercise abuse. *Int J Sport Psychol* 2000; **31**: 278–89.

60 Polivy J. Physical activity, fitness and compulsive behaviors. In: Bouchard C, Shephard RJ, Stephens T, eds. *Physical activity, fitness and health*. Champaign: Human Kinetics Publishers, 1994: 884–97.

61 Morgan WP, Brown DR, Raglin JS *et al.* Psychological monitoring of overtraining and staleness. *Br J Sports Med* 1987; **21**: 107–14.

62 Morgan WP, Costill DL, Flynn MG *et al.* Mood disturbance following increased training in swimmers. *Med Sci Sports Exerc* 1988; **20**; 408–14.

63 O'Connor PJ, Morgan WP, Raglin JS *et al.* Mood state and salivary cortisol level following overtraining in female swimmers. *Psychoneuroendocrinology* 1989; **4**: 303–10.

64 O'Connor PJ, Morgan WP, Raglin JS. Psychobiologic effects of three days of increased training in female and male swimmers. *Med Sci Sports Exerc* 1991; **23**: 1055–61.

65 Raglin JS, Morgan WP, O'Connor PJ. Changes in mood states during training in female and male college swimmers. *Int J Sports Med* 1991; **12**: 585–9.

66 Little JC. The athlete's neurosis — a deprivation crisis. *Acta Psychiatr Scand* 1969; **45**: 187–97.

67 Little JC. Neurotic illness in fitness fanatics. *Psychiat Annals* 1979; **9**: 49–56.

68 Carmen LR, Zerman JL, Blaine GB. Use of the Harvard psychiatric service by athletes and non-athletes. *Ment Hyg* 1968; **52**: 134–7.

69 Baekeland F. Exercise deprivation: sleep and psychological reactions. *Arch Gen Psychiat* 1970; **22**: 365–9.

70 Chan CS, Grossman HY. Psychological effects of running loss on consistent runners. *Percept Mot Skills* 1988; **66**: 875–83.

71 Morris M, Steinberg H, Sykes EA, Salmon P. Effects of temporary withdrawal from regular running. *J Psychosom Res* 1990; **34**: 493–500.

72 Thaxton L. Physiological and psychological effects of short-term exercise addiction on habitual runners. *J Sport Psychol* 1982; **4**: 73–80.

73 Robbins JM, Joseph P. Experiencing exercise withdrawal: possible consequences of therapeutic and mastery running. *J Sport Psychol* 1985; **7**: 25–39.

74 Mondin GW, Morgan WP, Piering PN *et al.* Psychological consequences of exercise deprivation in habitual exercisers. *Med Sci Exerc Sports* 1996; **28**: 1199–203.

75 Morgan WP. Selected psychological factors limiting performance: a mental health model. In: Clark DH, Eckert HM, eds. *Limits of human performance (the academy papers)*. Champaign: Human Kinetics Publishers, 1985: 70–80.

New modalities in the management of running injuries

MR TREVOR PRIOR

CONSULTANT PODIATRIST, ST LEONARD'S PRIMARY CARE CENTRE, LONDON, UK

Over the past 20 years, advances in medicine and new technologies have resulted in a greater understanding of running injuries. Diagnosis of these injuries involves the specific identification of the presenting pathology, and encompasses the mechanism of injury and contributing factors. This chapter aims to outline some of these advances and potential future developments.

Injury diagnosis

The single greatest advance in the diagnosis of running injuries may be the ability to identify the presenting pathology. This has become possible as a result of greater understanding of the types of pathologies, coupled with advanced imaging and other techniques.

Investigations such as X-rays, bone scans and computerized tomography (CT) scans are particularly useful in the diagnosis of bone injury. The combined use of these modalities enables identification and management of conditions that previously would have curtailed activity. However, advances in the use of ultrasound, magnetic resonance imaging (MRI) and compartment pressure provide a more detailed analysis of soft tissue conditions.

Ultrasound uses high-frequency sound waves that are reflected at tissue interfaces to identify structures. Although this method is relatively low-cost with low patient risk, the scans provided lack detail, are difficult to interpret and, thus, require an experienced practitioner. Furthermore, it does not allow assessment of bony injury. In contrast, MRI is a relatively expensive modality but allows a detailed analysis of both bone and soft tissue. The detail is of high quality, although in some areas (ie the foot) the anatomical complexity may make interpretation more difficult. This technique is also associated with low patient risk, but many implants may prevent examination.

A few study centres have attempted to correlate MRI findings with those found at surgery and clinical outcomes. Some conditions have a classification system based on MRI findings. Wainwright *et al* demonstrated the benefit of such a system for tibialis posterior muscle dysfunction[1], as their MRI findings in 29 feet correlated well with those at surgery with only one false negative. The authors recommended a treatment protocol based on the classification system. Wainwright *et al* also reviewed 126 consecutive MRI scans of the ankle and hind foot and concluded that this technique was most commonly used for flexor tendon dysfunction, recurrent ankle instability and Achilles tendon pathology, with the scan confirming diagnosis or influencing management in 73%, 86% and 84% of cases respectively[2]. However, they noted that MRI was less useful for diffuse, painless swellings around the ankle, suspected loose bodies of the ankle joint, arthritis and nonspecific hind foot pain.

Further MRI studies need to be carried out so that investigations can be used as effectively as possible to help diagnosis and guide management.

Analyses of pressures obtained in the lower leg muscle compartments during exercise have been available for several years; however, this investigative technique has only recently been widely appreciated, which may reflect the failure of traditional therapeutic techniques in the management of lower leg exertional pain conditions. It is a specialized technique that is still relatively inaccessible. Well-controlled studies using this technique have enhanced our knowledge and management of compartment syndrome. Padhiar has demonstrated that orthoses are not beneficial in the management of compartment syndrome and, if anything, increase compartmental pressures[3].

Aetiology and contributing factors

The factors causing and contributing to running injury are still not clearly defined. Although the roles of foot and leg function, muscle function and running shoes have been investigated, a clear picture has yet to be established that may represent an inability to analyse and define normal foot function. Advances in technology and our ability to manage injuries with, for example, appropriate exercises and orthoses have greatly improved.

Traditional podiatric biomechanical theory

Root *et al*, who proposed the concept of a neutral foot position, developed podiatric biomechanics in the 1960s[4]. This involves the subtalar joint (STJ) being in a neutral position when it is neither pronated nor supinated, and the midtarsal joint maximally pronated. In this model, the perfect foot, when placed into neutral position during walking, would have the posterior bisection of the heel and lower one-third of the leg perpendicular to the weightbearing surface and the forefoot flat on the surface. Various conditions were identified (mainly by eversion or inversion of the heel), which resulted in pronation or supination of the foot, thus predisposing to overuse and injury. Orthoses to control these positions were used in conjunction with appropriate flexibility and strengthening exercises. However, there is no significant research to validate this model; this is further complicated by the lack of repeatability and reliability of measurements of the foot and leg.

New developments in podiatric biomechanics

The traditional biomechanics theory described normal podiatric function during walking. Initial pronation of the foot following heel strike was thought necessary to allow the foot to become a mobile adaptor for various terrains, while supination in late stance was thought important for the foot to be a rigid lever for propulsion. Root *et al*, therefore, surmised that the foot must pass through neutral between these two positions[4], and suggested that this should occur in the middle of midstance (ie when the malleoli of the swing and stance limb are level). More recent studies have demonstrated that the heel remains everted (pronated) throughout its contact period, thus refuting the previous proposal[5,6]. Although this suggestion supports clinical observations, there have been some concerns relating to the normality of the subjects involved in these studies. As a result, other models of foot function have been considered.

In 1954, Hicks detailed the role of the plantar fascia (plantar aponeurosis)[7,8]. He demonstrated how dorsiflexion of the toes at the metatarso-phalangeal joints (MTPJs) caused tension in the fascia resulting in metatarsal plantar flexion and called this the 'tie bar mechanism'. As there is greater motion at the first metatarsal, plantar flexion is seen to be greater here, causing raising of the arch and thus inversion of the heel and external rotation of the leg. As the foot dorsiflexes over the toes during activity, this mechanism is initiated in latter stance and was demonstrated in patients with paralysis, indicating that it is independent of muscular control.

Bojsen-Moller has described the role of the MTPJ axes during function, where toe off through the first/second MTPJ axis initiates the tie bar mechanism and increases foot stability, and toe off through the second to fifth MTPJ axis reduces stability[9]. Conversely, Kirby has described a technique for determining the position of the STJ axis on the plantar aspect of the foot[10,11]. With the use of physical principles, he has described how varying positions of this axis affects structure and function and, thus, advocates the concept of rotational equilibrium about this axis position for controlling foot function. This technique still needs validation.

A further concept of function has been developed by Dananberg[12–4], which combines well with Perry's model[15]. Dananberg reports that motion is greatest in the sagittal plane (when first MTPJ, ankle, knee and hip joints are combined) and that this is the dominant plane for assessing function. During normal walking, approximately 20° of hip extension are needed towards the end of stance to place the leg in the required position for propulsion and subsequent swing. For this to occur, adequate first MTPJ dorsiflexion, mirrored by ankle joint plantar flexion, is important. If this does not take place within the foot and ankle, early knee joint flexion is needed which reduces hip joint extension. This alters normal gait and results in instability and dysfunction. It has been demonstrated that patients with lower back pain who have been provided with orthoses designed to improve this function have a significantly better outcome than controls[16].

The net result of these concepts is a complex set of proposals for foot function, which still require significant research and validation.

Running shoes

The role of running shoes in the aetiology of injury has become more apparent over the past 20 years, with most practitioners advocating the appropriate shoe for the appropriate activity. As a result, many shoe manufacturers are purporting to have specific technology incorporated into their shoes to either control pronation or facilitate function, depending on foot type and activity level. It is difficult to obtain scientific data relating to these technologies. One aspect of function that is promoted by companies is shock absorption. It is easy to demonstrate the basic rearfoot control provided by different shoes with simple video technology. However, Robbins and Gouw suggest that cushioning reduces plantar loads and may result in perceived impact being less than actual impact, predisposing to injury[17].

Scientific evaluation

Scientific evaluation has studied the effect of function in terms of kinematic and kinetic analysis. Kinematic analysis involves the measurement of linear and angular displacement, velocity and acceleration, centre of rotation and joint angles. One example is Milliron and Cavanagh's work, which describes thigh-knee angle-angle diagrams at different speeds[18]. Kinetics analyses the forces that cause movement which may be internal (eg muscle activity, ligamentous function and joint friction) or external (eg ground reaction, active and passive bodies). The joint movements reported by Eng and Winter are an example of this type of analysis[19].

Developments in equipment for analysing the motions have had a profound effect on the ability of researchers to collate this information. This includes the use of video analysis, goniometers, accelerometers, stroboscopy, force platforms/in-shoe analysis, electromyography and mathematical modelling.

Video analysis is perhaps the most widely used analysis modality with single and multi-camera systems. A minimum of three cameras is needed to adequately record rotational activity. The use of reflective markers to identify body landmarks is commonplace, although pins inserted into bone have been used to minimize the effect of skin movement and placement. The latter technique is less frequently used due to its invasive nature and because its effect on normal function is difficult to quantify.

The forces exerted on the plantar region of the foot are now commonly assessed both by force platforms fixed to the floor/walkway and specialized insoles within shoe. Most of these systems record vertical reaction forces, although some plates have the ability to record shear force. Generally, a minimum sampling frequency of 100 MHz is needed for running assessment.

Although much data is available from these studies, a clear picture of normal and abnormal function has yet to be developed. Collation of data from these studies can assist in the formulation of concepts. For example, Eng and Winter have demonstrated that most joints within the leg work primarily within the sagittal plane, although substantial frontal plane work occurs at the hip[19]. This correlates well with Lafortune *et al*'s conclusion that, while shoes with a valgus wedge in the sole cause 4° more internal tibial rotation, shoes with either a varus or valgus wedge do not alter the kinematics at the knee[20] — this motion is resolved at the hip. Thus, an understanding of hip function is needed to assess a runner's ability to compensate for foot/leg function.

Lack of a clear model for foot function has prevented the development of standards for orthotic manufacture, even though the ability of these devices to modify function has been demonstrated. Cornwall and McPoil have demonstrated that rearfoot and tibial rotation correlate well (0.95)[21] and, by measuring tibial rotation, have concluded that shoes and soft orthoses reduce rotation, velocity and acceleration. Orthoses made from rigid materials, however, increase rotation and acceleration. Nigg *et al* also found that soft orthoses were more effective at altering rotation, although tibial rotation was reduced in flexible feet but increased in stiff feet[22]. This suggests that soft orthoses are more effective than rigid devices for reducing tibial rotation in runners. Similarly, stress to the limb can be reduced by shoes/orthoses as the moment of ground reaction force is reduced with shoes with a varus wedge[23], as were the vertical forces in a runner with a history of stress fractures provided with soft orthoses[24].

The latter two studies used ground reaction forces by analysing the degree of load. However, improved software enables the assessment of the direction and velocity of motion and may provide greater insight to function. Furthermore, the ability to correlate this to the joint position from video analysis may result in a greater understanding of function.

Future developments

It is inevitable that continued development of examination and investigative equipment would enable a greater understanding of function and injury. Correlation between video and force analysis is likely to further enhance this.

However, in order to determine the relevance of foot function to injury, normal ranges over a wide age spectrum are required — simply assessing runners at different speeds may be insufficient. Individuals with similar pre-determined running velocities should be compared and then analysed at varying velocities.

Given the advances in investigative techniques, it is likely that further developments will be seen in the technologies produced by running shoe companies. Several companies are starting to develop a system whereby the running shoe is customized to the individual needs by compiling the shoe from varying component parts.

In addition, a greater understanding of MRI, coupled with the development of dynamic MRI, will further enhance practice. There is a need for more well-structured studies to relate these findings to pathology, management protocols and outcomes.

Conclusions

The diagnosis of running injury is excellent and our understanding of function has improved and scientific modalities advanced. However, there is still a lack of data pertaining to normal function and the relationship of function to injury remains largely unproven. Further development and research are, therefore, needed to enable improved patient management in terms of prevention and treatment on a truly evidenced based foundation.

References

1 Wainwright AM, Kelly AJ, Glew D *et al.* Classification and management of tibialis posterior tendon injuries according to magnetic resonance imaging findings. *Foot* 1996; **6**: 66–70.

2 Wainwright AM, Kelly AJ, Glew D *et al.* Clinical application of ankle and hindfoot magnetic resonance imaging. *Foot* 1996; **6**: 126–33.

3 Padhiar N, King JB. Foot orthoses can change compartmental pressures in the leg. *Br J Sports Med* 1998; **32**: 89.

4 Root ML, Orien WP, Weed JH. *Clinical biomechanics: normal and abnormal function of the foot.* Vol 2. Los Angeles, Clinical Biomechanics Corp., 1977

5 McPoil T, Cornwall MW. Relationship between subtalar joint neutral position and pattern of rearfoot motion during walking. *Foot Ankle Int* 1994; **15**: 141–5.

6 Pierrynowski MR, Smith SB. Rearfoot inversion/eversion during gait relative to the subtalar joint neutral position. *Foot Ankle Int* 1996; **17**: 406–12.

7 Hicks JH. The mechanics of the foot; I. The joints. *J Anat* 1953; **87**: 345–57.

8 Hicks JH. The mechanics of the foot; II. The plantar aponeurosis and the arch. *J Anat* 1954; **88**: 25–31.

9 Bojsen-Moller F. Calcaneocuboid joint and stability of the longitudinal arch of the rearfoot at high and low gear push off. *J Anat* 1979; **129**: 165–76

10 Kirby KA. Methods for determination of positional variations in the subtalar joint axis. *J Am Podiatr Med Assoc* 1987; **77**: 228–34.

11 Kirby KA. Rotational equilibrium across the subtalar joint axis. *J Am Podiatr Med Assoc* 1989; **79**: 1–14.

12 Dananberg HJ. Functional hallux limitus and its relationship to gait efficiency. *J Am Podiatr Med Assoc* 1986; **76**: 648–52.

13 Dananberg HJ. Gait style as an etiology to chronic postural pain. Part I. Functional hallux limitus. *J Am Podiatr Med Assoc* 1993; **83**: 433–41.

14 Dananberg HJ. Gait style as an etiology to chronic postural pain. Part II. Postural compensatory process. *J Am Podiatr Med Assoc* 1993; **83**: 615–24.

15 Perry J. *Gait analysis: normal and pathological function.* Thorofare, New Jersey: Slack Inc, 1992.

16 Dananberg HJ, Guiliano M. Chronic low-back pain and its response to custom-made foot orthoses. *J Am Podiatr Med Assoc* 1999; **89**: 109–17.

17 Robbins SE, Gouw GJ. Athletic footwear: unsafe due to perceptual illusions. *Med Sci Sports Exerc* 1991; **23**: 217–24.

18 Milliron MJ, Cavanagh PR. Sagittal plane kinematics of the lower extremity during distance running. In: Cavanagh PR, ed. *Biomechanics of distance running*. Illinois: Human Kinetics Books, 1990: 65–99.

19 Eng JJ, Winter DA. Kinetic analysis of the lower limbs during walking: what information can be gained from a three-dimensional model? *J Biomech* 1995; **28**: 753–8.

20 Lafortune MA, Cavanagh PR, Sommer HJ 3rd, Kalenak A. Foot inversion-eversion and knee kinematics during walking. *J Orthop Res* 1994; **12**: 412–20.

21 Cornwall TG, McPoil MW. Footwear and foot orthotic effectiveness research: a new approach. *J Orthop Sports Phys Ther* 1995; **21**: 337–44.

22 Nigg BM, Khan A, Fisher V, Stefanyshyn D. Effect of shoe insert construction on foot and leg movement. *Med Sci Sports Exerc* 1998; **30**: 550–5.

23 Holden JP, Cavanagh PR. The free moment of ground reaction in distance running and its changes with pronation. *J Biomech* 1991; **24**: 887–97.

24 McPoil TG, Cornwall MW. Rigid versus soft orthoses. A single subject design. *J Am Podiatr Med Assoc* 1991; **81**: 638–42.

DISCUSSION

Attendee: Are you able to determine whether or not an athlete will perform poorly?

Mr Trevor Prior: No, but I can study the individual's foot type and his or her muscle flexibility and strength, and advise the person not to become a marathon runner if he or she appears to be prone to injury. Some top performers have fairly bad mechanics but are able to cope with it. Data on foot physiology are still sparse, and an objective measure for assessing foot function and one that can be applied easily to a clinical situation is not yet available.

Attendee: Are there any studies of different injury rates on varying surfaces, such as running on a treadmill?

Mr Trevor Prior: Not as far as I know. A treadmill is an artificial situation — it imparts a degree of power and spring but training solely on it would not prepare you for running 42.2 km of road. Training patterns need to be mixed, even to the extent that you alternate your preferred route so that the camber is varied. The forces beneath the foot on different surfaces can be studied, as can the relative angles of limbs/joints. Your question would make an interesting study, although the types of runners on each surface would need to be controlled or at least compared to ensure it was the surface rather than individual characteristics of the runner that caused the injury patterns.

Should I run tomorrow?

DR RANDY EICHNER

PROFESSOR OF MEDICINE, HEMATOLOGY-ONCOLOGY SECTION,
UNIVERSITY OF OKLAHOMA HEALTH SCIENCES CENTER, OKLAHOMA, USA

Regular running provides numerous benefits, many of which have been discussed in detail in earlier chapters. Even marathon running promises several benefits, especially if the psychological benefits of striving towards and achieving a high goal are included. Endurance running, however, does confer a few risks including heat stress, immune perturbations, overtraining problems and even sudden death.

Endurance exercise has also been shown to affect blood and the gastrointestinal (GI) tract. In this chapter, the problems of GI bleeding and ischaemic colitis will be discussed, as well as muscular cramps and hyponatraemia. The chapter will also indicate whether and how these conditions may be reversed, and will refer to real-life cases — it aims to help individuals decide whether or not they should participate in a running event.

Nature's anticoagulant

Physical inactivity impairs blood rheology and haemostatic function to promote unwanted clotting. In a recent study, patients suffering from acute myocardial infarction (AMI) triggered by physical exertion were compared with those with non-exertional AMI[1]. The results revealed that patients who experienced exertional AMI were mainly male, smokers, hyperlipidaemic, obese and habitually inactive. Inactive men with exertional AMI were nearly twice as likely to have a large thrombus in the infarct artery, suggesting that unaccustomed exertion caused coronary artery plaque rupture and formation of a large clot. The clot appeared to be the proximate cause of the AMI. These findings suggest that inactive men with multiple cardiac risk factors should not participate in any race.

It has been proposed that a proximate cause of clotting in many exertional AMIs is 'couch potato' blood. A 'couch potato' is an informal term defined as an inactive person whose recreation consists mainly of watching television[2]. Such physical inactivity has a fourfold effect on blood by causing:

- elevated haematocrit, or 'thick blood'
- elevated plasma fibrinogen levels
- hyper-reactive or 'sticky' blood platelets
- reduced fibrinolysis.

Concurrently, these problems make blood more difficult to pump and prone to clotting; they can, however, be reversed by regular exercise, eg running[3].

Since the late 1970s, it has been well established that regular aerobic exercise is a 'plasma-builder', with the baseline plasma volume increasing and decreasing rapidly according to the level of physical activity[4]. Haemoconcentration from a workout results in the addition of salt, water and albumin to the blood, expanding plasma volume. A brief vigorous, upright workout can expand the baseline plasma volume by 10% within one day, in which time the albumin synthetic rate may be increased as much as 50% from baseline[5]. Some researchers believe regular aerobic exercise also increases the production of erythrocytes[6], but the few longitudinal studies have presented mixed results. Studies on whether or not acute exercise increases plasma erythropoietin levels also reveal varied conclusions, although most studies are negative. For example, when 10 competitive male distance runners ran at high intensity for 60 minutes in a recent study, no change was observed in erythropoietin plasma levels during the run or over the following two days[7].

Similarly, longitudinal studies show mixed results on the effect of exercise on fibrinogen levels, but most suggest that exercise training lowers baseline fibrinogen, perhaps merely by dilution as with haematocrit[3]. Three longitudinal studies agree that aerobic exercise reduces platelet reactivity[8], and it is clear that exercise acutely increases fibrinolysis by releasing tissue plasminogen activator from muscles[9]. Endurance training also appears to enhance fibrinolysis. For example, when endurance training and stretching were compared in older men and women for six months, the training enhanced fibrinolysis in men by reducing plasma levels of plasminogen activator inhibitor, and in women by increasing plasma levels of tissue plasminogen activator[10]. Thus, regular physical activity, such as running, improves the blood in four ways that can prevent heart attack and stroke — exercise is nature's anticoagulant.

Gastrointestinal bleeding

'Two hours later, the elation had worn off. I was urinating large clots of blood, and was vomiting black mucus and had a lot of black diarrhoea.'
Derek Clayton, 1969 world-record marathon run

Although exercise has many benefits, it can be a stress test for the GI tract as much as for the heart[11]. Gut reactions are common in athletes. Marathon runners, for example, can suffer upper GI symptoms such as nausea, bloating and acid reflux, as well as lower GI symptoms such as cramp, bleeding and diarrhoea. Of these, bleeding is the main cause for concern. It can stem from either the upper or lower GI tract, and can range from occult and trivial to overt and grave. Data reveal that about 2% of marathon runners or triathletes have noted blood in their stool after a race, and about 20% of distance runners have occult blood in the first stool post-race[12]. The incidence of occult GI bleeding has been shown to be even higher (up to 85%) after a 100-mile race.

Frequency

The frequency of GI bleeding over a competitive season was investigated by the Health Sciences Center of the University of Oklahoma, US, where a cross-country team was studied over a four-month period. Eleven runners kept training records and submitted stool specimens on guaiacum cards two to three times a week. Of 190 specimens (six to 26 per athlete), 33 (17%) were positive for occult blood; none had visible bleeding. Six runners were positive twice or more during the season. The bleeding was always minor and brief, did not cause iron depletion or anaemia, and was found to

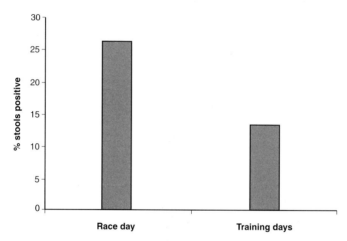

Figure 1

Percentage of stools positive for occult blood on race day and routine training days in 11 college cross-country runners

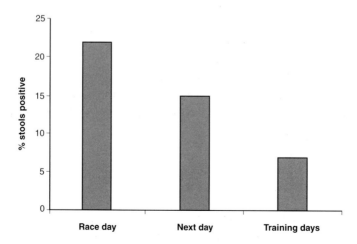

Figure 2

Percentage of stools positive for occult blood on race day, on the first day post-race and on routine training days in 12 community cyclists

occur most commonly after hard runs or races than after easy training runs (Figure 1). This pattern of exertional GI bleeding was confirmed in a similar prospective study of 12 community competitive cyclists, who kept training records and submitted stool specimens over a season. Occult GI bleeding was found to be more frequent on the day of the race than on the following day or on routine training days (Figure 2).

Other researchers measured GI blood loss by iron radiolabelling erythrocytes and collecting stools in a group of elite German male runners with low iron stores. On rest days, GI blood loss was 1–2 ml/day; on running days, however, this increased to an average of 5–6 ml/day. These results also revealed that GI bleeding was related to the intensity of running rather than the distance run[13].

Main causes and effects

From where does the bleeding originate? One source in marathon runners is gastritis; this was demonstrated in endoscopy studies carried out after the 1990 Chicago marathon, which revealed post-race congestion, haemorrhage or shallow erosions of the gastric mucosa[14]. More recent research suggests that prolonged running may interact with aspirin to increase GI permeability to marker sugars that are then excreted in the urine, but the clinical relevance remains unclear[15].

Repeated bouts of running related GI bleeding may contribute to iron deficiency anaemia in women. Because women in general have lower iron stores than men, women marathon runners are more apt than men to develop anaemia if they bleed small amounts over time.

Ischaemic colitis

Perhaps the most ominous cause of GI bleeding in marathon runners or triathletes is colitis, often heralded by lower abdominal cramp and bloody diarrhoea during the race or a hard training run. Although the cause of haemorrhagic colitis in runners is not clear, most experts consider it to be ischaemic and associated with severe dehydration that increases the physiological diversion of blood from the intestines to working muscles during intensive exercise. Cases of ischaemic colitis have been reported during or after triathlons, marathons, half marathons and 15-km road races[16].

Severe ischaemic colitis can require subtotal colectomy, as was the case in a female distance runner[17] and in two elite triathletes in the Hawaii Ironman triathlon[11]. Anecdotal reports suggest that mild or moderate ischaemic colitis that responds to conservative therapy is more common.

If you should run tomorrow, it may be worth thinking about the recent case report of Uta Pippig, an elite class female runner who won the 100th Boston marathon[16]. At the four-mile point of the race, she developed cramp-like pain at the lower abdomen followed by several bouts of bloody diarrhoea. Although her symptoms improved mid-race, they began to deteriorate towards the end of the race. After winning, she passed frank blood without stool and was hospitalized. A sigmoidoscopy revealed severe segmental ischaemic injury of the sigmoid mucosa and milder ischaemic changes in the rectum. Her symptoms resolved in one day following supportive therapy, and repeat sigmoidoscopy after six weeks was normal. She resumed graduated training; sigmoidoscopy during the most rigorous phase was also normal. This suggests that, with prudent training and racing (including good hydration), marathon runners can avoid ischaemic colitis.

Foot strike haemolysis

Marathon runners often suffer foot strike haemolysis. This intravascular haemolysis involves the rupture of erythrocytes in the bloodstream as the foot strikes the ground — this has the potential to drain iron stores and contribute to anaemia in certain runners. Following haemolysis, the free haemoglobin enters the plasma where it binds to haptoglobin and is delivered to the liver for salvage. The levels of plasma haptoglobin, however, can drop to zero if sufficient erythrocytes undergo haemolysis. When this occurs, some haemoglobin and its iron are lost in the urine.

Fortunately, the foot strikes of most runners are not forceful enough to exhaust haptoglobin, even during marathons or triathlons. For example, in a study carried out at the University of Oklahoma, US, we sampled blood from 25 triathletes before and after a minitriathlon. Levels of albumin, transferrin and ferritin increased during the race, mainly because of dehydration (haemoconcentration), while haptoglobin levels decreased due to exertional haemolysis — the mean haptoglobin reduction equalled about 5 ml blood that had undergone haemolysis (Figure 3). Researchers at the Hawaii Ironman triathlon have obtained similar data[18]. If a marathon runner was to exhaust haptoglobin in a race, only very small amounts of iron would be lost in the urine because haptoglobin is regenerated quickly. The regimens of even elite marathon runners, thus, do not appear to exhaust haptoglobin. Foot strike haemolysis is, therefore, apt to be only a negligible drain of iron stores and should not lead to anaemia in marathon performers.

Foot strike haemolysis, initially attributed to impact, may be better termed as 'exertional haemolysis', because it has been shown to occur in rowers and distance swimmers whose sports do not involve impact[19]. Further study has also found its occurrence in aerobic dancers and weight lifters. Exertional haemolysis in athletes may derive from impact or from other physical forces, possibly turbulent blood flow in the microvasculature of working muscles, along with the exposure of red cells traversing such muscles to the rigours of dehydration, acidosis and high temperatures. Exertional haemolysis removes the oldest, most rigid erythrocytes in world-class cyclists[20,21] and stimulates increased production of young, easily deformable erythrocytes that negotiate the microvasculatures.

The diagnostic triad of exertional haemolysis is:

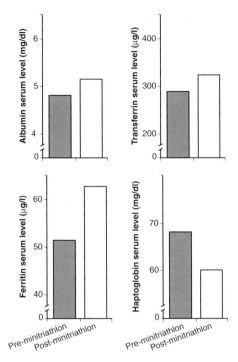

Figure 3

Comparison of serum levels of albumin, ferritin, transferrin and haptoglobin before and after a minitriathlon race in 25 athletes

- slightly elevated mean red cell volume (MCV), reflecting an increase in young red cells that are larger than older red cells
- slightly elevated reticulocyte count, reflecting increased production of red cells
- subnormal serum haptoglobin level.

Exertional haemolysis can be minimized in runners by wearing well-cushioned shoes, running lightly, and by running on soft surfaces as much as possible.

Muscle cramp

Muscle cramp is another hazard for marathon runners, especially in hot, humid races. These painful spasms can lead to runners or triathletes hobbling to the finish line or can force them to withdraw from the race. Severe heat cramps are also common in football 'two-a-days' (the first two weeks of football training in the summer, where players have two training sessions daily) and in long, tense tennis matches.

Causes and prevention

Although muscular fatigue and dehydration are thought to play important roles in initiating cramps in the heat, the exact causes are not fully understood. The theories compete with each other and the therapies vary. For example, some marathon runners and triathletes eat bananas to replace the potassium lost during performance, although only small amounts of potassium are lost in sweat. Others inject themselves with magnesium sulphate or calcium gluconate, as both magnesium and calcium may mitigate cramp via direct actions on nerves and/or muscles. Noakes *et al* have carried out much esteemed clinical research on cramp and hyponatraemia, and argue that there is no reliable evidence to support existing theories of muscular cramp. They have, therefore, proposed a novel hypothesis for exercise-associated muscle cramp — sustained α-motor neurone activity, stemming from aberrant control at the spinal level[22].

Sodium depletion

Setting this new hypothesis aside, I believe three lines of evidence implicate sodium depletion in heat cramps: history, published research on sodium loss, and the University of Oklahoma's data.

History

Knowing that stokers on ocean liners mixed sea water with their regular drinking water, a London doctor prevented cramps in industrial stokers via a saline drink. The US military began to follow this method[23], and a few years later drinking salty milk was shown to relieve cramp[24]. Also, in British coal mines, where a man could produce 20 g salt in his sweat in one shift, cramp was shown to be reduced by 'salt in water, about the composition of sweat'[25].

Research on sodium loss in athletes

As athletes acclimatize to heat, they generally sweat much earlier (at a lower body temperature) and heavier, and lose less sodium in their sweat. But the sodium content in sweat varies even in acclimatized athletes. And all athletes lose more salt as their sweat rate increases; this is because, at high sweat rates, sweat travels through the follicle too rapidly to allow maximal resorption of its sodium. Thus, athletes in the heat lose large amounts of sodium. This contributes to cramp if left uncompensated. Bergeron studied a tennis player with a high sweat rate (2.5 l/h), a high sweat sodium loss rate (90 mmol/h), and disabling muscular cramp. The cramps ceased when his salt intake was increased from 5–10 g/day to 15–20 g/day[26].

These findings have also been observed in football players. Davis *et al* carried out water turnover studies during collegiate 'two-a-days'[27]. Daily turnover of fluids averaged 11 l. Assuming a normal sweat sodium concentration of 40 mmol/l, this equates to losing 25 g salt per day. Using the typical American salt intake of about 10 g/day, even after five days of heat acclimatization, young men can still average a sweat sodium concentration as high as 40 mmol/l[28].

Research at the University of Oklahoma, US

Although our research at the University of Oklahoma, US, is only empirical and not a controlled clinical study, we have recently reduced muscular cramp in our football team by increasing salt intake. Team members are encouraged to add salt to their food, drink tomato juice and eat pretzels. They ingest a sports drink before, during and after practice. However, the sports drink contains insufficient sodium levels for the most cramp-prone players. These individuals tend to be the most fit and active players at their position. They sweat early and heavily, and tend to have a history of heat cramps, a low-salt diet, or sweat that burns the eyes (high salt). On the field, they rotate our regular sports drink with an oral electrolyte rehydration solution that has four times more sodium than the sports drink. Muscular cramps and 'locks' can usually be reversed in an hour with the rehydration solution and about 2 l normal saline intravenously. Individuals do not tend to suffer cramp again if they follow our guidelines. Our approach may not be ideal, and it is not the only one as other football teams use low-dose salt tablets. However, the common belief is that the threefold cause of heat cramps in football players is muscle fatigue, dehydration and salt depletion, and the common solution is salt.

Hyponatraemia

Why do some marathon runners and ultra-endurance athletes develop hyponatraemia? Noakes and colleagues have shown that symptomatic hyponatraemia in endurance athletes is due to fluid overload, either from overdrinking or from an abnormality in renal handling of a fluid load[29]. They studied 330 athletes who had completed the 1997 New Zealand Ironman triathlon and found that hyponatraemia was the most common serious medical complication. An intriguing gender difference was also observed, where 45% of female race finishers were hyponatraemic compared with only 14% of male race finishers[30]. A similar gender difference has been seen in Grand Canyon hikers with hyponatraemia and in those who became hyponatraemic after the inaugural San Diego Rock 'n' Roll marathon[31]. This gender difference may be both biological and behavioural. Compared with men, women tend to be smaller, on the racecourse for longer periods of time, and drink as directed. As a result, they may drink too much water and/or other sodium-poor beverages. According to press accounts, a woman who drank a lot of water before and during a recent Chicago marathon died in part from hyponatraemia.

In the 1998 New Zealand Ironman triathlon, preventive measures — eg educating athletes on hyponatraemia, advising them to drink only 500–1,000 ml/h, and reducing the number of drink stations — lowered the incidence of symptomatic hyponatraemia; this, however, resulted in a slightly increased incidence of major dehydration[29].

Overdrinking, or other forms of overhydration, can cause hyponatraemia especially if the levels of anti-diuretic hormone (ADH) remain too high, perhaps due to pain, fear, anxiety, or nausea during a race. This prevents the kidneys from removing the excess free water; this has been observed in the research laboratory when one of 10 soldiers drank and retained too much water during a day-long exercise study in the heat[32]. It has also occurred in the field, when a soldier drank 20 l water over the course of a few hours in order to ward off heat stress[33].

Symptomatic hyponatraemia (sometimes referred to as acute water intoxication) has also occurred as a complication of drug testing in the workplace[34], or after a football player with heat cramps was treated with excess hypotonic fluid orally and intravenously[35]. Hikers in the Grand Canyon are also vulnerable[36]. In addition, an ultra-distance triathlete was recently reported to have drank 23 l during the race, gained 5% in body weight, and had seizures from a serum sodium of 116 mmol/l[37].

Hyponatraemia may also be caused by loss of large amounts of sodium (and water) in sweat and replacing the losses mostly with water or other sodium-poor fluids. In Hawaii[38] and New Zealand[29,30], most competitors lose weight during the race. A few severe cases of hyponatraemia in Hawaii — some even involving seizures or coma — have involved dehydration but free-water excess. In both triathlons, hyponatraemic athletes lose less weight than non-hyponatraemic athletes[29,38].

If overdrinking is a root cause of many cases of hyponatraemia, it seems that sodium ingestion, in any form, reduces the risk of its development. Laboratory research has shown that ingesting a sports drink during endurance cycling in the heat maintains plasma sodium level better than ingesting water[39].

Hyponatraemia may not be a great threat in races held in cooler environments, ie the London marathon. In marathons or triathlons performed in warmer conditions, however, it can be avoided by: drinking no more than you sweat; favouring sports drinks, which contain sodium, over water which does not; consuming a salty diet in the days before the race; and eating pretzels in the last half of the race.

Conclusions

So, should you run tomorrow? Yes, of course, if you have trained properly for the marathon and if you keep your head about you as you run. You have set yourself a high and worthy goal; now achieve it and reap the benefits. As long as you never take your heart by surprise — and never lose your head — running offers far more benefits than risks. And in the general sense of tomorrow, yes, of course keep running. After all, we are given only so many tomorrows. In essence, life is motion. Stay fit and live each tomorrow more fully.

References

1 Giri S, Thompson PD, Kiernan FJ et al. Clinical and angiographic characteristics of exertion-related acute myocardial infarction. *JAMA* 1999; **282**: 1731–6.

2 *Collin's English Dictionary. Millennium Edition.* Glasgow: HarperCollins, 1998: 361.

3 Eichner ER. Physical activity, coagulability, and fibrinolysis. In: Leon AS, ed. *Physical activity and cardiovascular health: a national consensus.* Champaign IL: Human Kinetics, 1997: 120–6.

4 Eichner ER. Sports anemia, iron supplements, and blood doping. *Med Sci Sports Exerc* 1992; **24**: S315–8.

5 Nagashima K, Cline GW, Mack GW *et al*. Intense exercise stimulates albumin synthesis in the upright posture. *J Appl Physiol* 2000; **88**: 41–6.

6 Sawka MN, Convertino VA, Eichner ER *et al*. Blood volume: importance and adaptations to exercise training, environmental stress, and trauma/sickness. *Med Sci Sports Exerc* 2000; **32**: 332–48.

7 Bodary PF, Pate RR, Wu QF, McMillan GS. Effects of acute exercise on plasma erythropoietin levels in trained runners. *Med Sci Sports Exerc* 1999; **31**: 543–6.

8 Wang J-S, Jen CJ, Chen H-I. Effects of chronic exercise and deconditioning on platelet function in women. *J Appl Physiol* 1997; **83**: 2080–5.

9 Szymanski LM, Pate RR, Durstine JL. Effects of maximal exercise and venous occlusion on fibrinolytic activity in physically active and inactive men. *J Appl Physiol* 1994; **77**: 2305–10.

10 Chandler WL, Schwartz RS, Stratton JR, Vitiella MV. Effects of endurance training on the circadian rhythm of fibrinolysis in men and women. *Med Sci Sports Exerc* 1996; **28**: 647–55.

11 Eichner ER, Scott WA. Exercise as disease detector. *Phys Sportsmed* 1998; **26**: 41–52.

12 Eichner ER. Gastrointestinal bleeding in athletes. *Phys Sportsmed* 1989; **17**: 128–40.

13 Nachtigall D, Nielsen P, Fischer R *et al*. Iron deficiency in distance runners. A reinvestigation using Fe-labelling and non-invasive liver iron quantification. *Int J Sports Med* 1996; **17**: 473–9.

14 Schwartz AE, Vanagunas A, Kamel PL. Endoscopy to evaluate gastrointestinal bleeding in marathon runners. *Ann Intern Med* 1990; **113**: 632–3.

15 Ryan AJ, Chang R-T, Gisolfi CV. Gastrointestinal permeability following aspirin intake and prolonged running. *Med Sci Sports Exerc* 1996; **28**: 698–705.

16 Lucas W, Schroy PC 3rd. Reversible ischemic colitis in a high endurance athlete. *Am J Gastroenterol* 1998; **93**: 2231–4.

17 Beaumont AC, Teare JP. Subtotal colectomy following marathon running in a female patient. *J R Soc Med* 1991; **84**: 439–40.

18 O'Toole ML, Hiller DB, Roalstad MS, Douglas PS. Hemolysis during triathlon races: its relation to race distance. *Med Sci Sports Exerc* 1988; **20**: 272–5.

19 Selby GB, Eichner ER. Endurance swimming, intravascular hemolysis, anemia, and iron depletion. New perspective on athlete's anemia. *Am J Med* 1986; **81**: 791–4.

20 Eichner ER: Runner's macrocytosis: a clue to footstrike hemolysis. Runner's anemia as a benefit versus runner's hemolysis as a detriment. *Am J Med* 1985; **78**: 321–5.

21 Smith JA, Martin DT, Telford RD, Ballas SK. Greater erythrocyte deformability in world-class endurance athletes. *Am J Physiol* 1999; **276**: H2188–93.

22 Schwellnus MP. Skeletal muscle cramps during exercise. *Phys Sportsmed* 1999; **12**: 109–15.

23 McCord CP, Ferenbaugh TL. Fatigue in soldiers due to chloride losses. Replacement through the use of sodium chloride in drinking water. *Mil Surg* 1931; **lxix**: 608–14.

24 Talbott JH, Michelsen J. Heat cramps. A clinical and chemical study. *J Clin Invest* 1933; **2**: 533–49.

25 Brockbank EM. Miner's cramp. *BMJ* 1929; **1**: 65–6.

26 Bergeron MF. Heat cramps during tennis: a case report. *Int J Sport Nutr* 1996; **6**: 62–8.

27 Davis, MJ, Gentry M, Kennedy D *et al*. Helping athletes survive two-a-day practices. *Gatorade Sports Science Exchange Roundtable* 1999; **10**: 1–4.

28 Allsopp AJ, Sutherland R, Wood P, Wootton SA. The effect of sodium balance on sweat sodium secretion and plasma aldosterone concentration. *Eur J Appl Physiol* 1998; **78**: 516–21.

29 Speedy DB, Rogers IR, Noakes TD *et al*. Diagnosis and prevention of hyponatremia at an ultradistance triathlon. *Clin J Sport Med* 2000; **10**: 52–8.

30 Speedy DB, Noakes TD, Rogers IR *et al*. Hyponatremia in ultradistance athletes. *Med Sci Sports Exerc* 1999; **31**: 809–15.

31 Davis D, Marino A, Vilke G *et al*. Hyponatremia in marathon runners: experience with the inaugural Rock 'n' Roll Marathon. *Ann Emerg Med* 1999; **34**: S40.

327

32 Armstrong LE, Curtis WC, Hubbard RW *et al.* Symptomatic hyponatremia during prolonged exercise in the heat. *Med Sci Sports Exerc* 1993; **25**: 543–9.

33 Garigan TP, Ristedt DE. Death from hyponatremia as a result of acute water intoxication in an army basic trainee. *Mil Med* 1999; **3**: 234–8.

34 Klonoff DC, Jurow AH. Acute water intoxication as a complication of urine drug testing in the workplace. *JAMA* 1991; **265**: 84–5.

35 Herfel R, Stone CK, Koury SI, Blake JJ. Iatrogenic acute hyponatremia in a college athlete. *Br J Sports Med* 1998; **32**: 257–8.

36 Backer HD, Shopes E, Collins SL, Barkan H. Exertional heat illness and hyponatremia in hikers. *Am J Emerg Med* 1999; **17**: 532–9.

37 Speedy DB, Rogers I, Safih S, Foley B. Hyponatremia and seizures in an ultradistance triathlete. *J Emerg Med* 2000; **18**: 41–4.

38 O'Toole ML, Douglas PS, Laird RH, Hiller DB. Fluid and electrolyte status in athletes receiving medical care at an ultradistance triathlon. *Clin J Sport Med* 1995; **5**: 116–22.

39 Vrijens DMJ, Rehrer NJ. Sodium-free fluid ingestion decreases plasma sodium during exercise in the heat. *J Appl Physiol* 1999; **86**: 1847–51.

DISCUSSION

Dr Dan Tunstall Pedoe: Four cases in the London marathon with hyponatraemia have been hospitalized with fits (two men and two women) one of whom was a woman with 126 mmol/l Na, with no other cause for her fits — she had a normal CT scan. However, in my role as a physician, I admitted a young man who had been to Paris in mid-summer for his honeymoon. He came back severely hyponatraemic and in a state of collapse. We found that his siblings and himself, who had similar heat intolerance, were affected with a gene mutation which is sometimes found in fibrocystic disease. They had an incomplete form with hypertonic sweat. The trouble with 30,000 runners running in a marathon is that you do not know what sort of gene mutations you are encountering. They cannot all be normal! It is a huge uncontrolled experiment. I wonder if some of the cases we are seeing in marathons after just a few hours, much earlier than you would expect on conventional theory, are producing more sodium in their sweat than is normally measured.

Dr Randy Eichner: Yes, roughly one out of 20 or 25 Caucasians is heterozygous for cystic fibrosis and he or she is likely to have a higher than normal level of sweat sodium.

Attendee: In relation to the 30,000 runners tomorrow, I suspect a number will be normally hypertensive. Treatment for hypertension is diuretic and angiotensin converting enzyme inhibitors. Should they be recommended to continue taking those medications before the event?

Dr Randy Eichner: If they train on it, maybe they should race on it. But in one of the female Grand Canyon hikers, a diuretic was thought to have contributed to her very low sodium of 108 mmol/l.

Dr William Roberts: I would use the same guidelines if they have been training on these agents.

Dr Dan Tunstall Pedoe: I do not give general advice to people; they should go to their own doctor for that. If I see a patient who is being treated for hypertension with a diuretic and/or angiotensin converting enzyme inhibitor and is running a marathon or half-marathon, I usually tell them not to take the medication on the day as it might be dangerous if they become severely hypovolaemic.

Attendee: Do runners benefit from taking aspirin?

Dr Randy Eichner: If they have coronary risk factors, I advise one 'baby' aspirin per day because aspirin 'thins the blood' in a way different than exercise. Aspirin, even in low doses, increases the risk of bleeding.

Dr Dan Tunstall Pedoe: Would you tell them not to take it on the day of the marathon?

Dr Randy Eichner: Yes, I would stop aspirin a few days before the race, so as not to increase the risk of gastrointestinal bleeding on race day.

Dr Dan Tunstall Pedoe: With regards to the red cell deformability, I have always quoted that lower blood viscosity because of the increased plasma volume, decreased fibrinogen and increased red cell deformability are benefits of exercise. Is this the only cause that there are newer red cells or is there another feature of exercise that increases red cell deformability?

Dr Randy Eichner: The only well-supported cause is that they are younger.

Dr Dan Tunstall Pedoe: So if you do not get foot strike haemolysis, you are not increasing deformability in the red cells?

Dr Randy Eichner: That is probably correct.

Professor Eric Newsholme: A calculation shows that using E-mail several times a day to contact a colleague whose office is up two flights of stairs, in comparison with walking up the stairs, saves energy that is equivalent to about 1 kg fat over a year!

Dr Dan Tunstall Pedoe: I am sure everyone appreciates that the biggest difference in the population that we have now compared with 50 years ago is not their caloric intake, but their caloric expenditure. People are eating fewer calories but becoming obese because of their non-exercising lifestyles. Marathon runners are, of course, the extreme exception. This seems an appropriate note on which to end the discussion.

Glossary

AED: automated electric defibrillator — an apparatus for stopping fibrillation of the heart by application of an electric current to the chest wall

Allele: one of the alternative forms of a gene

Anhidrosis: failure to sweat

Autosomes: paired chromosomes other than the sex chromosomes; 22 pairs in man

Clo: the insulation required to maintain thermal comfort in a resting subject in a normally ventilated room at a temperature of 21 °C and humidity of <50%. It is a pragmatic definition and standard office dress is approximately 1 clo

Collagen: a protein structure of skin, tendon, bone, cartilage and other connective tissue

Concentric muscle contraction: muscular contraction that occurs as the muscle shortens

Core temperature: temperature of the central circulation and hypothalamus; the size of the core depends on climatic conditions and metabolic rate

Desmin: a structured protein in skeletal muscle that links Z discs of adjacent fibres

Dizygotic (DZ) twins: non-identical twins

EAC: exertion-associated collapse

Eccentric muscle contraction: a muscular contraction that occurs as the muscle lengthens

EHS: exertional heat stroke — a condition that occurs when endogenous heat production and exogenous heat gain are greater than heat dissipation to the environment

EMG: electromyography — an apparatus used to record electric currents generated in active muscle (muscle potentials)

EPO: erythropoietin — a hormone secreted in the kidney in response to a lowered oxygen content in the blood. It acts on the bone marrow to stimulate red blood cell production

F ratio: comparison of the between-family and within-family variance for VO_{2max}

Fast-twitch (FT) muscle fibre: type 2 muscle fibre

Gamow bag: a lightweight, portable, airtight bag in which a victim with altitude sickness can be repressurized using a foot pump similar to that used in rubber boats. The design includes a clear plastic observation window

Genotype: the genetic constitution of an individual

Haematocrit: red cell fraction of whole blood

Haptoglobin: a protein that binds haemoglobin of damaged red blood cells and is then removed from the circulation. A low or absent amount indicates red blood cell haemolysis or fragmentation

HCM: hypertrophic cardiomyopathy — a cardiac disease characterized by a hypertrophied and non-dilated left ventricle

HSPs: heat shock proteins — a family of proteins which acts as immunodominant antigens

Isometric muscle contraction: a muscle contraction that occurs with no change in muscle length

MASL: metres above sea level

Master's athlete: an adult individual who competes in events categorized by age, usually in five-year age bands. The lower limit varies to some extent by country and sport, but in the marathon it is often taken to be from age 40 in both genders. However, the World Veterans games is a biennial track-and-field championship for women >35 and men >40 years, which has been staged since 1975. *National Masters News*, the 'official world and US publication masters track and field, long distance running and race walking', defines masters as 'age 30+'

MET: metabolic equivalent. Multiple of resting metabolic rate

MET-hours: sum of average time per week spent in each activity x MET value of each activity

Monozygotic (MZ) twins: identical twins

Nebulin: a muscle structural protein

Phenotype: a set of observable characteristics of an individual as determined by genotype and environment

Polymorphism: the occurrence in the same population of two or more genetically determined phenotypes in such proportions that the rarest of these cannot be maintained purely by mutation

Respiratory exchange ratio (RER): the volume of carbon dioxide released during respiration compared to the volume of oxygen consumed

Respiratory quotient (RQ): the ratio of carbon dioxide produced to oxygen consumed; an old term now used for tissues or organs

Sarcolemma: the cell membrane of the muscle fibre

Sarcomere: the basic contractile unit of the myofibrils which are arranged end-to-end at the Z line and are composed of thin filaments (actin) and thick filaments (myosin); the thick and thin filaments slide over each other during contraction. Each muscle cell (fibre) contains up to several thousands myofibrils

Secular: occurring once in an age or century

Shell temperature: temperature of the skin and superficial tissues. The size of the shell depends on climatic conditions and metabolic rate

Sib: brother or sister

Slow-twitch (ST) muscle fibre: type 1 muscle fibre

STPD: standard temperature pressure dry — a means of normalizing samples of expired air to reference values

Telomere: end region of chromosomes

Titin: a large protein that links the end of the thick filament to the z disk in a muscle fibre

VO$_2$: oxygen uptake

VO$_{2max}$: maximal oxygen uptake

Wall ('hitting the wall'): a mythical barrier in marathon running describing a point at about 20 miles where many runners suddenly slow down and experience intense fatigue. This is probably multifactorial but can be caused by glycogen depletion of muscle

WBGT: wet bulb globe temperature — an index of heat stress

Index